DEATH FORETOLD

NICHOLAS A. CHRISTAKIS

DEATH

foretold

PROPHECY AND PROGNOSIS
IN MEDICAL CARE

THE UNIVERSITY OF CHICAGO PRESS

CHICAGO AND LONDON

Nicholas A. Christakis, M.D., Ph.D., M.P.H., is associate
professor of medicine and sociology at the University
of Chicago.

The University of Chicago Press, Chicago 60637
The University of Chicago Press, Ltd., London
© 1999 by The University of Chicago
All rights reserved. Published 1999
08 07 06 05 04 03 02 01 00 99   5 4 3 2 1

ISBN (cloth) : 0-226-10470-2

Library of Congress Cataloging-in-Publication Data

Christakis, Nicholas A.
    Death foretold : prophecy and prognosis in medical care / Nicholas
A. Christakis.
        p.   cm.
    Includes bibliographical references and index.
    ISBN 0-226-10470-2 (alk. paper)
    1. Prognosis.   I. Title.
RC80.C48   1999
362.1—dc21   99-16442
                                                         CIP

⊗The paper used in this publication meets the
minimum requirements of the American National Standard
for Information Sciences—Permanence of Paper for
Printed Library Materials, ANSI Z39.48-1992.

When I was six, she was given a 10 percent chance of living beyond three weeks. She lived for nineteen remarkable years. This prognosis, the physician's courage in making it, and the fact that it proved to be in error were consequential indeed. I spent my boyhood always fearing that her lifelong chemotherapy would stop working, constantly wondering whether my mother would live or die, and both craving and detesting prognostic precision. This ambivalence did not change when I became a physician myself.

Patients, when their illness has been given a name, usually ask next: And how long will it take? How long will it be before . . . ? How long? How long? And the doctor replies that he cannot promise but . . . He can appear to be the controller of time, as, on occasions, the mariner appears to rule the sea. But both doctor and mariner know this to be an illusion.

—J. BERGER AND J. MOHR,
A Fortunate Man: The Story of a Country Doctor

Contents

I am concerned here with the use physicians make of prognosis, the symbolism it contains, and the practical and emotional difficulties it involves. These difficulties have been more than abstract for me. On numerous occasions, patients have asked me if they would be cured of their cancer, if their pain would ever stop, if they would live until the end of the week, or until their next Christmas, their next anniversary, their next child's graduation from high school. These questions pained me, and not just because they touched on the ineffable sadness of deadly disease or the efforts the dying often make to stay connected to the living. They pained me as well because it was so difficult, yet at the same time so essential, to answer them.

Over the course of my clinical training, I came to regard explicit, precise, and compassionate responses to patients' requests for prognosis to be a key part of my role as a physician. I came to see the deliberate assessment of prognosis as absolutely obligatory, even if patients did not happen to ask. I became convinced that establishing the patient's prognosis, at least in my own mind, should be as routine for me as evaluating diagnostic possibilities or considering therapeutic options. Yet I found that I had been poorly trained for this.

I also found that the prospect of predicting the death of a patient to myself, let alone to the patient's face, was something frightening that I wished to avoid. Yet, like other physicians, I was obliged to perform many unpleasant tasks: I had roused families in the middle of the night and told them that their loved one had died. I had put needles the length of knives into people's necks, transported coolers with eyes and kidneys destined for transplantation, wheeled still-warm bodies to the morgue. I had asked patients questions that in a nonclinical situation would be considered indecent and shocking. I had been sworn at by psychotic patients, vomited on by intoxicated patients, kicked by seizing patients. I had stayed up forty hours without sleep on countless occasions. I had made desperate efforts to save an electrocuted young father's life and been deeply ashamed of my inability to do so. I had examined blood in the basement lab of the hospital and been the first to see signs of leukemia in a patient, the first with the secret, guilty knowledge about the elusive threat in the patient's body. So why was I hesitant to predict a patient's death? Why was it so hard to formulate, let alone communicate, prognoses?

As I looked around me, I found that other physicians also appeared to avoid prognostication and rarely talked explicitly with patients about their future. I began to ask my colleagues about this and learned that they avoided even thinking about prognosis explicitly, except occasionally, in the most benign and casual ways. I noticed that textbooks omitted prognosis, journals avoided it, and medical schools ignored it. The whole profession seemed to overlook prognosis. And few of my colleagues, I found, shared my conviction that this might be a problem. They even seemed bemused by my interest in this "marginal" topic, as if the proper and scientific role of medicine were only to diagnose and treat disease, not to predict its outcome.

Why was this? Was prognosis really so unimportant? Were the obstacles to it really insurmountable? When it came to prognostication, physicians appeared to speak hesitantly, softly, and ambiguously—if at all. This contrasted markedly with the confidence they exuded when making a diagnosis or prescribing a therapy.

I ultimately concluded that the muffled presence of prognosis had a lot to do with the raging authority of death. Prognostication and death are tightly interwoven. Although there certainly are more routine, less serious incarnations of prognostication, if one asks doctors to free-associate with the word *prognosis,* they are apt to say "death." And when physicians are asked to think about the role of prognosis in their practice, the question they imagine—and dread—is "How long do I have to live?" Like death, prognostication seems mysterious, final, powerful, and dangerous.

After I acquired sociological training, and over the course of more formal research into this topic, I came to regard the avoidance of prognostication as a sort of advertent and inadvertent self-deception, as an almost ideological, and not merely utopian, commitment in the medical profession. Physicians avoided prognostication, both consciously and subconsciously, because they did not want to deal with its unpleasant aspects or to think about the limits of their ability to change the future. But they also avoided it because they wanted to deceive themselves about death, as if in not predicting death they could avoid causing it or witnessing it.

Long ago, Aristotle was concerned with the ways human effort brought about ends.[1] The ends are products of an agent. But the agent is in turn defined by—and therefore brought about by—the ends. This type of reciprocal relation is troubling for physicians. Since, ultimately, all patients die, are physicians defined by this end, by death? If death can always be expected to occur, then is the way to avoid being defined by it to avoid predicting it?

On more than one occasion, I have seen the avoidance of prognostication, or needlessly incorrect prognoses, harm patients. A recent newspaper article entitled "For Cancer Patients, Hope Can Add to Pain" poignantly captured how such harm can come about. It quoted a patient's wife as saying:

> The Thursday before my husband died, I thought he was dying and he thought he was dying. But the doctor was talking about aggressive chemotherapy. I asked if this was palliative, and he said that he still hoped for a cure. I was with him at the time of his death [three days later], but the room was filled with eight other people hanging bags of blood and monitoring vital signs. It was about as horrifying as anything that could have happened. I don't think the [doctors] were trying to mislead us. They thought he might be the one case that would have a positive outcome. [But if I had been told the truth,] we could have spent days with the children, together, not filled with painful regimens in the hospital.[2]

The failure to predict this patient's death—in the sense of not thinking about the prognosis clearly, in the sense of not articulating it, and in the sense of encouraging an unduly optimistic expectation—was harmful. Such a failure can contribute to a therapeutic imperative that prevents families from taking steps to prepare for death. The physicians did not want to see that the therapy would not result in the desired outcome. They did not want to predict that the patient was about to die. And they did not want to take action, such as limiting therapy, based on such a prediction. If doctors were to think more cogently about the outcomes of their actions, if they were to develop prognoses more consciously (even in all their uncertainty), and if they were to share their prognostic estimates sensitively with patients to the extent that patients were interested, it would help them to avoid such outcomes. My feeling is that the problem in this case, and countless other cases like it, arises more from errors in prognosis than from errors in therapy. In our rush not to abandon patients therapeutically at the end of life, we abandon them prognostically.

Some awareness of this propensity to avoid prognosis, or to misjudge it, is reflected in a sort of self-mocking humor; physicians frequently refer to "flogging" patients with the painful administration of futile therapy. Yet this awareness fails to change the behavior. As one physician described it:

> We don't step back and say, "We've lost all perspective and we're using up resources and we're torturing this patient." In the intensive care unit especially, you find yourself putting in swans [a type of intravenous catheter that is threaded into the heart] and doing CPR and flogging people with lung failure and liver failure and kidney failure for days and days and days. The junior physicians lose the forest for the trees and are concentrating on the numbers, whereas the senior physicians with experience should stand back and say, "This is absurd. We should stop!" But they usually don't.

The ability of physicians to prognosticate is equated here with showing restraint, maintaining a sense of perspective, and knowing one's limits. Acting on predictions to avoid such disrespectful overtreatment requires assiduous data collection, substantial learning, excellent judgment, and considerable courage. It also requires a commitment not to abandon the patient.

Of course, patients might also be harmed if erroneous predictions of imminent death resulted in the withholding of interventions that would otherwise save a life. But my study has convinced me that, most of the time, the problem is the other way around. Rare are the cases where making or offering a carefully considered and framed prognosis results in choices that are harmful to a patient. Neglecting prognosis simply to avoid those cases may not be worth the cost. As a result of a failure to prognosticate, let alone prognosticate accurately, patients may die deaths they deplore in locations they despise. They may seek noxious chemotherapy rather than good palliative care, enroll in clinical trials of experimental therapy that offer more benefit to researchers than to themselves, or reassure loved ones that it is not yet time to pay a visit—only to lapse into a coma before having a chance to say good-bye.

There are many documented deficiencies in the experience of patients at the end of their lives: the great majority of Americans die in institutions rather than at home as many would prefer; most die in pain despite being in the care of health providers; many die alone; and many have deaths that are financially devastating for their families. These problems persist even in the face of enormous public and private expenditures in the last year of life. They persist, moreover, despite the fact that we all must die; all of us should thus have a stake in improving end-of-life care. I find the most disheartening indication of Americans' feelings about the care we give the dying to be the currently widespread interest in euthanasia.[3]

I am convinced that some (though certainly not all) of the problems people have with terminal care result from the absence or poor quality of prognostic information they are given. If seriously ill patients had better information about their chances of survival and about the likely success and implications of proposed treatments, and if they were supported by their physicians in how they chose to use this information, they might make different choices at the end of their lives. As we shall see, patients often desire such information. With it, they might be empowered to plan for, and achieve, the kind of good death most Americans say they want: free of pain, at home, with loved ones, having said good-byes and put their affairs in order. Moreover, if physicians were more thoughtful, deliberate, and self-aware in their formulation of prognoses; if they formulated more accurate prognoses; if they talked more deliberately among themselves about prognosis; and if they made these cognitive adjustments regardless of whether they communicated prognoses to patients—then they might find *themselves* behaving differently, choosing, for example, to forgo futile therapy or choosing to engage in more timely discussions with patients about optimal terminal care. They might even find this style of practice more rewarding.

Cogent and compassionate prognostication, I believe, could decrease the prevalence of bad deaths in our society. For me, such prognostication is a sensitively delivered and well calibrated best guess about the patient's future. It requires physicians to be as versed in the art and science of prognosis as they are in diagnosis and therapy, to make strenuous efforts both to learn the state of the art with respect to the prognostic problem presented by the patient and to communicate that knowledge in a way that the patient can comprehend, to the extent that the patient wants this. Moreover, it requires physicians to adopt a broader view of the meaning of hope and to realize that there is much patients can realistically hope for even if death is imminent and unavoidable. The kind of prognostication I have in mind includes physicians' willingness to spend time talking with patients, assuring them that they will not be abandoned. It entails, finally, the willingness of physicians to *act* on predictions, despite the risk of error. Such behavior by physicians would reflect the realization that temporizing or self-delusion in prognosis can be as harmful to patients as an incorrect diagnosis or a mistaken treatment. And such behavior would, ultimately, reflect what I think are the very real *moral* aspects of prognostication.

These are not easy things to do, of course, and there is good reason that physicians avoid prognostication, beyond the fact that it is technically difficult and emotionally frightening. Prognostication can hurt patients, and not just when it is inaccurate. Some patients do not wish to be provided with prognostic information. And I am deeply empathetic to the complexity of prognostication. What I am suggesting, therefore, is an approach that balances the benefits of prognostication against the benefits of avoiding it, an approach that realizes that unfavorable predictions do not mean physicians have nothing to do and patients nothing to hope for, an approach that recognizes that acting on an uncertain prediction may be better than making no prediction at all. I am also arguing for much greater attention to prognosis, in research and in teaching, at the level of the medical profession as a whole. My impression, from both clinical experience and my study of the issue, is that we are leaning too far toward the avoidance of prognosis and that we are causing harm as a result.

A better understanding of how physicians prognosticate is justified not only by the prospect of enhancing patient care, but also by contemporary developments that are increasing the importance of prediction. Physicians will increasingly be expected to prognosticate—they may be reluctant prophets, but they will be prophets nonetheless. For example, the increasing public interest in humane terminal care requires that medical professionals be more willing to make and act on predictions about the imminence of death. A physician's prognostic assessment that a patient is "terminally ill" is an essential element in the withdrawal or withholding of life support,[4] in proposals regarding physician-assisted suicide,[5] and in patients' qualifying for hospice entry.[6]

It is also clear, however, that it will not be easy to change physicians' care at the end of life, and that the problem is not simply that physicians have inadequate information about prognosis. A recent five-year, thirty-million-dollar study showed, sadly, that even physicians who were given accurate prognostic data developed with statistical models did not change their practice.[7] In one phase of this so-called SUPPORT study (Study to Understand Prognoses and Preferences for Outcomes and Risks of Treatment), physicians treating a randomly chosen half of a population of 4,804 seriously ill patients were provided with comprehensive information on each patient's prognosis and preferences for care. Comparing the group of patients and doctors that received this information with the control group that did not, the investigators concluded that the intervention did not have an impact on any of the several prognostically relevant outcomes it sought to influence (such as the quality of care at the end of life) or on physician-patient communication about prognosis. The study findings and the authors' conclusions were widely reported in the popular press.[8]

In my view, however, certain findings of this study did not receive the attention they deserved. The investigators noted, for example, that although the patient's physician was provided with prognostic information 94 percent of the time, the physician acknowledged or remembered receiving the information only 59 percent of the time, and, more remarkably, the physician reported having discussed this specific prognostic information with patients or their families only 15 percent of the time! The patients themselves confirmed a low rate of discussion with their doctors about their prognosis and their preferences for care; only a minority reported having had a prognostic discussion with their doctor—despite the fact that the patients examined in this study were seriously ill with a high risk of death and despite the fact that a majority said they would have welcomed such a discussion. For me, this was the most astounding finding of this remarkable study. Sadly, most of the patients in this study went on to experience deaths that, as the investigators documented in rich detail, were very unsatisfactory.

It is not surprising that giving physicians prognostic information failed to change patients' care or experience of dying since it failed to change physicians' behavior in communicating with patients about their prognoses. The failure of the intervention highlights how ingrained are physicians' patterns of practice. My hope is that this book will offer a subtle understanding of physicians' aversion to prognostication and their biases in generating and using prognostic information. My hope as well is that this book adequately explores two fundamental paradoxes about prognostication. The first is that physicians both fear prognosis and desire it; they avoid it but (in specific ways at specific times) engage it. The second is that even as the uncertainty in prognosis leads to the avoidance of prognosis, it also leads to a feeling of control and of hope; like prognosis itself, the unpredictability of the future is both repulsive and attractive.

When prognosticating is unavoidable, physicians cope with the difficulty it presents in a number of ways, including recourse to certain cognitive biases, magical ideas, and religious sentiments. Most, for example, develop a ritualistically optimistic attitude when it comes to foretelling the future. Identifying such aspects of physicians' thinking has several implications, in some cases suggesting corrective techniques. For example, disinterested parties might be sought to render prognoses, prognoses might be elicited in methodologically superior ways (e.g., in probabilistic rather than temporal terms), prognostic estimates might be averaged across physicians, or prognoses might be supplemented (though not replaced) by computer assessments—four techniques that have been shown to enhance the accuracy of prognostic estimates.[9] There is a broader implication, however. Identifying "nonrational" elements of physicians' thinking may serve to make physicians more empathetic to patients' own nonrational thoughts about their illnesses. In fact, patients' ideas about the causation and meaning of their illnesses may be seen as a competing rationality, and doctors' claim to objectivity may be subverted. Doctors too are situated in a domain of subjective experience and subjective ideas about illness; they too have a view from somewhere rather than a view from nowhere.

Prognosis gives diagnosis and therapy their affective components, for physicians and patients alike. When patients, or physicians, fear a diagnosis, the reason is that they fear its prognosis. As a consequence, prognosis is responsible for much of the *meaning* in diagnosis and therapy. What are the implications of the diagnosis? Will the treatment be effective? Will the patient live or die? These are fundamental questions in medical practice, and they are fundamentally prognostic.

In its ability to induce emotions and change behaviors, prognosis, I will argue here, resembles prophecy and, as such, casts the physician in the role of prophet. I invoke this analogy for three reasons. First, it sheds light on aspects of the prognostic role of the physician, a role that has heretofore been relatively overlooked. Second, prediction in medical practice instantiates and therefore illuminates a fundamental social relation between a "prophet" and a "supplicant." And third, the resemblance between prognosis and prophecy highlights the moral dimension of prognosis and therefore physicians' duty to engage in it.

This book focuses largely on internists. Most of the physicians interviewed and surveyed, and most of the clinical problems considered, are drawn from internal medicine (including oncology, cardiology, intensive care, general internal medicine, and other of its subspecialties). As a specialty, internal medicine accounts for 25 to 35 percent (the largest fraction) of the country's practicing physicians, and it covers the vast majority of the causes of death, including cancer, heart disease, and infection. This focus also reflects my own clinical training and the type of deadly illness I am interested in. Surgical, psychiatric, and pediatric concerns are much less represented here, though they do appear; sometimes these appearances illuminate contrasts with internal medicine, but usually they demonstrate the consistency of the patterns I identify across much of the practice of medicine. Inasmuch as death, and the "serious" kind of prognostication that concerns death, is my focus, I believe my findings have implications for other medical specialties.

This book draws on both social scientific and medical perspectives to illuminate the problem of prognosis. Taking advantage of my position within both sociology and medicine, I draw on the methods, the ideas, and the literatures of both. Multiple and heterogeneous sources of data (both qualitative and quantitative), mostly from my own studies, are used for the main arguments. I ask the reader's forbearance if any one method seems too abstruse or marginal, but I am hoping the preponderance and variety of the evidence will be persuasive.

My most important caveat is that this book is about doctors themselves. To the extent that patients appear, it is only through the eyes of doctors. I do not mean to privilege the role of the physician in confronting the necessity and strain of prognosis at the expense of the patient. Clearly, seriously ill patients suffer immensely with their desire for prognostic information, their inferior medical knowledge relative to that of the physician, their uncertainty regarding their future, and their experience of events that confound their expectations and hopes. Another book could, and should, be written about how patients experience and cope with prognosis. I focus on physicians here because they provide a clear window into this topic and because I believe they have both the duty and the capacity to change their prognostic behavior for the better.

This book begins, in chapter 1, by documenting the ellipsis of prognosis from contemporary medical thought and practice, despite a prominent position in medicine at the turn of the century. I show that there is a complementary, reciprocal relationship between prognosis and therapy—that when therapy is available, physicians will blithely neglect prognosis. Because modern medicine has numerous effective treatments at its disposal, it has tended, I argue, to overlook prognostication as a way of coping with illness. I then examine why I believe prognostication is increasingly relevant. I also argue that prognosis is socially constructed, and I lay the groundwork for the link between prognostication and death.

In chapter 2, I analyze the uses of prognosis, both implicit and explicit. I show that physicians make use of prognosis to achieve several clinical, interactional, and symbolic objectives. In clinical care, they use prognosis to help guide the choice of therapy or to encourage patients to comply with it. But they also use prognosis, for example, in evaluating the performance of their colleagues and in supporting ethical decision making. Prognostication is filled with uncertainty, however, and physicians must cope with this fact. I examine some of the ways they respond to unpredictability, and I argue that, paradoxically, this unpredictability is both deplored in its own right and manipulated as a predicate for hope.

In chapter 3, I examine the level of accuracy in physicians' prognoses and show that it is quite poor. This inaccuracy is manifested in two ways. First, physicians' prognoses are prone to error, meaning that they tend not to be correct for any given individual. Second, their prognoses are prone to bias, meaning that they err in a systematic way—exhibiting, for example, a tendency to overestimate survival in both their inward and outward prognoses. I then examine physicians' responses to prognostic error. I show that physicians believe that patients and colleagues will hold them accountable for error. In the opinion of physicians, the unavoidable presence of error in prognostication, as well as the fact that this error is felt to be consequential for patient care and for professional reputation, strongly encourage the avoidance of prognostication. Paradoxically, however, the presence of unavoidable error is also reassuring to physicians in that it can result in their not being held responsible for patients' outcomes. Finally, I show that the fact that physicians are fallible in prognosis engenders spiritual sentiments in them; this is not surprising in that religion is, after all, a fundamental way people cope with uncertain and important matters.

In chapter 4, I examine several additional sources of stress for physicians in prognostication, beyond its propensity to error. These sources include their inadequate training in prognosis; the uncertainty inherent in prediction; the dependence of prognosis on patients' social attributes; the emotional strain of communicating a prognosis; and the fear that explicit prognostication can harm patients. These factors lie behind a set of professional norms that encourage the avoidance of prognostication. I also show, however, that—again, paradoxically—prognostication can be embraced by physicians as a way to cope with the stress of their practice. I conclude with an examination of the ways that the norms stressing avoidance of prognosis are sustained in the medical profession.

In chapter 5, I show that physicians favor a staged, statistical, and optimistic form of prognostication when communicating a prognosis is unavoidable, and that they believe they should take into account patients' own prognostic estimates both in constructing and in presenting a prognosis. I argue that this type of communication reflects the ambiguity inherent in medical knowledge and that, furthermore, physicians see this ambiguity in communication as fostering hope and thus being beneficial.

In chapter 6, I turn to one of the main "nonrational" aspects of prognostication: physicians' belief in the self-fulfilling prophecy. After first defining various types of self-fulfilling prophecy, I show that physicians recognize that prognoses in and of themselves influence human action and, consequently and unavoidably, future events. Using material from in-depth interviews, I explore physicians' rationales for their perceptions of the way self-fulfilling prophecy works in medical situations. Physicians believe that predictions can work by changing patients' attitudes, behavior, and physiology; by changing physicians' attitudes and behavior; and by almost magical means. To validate these findings, I analyze experimental data from a national survey of internists. I establish that while physicians do, in fact, believe in the self-fulfilling prophecy, belief in the obverse phenomenon, self-negating prophecy, is not common. Finally I discuss the implications for the doctor-patient relationship of both belief in the self-fulfilling prophecy and beliefs regarding its mechanisms of action.

In chapter 7, I explore one of the main consequences of the belief in the self-fulfilling prophecy: the "ritualization of optimism." I also consider the complementary phenomenon of the "ritualization of pessimism." I examine the reasons that physicians ritualize optimism and pessimism, and I consider the practical and symbolic functions that each of these strategies serves. Then, I analyze how physicians choose between the two strategies and show how the belief in the self-fulfilling prophecy and physicians' desire to be held responsible for favorable, but not unfavorable, outcomes together strongly support these strategies. I argue that the tendency towards prognostic optimism complements the tendency towards diagnostic pessimism in medical thought and practice. And I conclude by examining some possibly adverse consequences of optimism, using hospice referral at the end of life as a primary example.

In chapter 8, I argue that prognostication among physicians resembles prophecy and that, as such, it has strong moral overtones. This observation implies that to avoid prognosis in medicine is to neglect an important responsibility. Both individual physicians and the profession as a whole, I argue, have a duty to prognosticate. I conclude with some observations about how physicians and the medical profession might best discharge this duty.

Prognostication is a troubling aspect of being a physician, but it need not and should not be as neglected as it is. The fact that prognosis was once a more prominent part of medical care, and the fact that it is occasionally still prominent, together suggest that it may be possible to rehabilitate prognosis and introduce it anew into medical practice. It is my hope that this book will prompt a reexamination of the justifications for the ellipsis of prognosis and, in so doing, help simultaneously to improve our understanding of medicine as a social form and to enhance our care of the seriously ill.

Chicago, July 1999

One

PROGNOSIS IN MEDICINE

Predicting the outcome of life-threatening illness is never inconsequential or insignificant, for the patient or for the doctor. Will the outcome be survival or death? What kind of death? When will it occur? How might therapy affect the outcome? The difficulty physicians face in addressing such questions is only magnified when it is presumed that they are both able and willing to make such predictions. Prognostication elicits potent and troubling attitudes and behaviors in physicians. And these in turn ramify widely through many aspects of medical practice.

When physicians prognosticate, they confront some of the most serious, emotional, and meaningful aspects of their professional practice. Doctors often characterize their experience with prognosis quite vividly:

> I had a patient who died of a progressive, degenerative neurological disease. And certain things started happening to this patient—like he couldn't speak, or he couldn't swallow, or he couldn't raise one eyelid, or he couldn't walk. Virtually every day something new would happen. Eventually, he stopped being able to see, he couldn't see his family, and then he got confused, and then he couldn't talk. And every time I went to see him throughout the course of his illness, he would ask: "Doctor, what is going to happen tomorrow? Will I wake up tomorrow and not be able to see? When is this going to end?" It was a horrible thing for me to see him go through this and not to be able to do anything.
>
> I would say, "I'm sorry, I can't tell you what's going to happen tomorrow, and I can't make these things go away. If you're in pain, we can do something about that, and if you're feeling dry in your mouth, we can do something about that. But I'm sorry, I can't tell you when it's going to end, and it's not going to get better."

This patient has a serious, life-threatening illness, and he is being buffeted by serious symptoms that occur unexpectedly. He wants to know when it will end—when he will die. His lack of foreknowledge intensifies his suffering.

The doctor, like the patient, does not know what to expect, and he also finds this very disturbing. He is limited both therapeutically and prognostically, and these distinct limitations are both problematic.

The patient's clinical state and the patient himself demand a prognosis, yet the situation seems to defy prognosis. What the doctor does know—that the patient will die, that the therapy cannot "make these things go away"—provides little comfort to either patient or doctor. Indeed, the doctor avers, he cannot tell the patient "what's going to happen tomorrow"; the predictions he can make are both disagreeable and vague. Predicting the future for such a patient may engender feelings of ignorance, impotence, sadness, guilt, or fear. Yet, with patients in different circumstances—patients for whom the future is more certain or more favorable or more modifiable—predicting the future may engender feelings of competence, confidence, or joy. In no case of serious illness, however, is predicting the future straightforward or meaningless.

When physicians tell patients that they cannot predict the future, they are eliding an important distinction between *inability* to predict and *unwillingness* to predict. Physicians themselves are often not conscious of which is the greater obstacle in a given situation. But the distinction is important because inability and unwillingness have different origins and different implications. Part of the problem is that even formulating, much less communicating, a prediction about death is unpleasant, so physicians are inclined to refrain from it. But when they are able to formulate a prediction and fail to do so, the quality of medical care that patients receive may suffer. For example, the lack of a prognosis (or the presence of a needlessly inaccurate one) may mean that physicians give seriously ill patients unnecessary treatments or, conversely, deny them beneficial ones. And patients who themselves lack critical prognostic information may make bad choices near the end of their lives.

Prognostication is an essential part of medicine. Patients often seek prognostic information from physicians, and patients and physicians require it when choosing among alternative therapies. But despite its being essential, it is usually, and somewhat paradoxically, implicit. Explicit prognostication about unfavorable outcomes, or even about favorable ones, evokes anxiety and dread in physicians; hence, whenever possible, they avoid it. How can prognostication be both essential and implicit? What cognitive, emotional, professional, and social factors lead physicians to avoid or engage prognostication? How should a physician respond to a prediction? In short, what is the role of knowledge of the future, and of claims to such knowledge, in medical care?

These questions touch on issues that transcend the merely technical aspects of prediction or the merely individual aspects of clinical care. They are fraught with meaning, have overtones of morality, and suggest lines of responsibility. As such, they cast the physician in the role of a prophet. To say that prognosis has prophetic elements is to say that it is often meaningful, mysterious, and influential. To say that physicians are like prophets is to say that, in rendering prognoses, they resemble the idealized image of prophets as selfless and reluctant sages engaged in a difficult, obscure, moral, and valuable activity.

The Neglect of Prognosis

There are three complementary ways in which physicians may understand and, in the broadest sense, control a patient's disease: they can identify it, eliminate it, or predict its course. All three—diagnosis, therapy, and prognosis—are means by which physicians come to terms, clinically and cognitively, with disease. These three means are clearly interconnected; nevertheless, physicians maintain rigid distinctions between them in their case presentations, notes, textbooks, and thinking. Of the three, diagnosis and therapy receive much more attention than prognosis—in patient care, medical research, and medical education. Prognosis is not merely neglected, however, it is avoided. Documenting the extent of this neglect and avoidance, and understanding the reasons for it, are two of my central concerns. When and why did prognosis come to be deemphasized in clinical practice? Is the ellipsis of prognosis uniform, or does it vary according to the clinical and social circumstances of the patient and physician?

The relative lack of explicit consideration of prognosis has been lamented by some physicians for a long time. In 1934, for example, one observed:

> Of the three great branches of clinical science—diagnosis, prognosis, and treatment—prognosis is admittedly the most difficult. It is also that about which least has been written and of which our knowledge is least systematized.[1]

In 1953, another wrote:

> [Prognosis] still remains a stepchild in medical advance partly because it is a difficult subject and partly because, for some reason or other, it has rarely been studied scientifically. The few sentences devoted to it in the account of almost any disease or condition in almost all textbooks and papers are little more than a sop to the conscience.[2]

A review of the content of clinical research published between 1946 and 1976 revealed that in 1976 diagnosis and treatment were the subject of 37 percent and 33 percent of published studies respectively, but prognosis was the subject of only 4 percent.[3] Moreover, although interest in diagnosis increased during this period, there was no change in the low percentage of studies devoted to prognosis. In 1981, this state of affairs led other physicians to observe: "Neglect of prognosis in standard medical texts is nearly complete; often the term does not even appear in the index."[4] A recent analysis of entries in contemporary textbooks confirms this. *Harrison's Principles of Internal Medicine,* a prestigious and widely used textbook, for example, has explicitly demarcated discussions of etiology, pathogenesis, clinical manifestations, diagnosis, and treatment for virtually all of the diseases it considers. However, only 27 percent of the entries contain discussions of prognosis, and such material, where it appears, is usually only one paragraph long.[5] This organization of modern textbooks mirrors modern medical practice, in which physicians focus on diagnosis and therapy and avoid explicit consideration of prognosis.

The relative absence of explicit prognostication in modern textbooks is partly a consequence of the contemporary dominance of an ontological view of disease—a view in which disease is seen as generic and generally independent of its expression in an individual. Making a diagnosis has become the central concern of the clinical encounter—in large measure because the prognosis and the therapy are seen to follow from it necessarily and directly. This perspective is reinforced when there is an *effective* therapy for a disease, because effective therapy further narrows the range of possible outcomes. Once a diagnosis is made and effective therapy initiated, the clinical course of a disease is often presumed to be relatively fixed—the same for everyone. A favorable outcome is presumed, so it does not need to be explicitly predicted. The conflation of diagnosis and prognosis, and the reduction of prognostic variability through the application of effective therapy, are complex phenomena that imply an evasion of the individual and the idiosyncratic. Yet, in another sense, it is the idiosyncratic, the individual, and the atypical that define the prognosis.

The Progressive Omission of Prognosis

If it is true that physicians presume that diagnosis and therapy dictate prognosis, we would expect that when diagnosis is straightforward and many effective therapies are available, prognosis should be relatively less prominent. Conversely, when therapeutic options and diagnostic knowledge are limited, physicians should deem prognosis to be a more central clinical task and should focus on it. An examination of entries in successive editions of *The Principles and Practice of Medicine*, another prestigious and widely used textbook, reveals that in the period from 1892 to 1988 there is just such a complementary, reciprocal relation between the clinical acts of prognostication and therapy—that as one increases in salience in the management of a disease, the other decreases.[6] In entries for a variety of conditions written in the earlier part of the twentieth century, in contrast to those in more recent editions and to current practice, prognosis was an important part of the clinical formulation of patients' cases. That is, when effective treatment for a given condition was unavailable, prognosis played a key role in clinical management.[7] However, with the advent of manifestly efficacious therapeutics, the ability to predict the "natural history" of a disease lost importance, if only because it was no longer observed.

Pneumonia provides an illustrative example. Pneumonia was a leading cause of death throughout the period from 1892 to 1947. In 1900 it was the leading killer in the United States, and it remained one of the top five killers well beyond 1947.[8] Indeed, during this period, many physicians regarded pneumonia as the prototypical condition they faced; in 1924, for example, a textbook referred to pneumonia as "one of the most widespread and fatal of all acute diseases" and "Captain of the Men of Death."[9] After antibiotic therapy for pneumonia was discovered in the late 1930s, however, the prognosis improved substantially—so much so that it became assumed and, consequently, neglected. The natural history of the disease was replaced by a clinical course, and the "unnatural history of disease" became the standard in clinical encounters.[10] Now the task of the physician was primarily to diagnose and treat the disease and only secondarily, if at all, to predict the future. Moreover, now the future was brought about not only by the disease itself but also by the beneficial or detrimental consequences of therapy.

Figure 1.1 shows the percentage of chapter length devoted to various aspects of the clinical management of pneumonia in various editions of *The Principles and Practice of Medicine*. The 1892 chapter gives more attention to the presentation of the disease than to anything else, but diagnosis, therapy, and prognosis receive roughly equal attention. By comparison, most of the chapter in 1988 is devoted to diagnosis, and there is no explicit discussion of prognosis at all. These proportions are relatively typical of modern textbook entries.[11] The 1947 entry is intermediate between those of 1892 and 1988; it shows increased attention to therapy, reflecting the emergence of effective antibiotic treatment in the late 1930s, and decreased attention to prognosis.

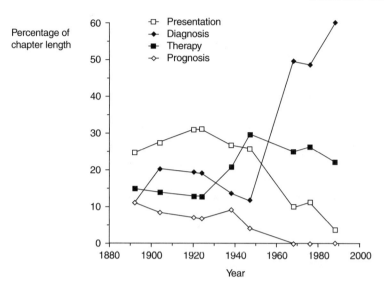

Figure 1.1. Percentage of chapter on pneumonia devoted to selected clinical tasks, *The Principles and Practice of Medicine*, 1892–1988. "Presentation" refers to symptoms and physical findings seen in the patient; aspects of the chapters that are not shown include etiology, pathology, and complications. Source: After N. A. Christakis, "The Ellipsis of Prognosis in Modern Medical Thought," *Social Science and Medicine* 44 (1997): 301–15, used with permission from Elsevier Science.

Another force, in addition to the emergence of effective therapy, has led to the relative absence of prognosis from modern textbooks: a fundamental change in the cognitive basis of medicine with respect to diagnosis over the course of the twentieth century. In the late nineteenth century, the outcome and course of a disease were believed to be determined largely by the "constitution" of the patient. If two individuals were exposed to a contagious ailment, for example, the one with the "firmer" constitution would be expected to have the more favorable outcome. The two individuals were seen, in some sense, as having different diseases, and their prognoses were believed to differ because of individual factors distinct from the diagnosis itself.

Around the turn of the century, however, physicians began to believe that different patients might have—in a fundamental sense—the *same* disease. Beginning at that time, medicine moved from an individualistic notion of disease to one concerned with the centrality of diagnostic categories based on specific causative agents. This development in clinical thought—the belief that conditions have identities independent of their existence in given patients—was associated with a substantial increase in attention to diagnosis and a relative decrease in attention to patient-specific factors, whether age, sex, occupation, or precise symptoms. A cognitive shift toward the notion that disease had a discrete existence that was not only ontological and etiological but also prognostic—that a disease had a "natural course" that was "typical"—had begun. Clinical thought progressively moved from an individual-based to a diagnosis-based conceptualization of disease, and prognosis increasingly was presumed to be intrinsic to the diagnosis.[12]

Effective therapy and nosologic systems thus both work to shift clinical attention from the individual patient. Attention is directed to what is deemed to be the essence of the patient's problem, the diagnostic category and the corresponding therapy, and this leads to a clinical view that looks *through* rather than *upon* the individual case. The patient becomes not so much a sick person as an "endlessly reproducible pathologic fact."[13] Prognosis is viewed as a simple extension of diagnosis and therapy, an extension no longer dependent on individual traits and typically not requiring explicit consideration.[14]

The Complementarity of Prognosis and Therapy

The complementary relation between prognosis and therapy holds both in the construction of theoretical knowledge, as reflected in textbooks, and in the actual treatment of patients. Some physicians are old enough to recall the historical transition that has occurred in this relationship; as one seventy-year-old physician noted:

> I think that fifty years ago, when their armamentarium was limited, physicians believed that the way one handled patients—the way one treated patients, the way one communicated with patients— was as important as whatever they had to do in the way of drugs or whatever. Indeed, often they had *nothing* they could do. Not only was communicating the prognosis important to the patient, but it also was important to the physician in that good communication with the patient meant that he became known as a good doctor.

Other physicians make this point about their current practice. When a patient is so sick that death seems certain, and when therapy is ineffective, they note a shift in their thinking and interactions toward predicting the course of the disease. That is, depending on the clinical circumstances of any given patient, prognosis may eclipse therapy as the focus of the clinical encounter.

This relation between prognosis and therapy is thus seen in several aspects of medical practice: at the level of epistemology, in the perception and representation of particular diseases, in the care of individual patients, and in the way particular specialties practice. Physicians rely on prognosis to "control" diseases for which they have no treatment—when a disease lacks effective treatment, prognosis occupies more space in textbooks and prognostication occupies more time in physicians' ministrations. Indeed, the very term *incurable disease* evinces the transmutation of a strictly therapeutic assertion into a prognostic pronouncement. In the care of individual patients, physicians may focus more attention on prognosis if therapeutic options are absent or diminishing; the proverbial (and inappropriate) statement "There is nothing more we can do" often suggests the question "What will happen next?" On a broader scale, medical specialties with many options for therapy will tend to neglect prognosis, while those with few options will attend to prognosis. For example, there is, in general, greater attention to prognosis in neurology than in the specialty of infectious disease.[15]

Sometimes, patients' actions too seem to reflect this complementary relation between therapy and prognosis. For instance, one physician contrasted two of his terminally ill patients as follows:

> One patient wanted me to do very little therapeutically and wanted to know what the time frame for survival was. The other wanted me to do everything conceivable and didn't want to know about timing. Although I think at some level both patients recognized and acknowledged that they had metastatic disease that would likely be the cause of their death, one recognized that it would do so in the short term, and the other one was not willing to accept that possibility.

Although both patients wanted their doctor to do something for them and to show mastery over the disease, they had different ideas about what this should be. Some patients strive for the elimination of their disease, others to know what will happen.[16]

The fact that prognosis and therapy are complementary, when coupled with the increasing prevalence of effective therapy, helps explain why modern clinical practice pays so little attention to prognosis. But there are many other reasons for the lack of attention. A close study of physicians' attitudes and behavior reveals a *dread* of prognostication—whether favorable or unfavorable, accurate or inaccurate. Physicians would rather not formulate or discuss prognoses. As we shall see, especially in chapter 4, a number of powerful professional norms have evolved that limit the explicit consideration of prognosis in clinical practice.

The Resurgent Relevance of Prognosis

Despite the reduced prominence, in recent decades, of explicit prognostication, several developments in contemporary medical practice, as well as broader cultural changes, are contributing to its renewed importance. These changes are occurring on three broad fronts: in the type of medical problems patients have, in the way health care is delivered, and in the philosophy and cultural outlook that guides health care delivery. We have seen increases, for example, in (1) the prevalence of chronic disease; (2) the bureaucratization of health care delivery; (3) the need to compare health care providers and rationalize expenditures; (4) the reliance on randomized, controlled trials to evaluate drugs and on health services research to evaluate other, nonpharmaceutical medical interventions; (5) the use of novel biomedical technologies; (6) the attention paid to patient self-determination and to other ethical issues in medical care, especially at the end of life; and (7) the expectations that patients express regarding access to information and respect for their "rights" (ranging from a "right to know" to a "right to die").[17]

Changes in Types of Diseases

The number and percentage of patients with chronic disease—for whom the diagnosis is already known and therapy is often simply the continuation of previously initiated interventions—are increasing.[18] In such cases, because curative therapy is limited and the course of the disease is long, prognostication can become especially prominent. The clinical encounter is focused on the anticipation, avoidance, and mitigation of complications of the underlying disease itself or of the treatment. Patients with long-standing diabetes, for example, do not need to be told their diagnosis (which is known to them) or their therapy (for example, insulin—also known to them). Rather, they and their physicians are concerned with such questions as "Will my kidneys fail, and if so, when?" "Will I become blind?" "How long will I be able to care for myself?" "How long do I have to live?" Moreover, in chronic conditions, there is more opportunity to revise previously rendered prognoses as, over time, the physician learns more about the patient.[19]

Changes in Health Care Delivery

Several developments in health care delivery and health care technology also support the increasing importance of prognosis in medicine. A

key factor is the increasingly bureaucratic structure of American medical practice. Physicians are increasingly becoming salaried employees
beholden to bureaucratic management or are otherwise losing their
economic independence and some of their professional autonomy.[20]
External review of physicians' clinical behavior often focuses on actions that are at least implicitly based on their prognostic judgments.
For example, administrative oversight plays an increasing role in therapy management. Physicians are being asked, in the context of cost-
effectiveness, to predict outcomes among a variety of (more or less
costly) treatment options or to estimate the length of the hospital stay
necessary for an anticipated medical outcome. Better prognostication, in
the sense of a superior ability to foresee the outcome of a patient's illness,
can help to optimize the choice of treatment and the timing of hospital
admission, thus reducing costs. Similarly, federal regulations dictate that
physicians wishing to refer Medicare patients for hospice terminal care
must certify that the patient has less than six months to live. Although
physicians are expected to make this serious prognostic determination,
which has significant administrative and clinical consequences, this
characterization of the terminal state has no real clinical basis. It was
adopted simply as a result of the original Medicare legislation.[21] Prognosis is also evoked when physicians' performance is evaluated through
the comparison of their patients' outcomes to "normal" standards, the
latter being implicitly prognostic. Bureaucratic superiors, for example,
may evaluate surgeons' success rates for certain types of procedures by
comparison to expected success rates.[22]

A greater focus on prognosis also results from the increasing need
to compare the quality of health care providers, along with a more
general societal interest in rationalizing health care expenditures by
directing resources to those most likely to benefit. Accurate and reliable
prognostic assessments are central to the identification, development,
and implementation of optimal health care delivery systems in that
they help patients and payers determine which systems lead to good or
bad outcomes. Moreover, comparison across systems should optimally
include a "risk adjustment" that takes into account the relative sickness
of patients in the systems—that is, whether the patients in one were
intrinsically sicker than those in another and thus might be expected
to do worse.[23] Health care providers must demonstrate that the care
they offer is effective and of good quality, after adjusting for their patients' "baseline" prognoses. Similarly, evaluating the cost-effectiveness
of different medical therapies relies on access to accurate information
about the probabilities of various outcomes, which are, in essence,

prognoses.[24] Some medical interventions may be cost-effective only in subpopulations where the patients are at particularly high or low risk of mortality, and payers may target interventions—conditional, again, on the patient's prognosis—to cases in which they feel the benefit justifies the cost. In each case, the ability to develop and analyze prognoses is essential to asking the right counterfactual questions and getting the right policy answers.

Another factor lending salience to prognosis is the increasing frequency of randomized, controlled clinical trials. The customary role of prognosis in clinical trials has been to ensure that patients of similar illness severity are compared, since groups of patients with an equivalent average prognosis (e.g., for death) are formed by the randomization process. However, prognosis is finding a new use: rather than waiting for uncommon or temporally distant outcomes to occur in long-term clinical trials, which can be difficult and expensive, investigators are increasingly making use of "intermediate endpoints," that is, findings that are taken to be *predictive* of long-term outcomes.[25] A decrease in a lab test value is taken to indicate a decreased risk of eventual death, making shorter and less expensive trials possible. The booming industry in clinical trials thus supports increasing interest in the development and use of various prognostic staging systems and clinical markers.[26]

The emergence of certain medical technologies also increases the relevance of prognosis. On the one hand, the evaluation of their effectiveness generally relies on the availability of prognostic information.[27] But, in addition, these technologies—although often directed at improving diagnosis and therapy—also provide, directly or indirectly, more accurate and earlier prognostic information and therefore foster the rendering of prognoses. One example is obstetrical ultrasound, which may *incidentally* reveal information about the internal anatomy of a baby that would not otherwise be detected until well after the baby was born. Thus, parents and physicians are made aware of conditions long before the child is able to present with the illness. Such early findings, not yet corresponding to any observed symptom, demand explanation: patients wish to know what the findings *will* mean, what the future has in store. One pediatrician gives a typical example:

> Nowadays, many kids come to our clinic when they're two weeks old because their kidneys were abnormal on *Mom's* prenatal ultrasound! In the old days when someone was diagnosed with polycystic kidney disease in the neonatal period, they died before they were one year old. But now there are so many much milder cases that only come to our attention because of an ultrasound that happens to have been

done for other [obstetrical] reasons. We have no idea what to tell the parents about what to expect. It used to be that the children came to our attention because they were failing to thrive or anemic or acidotic or any of the serious things that renal insufficiency causes, and all the information about prognosis used to be based on their features at that time. But now they're presenting much, much earlier and no one knows what to do with that.

The parents ask for predictions. They want to know when will the kid need dialysis, when will they have to start thinking about transplant, when will this kidney disease that we see on the ultrasound affect them. Because right now their kids are thriving, they're doing well. But at some point they're going to need erythropoeitin shots and growth hormone and vitamin D and all these different things that we see with renal failure. We have no idea when that will be.

New technology makes it possible to detect bodily aberrancies with prognostic significance, even before they are symptomatic.[28]

The advent of genetic testing technology provides yet another important new arena for prognostication. Analysis of a person's genes may reveal relevant medical outcomes years or decades in advance in what are generally termed "presymptomatic carriers." In contrast to other tests applied for diagnostic purposes, such genetic tests have specifically prognostic importance, which is made all the more apparent by the fact that, in most cases, no specific interventions are available to cure the condition so detected, or even to delay its onset. A prototypic example is Huntington's disease, a fatal, degenerative neurological disease that usually begins in the patient's forties. Tests can now reveal with certainty, decades before any symptoms are noted, whether asymptomatic individuals will or will not develop the disease.[29] Because no treatment is available for the condition, this is yet another example of the complementary relationship between therapy and prognosis, in that the prognostic significance of these tests eclipses their therapeutic utility. In other situations, genetic tests are used to develop prognostic information that does indeed have therapeutic implications. For example, some women, on the basis of the prognostic information provided by genetic tests to evaluate their risk for breast cancer, undergo prophylactic mastectomy—even though this prognosis is not certain.[30] As more studies reveal genetic bases for diseases as diverse as emphysema, diabetes, dementia, cognitive disability, and alcoholism, the prognostic use of genetic tests will certainly rise.[31] The use of such tests is also likely to rise outside of medical arenas, for example, in law.

The increasingly technological, "postclinical" nature of medical practice fosters the availability of information that is presymptomatic in nature, and thus *inherently* prognostic.[32] "Presymptomatic" illness is, indeed, the specifically prognostic analog of "asymptomatic" illness. The notion of asymptomatic or "occult" or "silent" illness is itself interesting in that it posits a phenomenological realm of disease of which the patient has no subjective experience. This realm requires the intercession of an expert, a physician, to be comprehended. Typically, the expert must use technology to approach this realm, as when the physician uses diagnostic tests to adduce the presence of disease even when the patient has no symptoms.[33] The implications of the term *presymptomatic,* however, extend even beyond those of *asymptomatic.* Rather than indications of an already present disease, the expert is said to have discovered indications of a disease that is not yet even present. Some physicians have even begun to call individuals whose genetic tests are positive for a worrisome gene "prepatients."[34] The notion of presymptomatic illness thus represents an even further distancing of the patient's subjective experience of disease from the everyday practice of medicine. Moreover, the term *presymptomatic* suggests an inexorable outcome: the patient *will*—eventually—develop symptoms.

The application of new technologies to patient care increases the importance of prognostication in one other way: it creates a whole new class of things about which to prognosticate, namely the complications of the technology.[35] Beneficial new technologies in medicine—from computed tomography to chemotherapy to open heart surgery—have not come without risk. Predicting their consequences is important, and doctors are frequently called upon to explain to patients a potentially confusing array of possible outcomes.

Changes in Ethical and Cultural Expectations

In addition to changes in the types of medical problems people face and in the ways physicians confront them, there have been changes in the way that patients and physicians think about the ethical duties of physicians to their patients. Prognosis is a fundamental, though implicit, basis for many theoretical and practical ethical decisions in medical care, and prognostic uncertainty may complicate such decisions considerably. Ethical decision making is increasingly finding its way to the bedside.[36] The elaborate informed consent process that patients undergo prior to having procedures or participating in research, for example, is predicated upon *predicting* risks and benefits.[37] Prognosis also profoundly affects decisions to initiate, withhold, or terminate life support for critically ill newborns and adults, and it figures in the discussions about these decisions that doctors have with patients' families.[38] Prognostication is critical when one must allocate scarce medical resources to those patients for whom they can do the most good. Finally, it is central to the notion of "futility," a concept usually invoked in situations where death is predicted to be imminent and inevitable.[39] The relatively recent emergence of futility as a theme in bioethics reflects the moral desirability of acknowledging medical limitations and the practical necessity of allocating scarce resources.[40] Futility is based on a prognosis not only that the patient is unlikely to recover spontaneously, but also that any intervention will likely be ineffective. As the avoidance of futile treatment has assumed increasing prominence, for reasons of justice, beneficence, or economy, prognostication—which is, after all, the fundamental and essential basis for a determination of futility—has increased in importance.[41]

Broad changes in American society are influencing the doctor-patient relationship and fostering an increased interest in prognosis. In areas ranging from childbearing to terminal care, patients want information about expected outcomes that they can use to manage their care actively. This is especially true with respect to care at the end of life. Beginning in the 1960s, and consistent with then-contemporary societal trends toward "consciousness raising" and the questioning of authority, a death awareness movement emerged. The way was led by books such as Herman Feifel's *The Meaning of Death* in 1959 and Elisabeth Kübler-Ross's *On Death and Dying* in 1969.[42] Kübler-Ross showed, among other things, that dying patients did not wish to be isolated, abandoned, or misled by their physicians. These books, both authored by psychiatrists, galvanized the public more than they changed the medical profession. Nevertheless, the sentiment that patients and physicians should discuss death more openly eventually gave way, in the 1970s and 1980s, to the obligation that they do so. Now, physicians have the *duty* to inform their patients about their illness, and patients have a *right* to know.

In recent years, the American public has become more focused on planning for death, a development reflected in the increasing interest in everything from living wills to physician-assisted suicide. There has been a profusion of books on caring for the terminally ill at home, which include vivid, nontechnical descriptions of what to expect and which document the impact of death on family members.[43] There have been best-selling how-to books on "self-deliverance."[44] And there have been books describing the process of dying, often using detailed and intimate case histories.[45] These latter books typically reflect an attempt to help people find meaning in dying, and they suggest that death is increasingly viewed as a passage that can be actively anticipated and therefore managed. To enact these popular visions of death, however, patients must rely on reasonably accurate prognoses from professional physicians.

In sum, ongoing changes in the nature of illness in contemporary American society as well as in the way medical problems are being confronted are resulting in a substantial increase in the relevance of prognostication in clinical care. Although it has typically been a less obvious part of medicine, prognosis has never been easily avoided, and several trends are converging to make it still harder to avoid.

The Social Construction of Prognosis

The foregoing factors suggest an increasing relevance for prognosis in medicine. But they also suggest the extent to which prognosis depends on context. Indeed, prognosis, like other forms of medical knowledge, may be seen to be socially constructed: it is not merely a function of patients' biology, but is influenced by physicians' and patients' beliefs and attributes and by social structures and organizations.

To begin with, social attributes of patients may influence the prognosis, affecting the biological prognosis itself, influencing the doctor's actual formulation of the prognosis, and determining whether the doctor communicates it to the patient. The impact of poverty, race, religion, and social support on medical outcomes, even after taking into account the patient's diagnosis and treatment, is well documented.[46] For instance, the actual, biological course of coronary artery disease may depend on such variables as whether the patient lives alone or has social contacts or economic resources.[47] The patient's capacity to interact socially may transcend its impact on biological course and come to influence how physicians formulate a prognosis. Patients who are disconnected from the physician or from their family are, according to physicians, more likely to have unfavorable outcomes. As sociologist Renée Anspach observes in her study of neonatal intensive care, this particular aspect of prognosis is social in that the relevant information is gleaned through interaction with the patient and in that the relevant information is interpreted by reference to "appropriate" social standards.[48] Thus, when strictly biological criteria for prognostication are absent, doctors may turn to social criteria in order to formulate the prognosis.[49]

Regardless of the true import of social factors, physicians *believe* that such factors can influence the prognosis. One physician characterized their role as follows:

> In prognosis, you have got the combination of a disease process and "host resistance." Host resistance probably accounts for why so many people die within a short period of time after the death of their spouses. They've had these chronic diseases or problems which have been stable for years; then their husband dies, and six months later they are dead because their resistance has been compromised. Or, right at the age of sixty-five, at retirement, you see the same type of thing. You have got a disease with a reasonably well known prognosis, for example, exercise-related angina pectoris. The patient retires, and two weeks later they have died of an infarct. Explain it! You can't, except that prognosis in an individual patient is a combination of disease-related factors and host-related factors. That is why prognosis has more inherent variability than diagnosis. Diagnosis is fixed to a disease process, tagging a label, but what happens in an individual patient is not only a function of the disease but also a function of them.

Another elaborated:

> Estimates of prognosis take into account a complicated set of factors, including the patient's own perceptions of what they have; the patient's social, economic, and support situation; their physical frailty; their emotional frailty; and the number of the problems and their severity levels. In an individual patient's situation, the set of variables that we use to estimate likely outcome is extremely complicated.

Physicians often characterize the use of such information as "knowing the patient and the patient's life situation," and they think that it is important for proper prognostication. However, physicians are much more likely to take certain types of social information into account than others when making predictions. For example, nearly all physicians believe that social support affects the course of illness, but smaller percentages believe that the patient's religion or income does.[50] Overall, however, physicians' acquisition of social information about patients meaningfully affects the survival predictions they make.[51]

Insofar as prognosis depends on patients' social attributes, physicians believe that prognosis may indeed be patient-specific. That is, although a patient's income or religion might not be so much a factor in the biological expression of a disease, they are likely to be a factor in the course of the disease. Although a diagnosis as an abstract concept does have a prognosis attached to it, the prognosis in a specific patient might still depend on individual factors, including social ones. Making a prognosis thus requires the physician to be more familiar with the particular and social circumstances of the patient than diagnosis does.[52]

Patients' social attributes can influence whether a prognosis is offered at all, and not just its content. For example, a study of routine prognostication revealed a broad pattern in which prognostic information was more likely to be shared with patients with privileged socioeconomic status, regardless of whether they asked for it; the physician, that is, was more likely to discuss prognosis with male, wealthy, college-educated, and white patients during routine clinical encounters.[53] Moreover, the patient's physical or emotional health was *not* associated with whether prognosis was discussed; that is, social attributes appear to be more important than clinical ones.

Not only may social attributes be used as *determinants* of prognosis (influencing the formulation and communication of the prognosis as described above), they may sometimes replace medical parameters as the *outcomes* of interest. For example, for a thirteen-year-old girl who is pregnant, the doctor might predict "social failure" despite an acceptable clinical outcome (i.e., the delivery of a healthy baby). Similarly, physicians may make prognoses about a patient's ability to fulfill professional obligations, such as returning to work.

Prognosis is also socially constructed in that the valence and nature of a prognosis may themselves be defined socially. For example, sociologist Fred Davis, in his remarkable analysis of the medical experience of polio patients in the 1950s, demonstrates that the same clinical outcome can be presented and perceived in different lights; a prediction that the patient will be left partially paralyzed can be presented with varying degrees of optimism.[54] Physicians might note that although the patient will have to wear braces for the rest of his life, he will be able to use his legs. More generally, institutional and social systems structure prognostication. The treatment that patients undergo and the rhythm of their care, especially in hospital settings, reshape and redefine their expectations. A patient who at first expects to recover from a paralyzing injury, for example, eventually realizes (even if not told explicitly) that he should instead hope for different outcomes. The perception of any particular outcome is thus socially contingent. Moreover, differently situated individuals regard prognoses for severe incapacity differently. People who are more familiar with disability, for example, tend to regard being disabled as less problematic than those who are not.[55]

Finally, prognosis is socially constructed in that the prognosis rendered depends on the social and occupational attributes of the physician and on structural and organizational factors of the physician's practice. One study found that the survival estimates given by physicians varied according to their specialty training.[56] Another noted that physicians' definitions of "terminal" illness varied with both their specialty and their clinical experience.[57] A study of the propensity to overestimate prognosis for survival, on the other hand, found that it tended to be associated not with the attributes of physicians but rather with the extent to which the physician was familiar with the patient.[58]

A study of 125 routine clinical encounters found that the most important factor accounting for whether prognosis was discussed was the specialty of the physician—surgeons were much more likely than primary care physicians to offer predictions.[59] Other physician attributes that were associated with whether prognosis was mentioned included the number of years in practice and the number of hours per week devoted to patient care; physicians who had been in practice longer and those who spent fewer hours per week in clinical practice were less likely to mention prognosis. Less experienced physicians appear to have had fewer opportunities to be humbled by their errors; older physicians are more cautious about offering predictions. This is a general pattern. Older physicians feel that, when it comes to prognosis, "you're more likely to be wrong than right, so keep quiet."

The setting in which physicians practice may also affect prognostic decision making. For example, Anspach observes that in life-or-death decision making in the neonatal intensive care unit, even if there is agreement about what to do given a particular prognosis (for example, with respect to withdrawing life support), there may still be disagreement about the prognosis itself. Such disagreement, she argues, may arise from the different social and professional positions of the various actors.[60] Moreover, in patients from whom the withdrawal of life support is contemplated, the dissent of a single physician regarding the prognosis is often sufficient to introduce uncertainty and thus to mandate continued treatment. In this sense, the rendering of a prognosis is truly a group process: a definitive prognosis—upon which action may be based—can be rendered only by the group as a whole. The uncertainty as to prognosis here arises from the organization of decision making rather than from conflicting clinical facts.[61] And the requirement for unanimity of opinion in part reflects the belief that the more people who agree with a prediction, the more likely it is to be correct and accurate.[62]

The institutional practice of medicine has an impact on prognosis in other ways as well.[63] The nature of the statistics that are collected by bureaucracies may structure the prognoses that are communicated to patients and may be used to rationalize treatment decisions. For example, partly for reasons of administrative simplicity, follow-up studies conducted by neonatal ICUs often collect data taking as an endpoint "survival to discharge." These statistics are then used to justify a strongly interventionist stance, guiding decisions about therapy and the provision of life support, even though statistics about longer-term survival, quality of life, or longer-term cognitive or physical deficits might not show such a favorable prognosis for these infants.[64] Similarly, as we have seen, the frequency and type of visits, examinations, and procedures indicates to patients which outcomes they should be interested in and what "recovery" means; institutional perspectives on what expectations are legitimate can supplement, if not supplant, the expectations of the patient or physician.[65] Patients come to realize, for example, that daily visits from the speech therapist suggest an outcome to focus on. Finally, the way prognoses are made and communicated can vary according to institutional settings (such as HMOs), which structure how well and how long the doctor knows the patient and the patient's family.[66]

In sum, social attributes of the patient and physician influence the actual and predicted course of illness. The importance of social factors in determining prognosis is another reason that physicians avoid prognosis, both because physicians consider social factors to be imponderable compared with the biological factors in a patient's illness (contributing to the greater uncertainty and complexity of prognostication compared to, say, diagnosis) and because the relevance of social factors is viewed as a threat to medicine's claims to scientific precision and legitimacy.

Attributes of Prognosis

Prognosis can have at least two meanings. First, prognosis can be what actually will happen—that is, the objective reality or "true prognosis," the actual prospect of recovery from a disease given the nature of the disease and the special features of the case in question. Second, prognosis can be a physician's impression of what will happen—that is, the subjective reality or "anticipated prognosis." The anticipated prognosis, which I will refer to as "prognostication," in turn includes the acts of both *foreseeing* and *foretelling* the course and outcome of a disease, which I also characterize as "inward" and "outward" prognostication.[67] Foreseeing the future and foretelling it are, however, distinct elements, the first act being to formulate a prognosis, the second to communicate it. The true prognosis is thus what actually happens to a patient in the course of a disease and is the patient's experience of it. The anticipated prognosis, on the other hand, is the physician's mode of understanding the patient's course (albeit in advance of its occurrence); it is a *professional* perception of the patient's experience of the disease.[68]

The notion of a "true prognosis" captures what is often termed the "natural history" or "clinical course" of a disease. The former is the typical course of an illness that is not treated (the "innate prognosis") and the latter is the typical course of a disease that is treated. Prognostication thus is equivalent to stating the natural history or clinical course of the given disease—in a sense, specifying its average prognosis in most patients—and then establishing its applicability to a particular patient, for whom particular treatment decisions have been made. In this light, prognostication is an intellectual process whereby the physician moves from knowledge about disease in patients in general to knowledge about its expression in an individual.

The true prognosis can never be known definitively in a specific patient. After the fact, a particular outcome may be observed, and we may speak of a "realized prognosis"—as when physicians say, "His prognosis was good, but he died anyway; the prognosis turned out to be bad."[69] Among other things, the outcome in any given patient can deviate from the true prognosis on the basis of the treatments that are (correctly or incorrectly) instituted; in other words, the realized prognosis is not necessarily the same as the true prognosis, though the two are empirically indistinguishable in a given patient.

"Natural history" is a problematic concept even without the implementation of an effective therapy that transmutes the natural history of a disease into a clinical course. Moving from the general to the specific and trying to sort out the likely course of an illness in a given individual is always fraught with uncertainty. Aside from the intrinsic variation in the expression of a disease, the trajectory of illness in a given person may depend upon a number of individual factors, as we have seen. In a sense, there is no such thing as a usual or natural illness trajectory because each patient's experience is unique and because each patient, in ways large and small, modifies the course of a disease both subjectively and objectively.[70] That is, there is a *personal*—and a *social*—course of a disease that fundamentally subverts, if not replaces, the natural—implicitly solely biological—course. When treatment is superimposed upon natural history, the task of prognostication can become even more difficult; doctors are then faced with the tasks of predicting not only the impact upon the patient of the underlying disease and the patient's underlying traits, but also the impact of the treated disease and, finally, of the treatment itself. Moreover, the institution of therapy magnifies the doctor's sense of responsibility for the course. The extent to which the physician believes that the prognosis does or does not depend on individual factors (whether social, biological, or therapeutic) is one of the key problematic aspects of prognostication. Prognosis is at once about the generic and the individual, the typical and the atypical, and the treated and the untreated course of disease. It touches on the difference between knowing and communicating knowledge, between personal and professional domains, and between subjective and objective realities.

Favorable, Optimistic, Certain, and Competent Prognoses

To say that a prognosis is "good" or "ideal" masks several important distinctions about prognoses that are important to both patients and physicians.[71] Certainly, a crucial attribute of an ideal prognosis is that its "valence" should be favorable, in the sense that the outcome will be salutary and the patient will recover. Patients with favorable prognoses reassure physicians that what they do is valuable and effective. Favorable prognoses are also pleasant to deliver and are generally unthreatening to the physician-patient relationship. For these reasons, they are desirable.

However, a prognosis may also be "good" if the anticipated outcome is simply more favorable than might otherwise be expected—that is, relative to the patient's illness. For example, physicians may say a patient with a particular type of cancer has a good prognosis and mean that the patient has only a 30 percent chance of death over five years. A 30 percent chance of death would not be a good prognosis for an individual with a less serious condition, such as pneumonia. In such circumstances, when physicians say that the prognosis is good they mean not so much that the valence of the prognosis is favorable, but that it is favorable compared with expectations. Hence, it is possible to be "optimistic." Optimistic prognoses can be offered when favorable outcomes are possible, relative to the seriousness of the diagnosis and relative to similar patients. Optimism may also refer, however, to situations where the prognosis being offered is *unduly* and not merely *relatively* favorable. That is, an optimistic prognosis may mean that, relative to the true prognosis, the physician is biased and is overestimating the prospects for recovery despite evidence to the contrary.

A prognosis may also be good if it is certain. Just as unfavorable prognoses challenge physicians' feelings of efficacy, uncertain prognoses challenge physicians' feelings of knowledge. Paradoxically, as we shall see, physicians find prognostic uncertainty to be both threatening and felicitous. Uncertainty leads to unavoidably unexpected results and can compromise perceptions of professional standing. But uncertainty may also lead physicians to the conclusion that they cannot be held responsible for ensuring that any particular outcome will occur.

Finally, a prognosis may be good if it is possible to formulate it easily and accurately. Such a prognosis, for example, might not require complex interventions or evaluations. To make a "good" prediction is to make an accurate prediction. In other words, a prognosis is good if a physician can develop if competently.

"Routine" versus "Serious" Prognoses

A key attribute of a prognosis is its object: about what is a prediction being made, and in what clinical situation? In everyday clinical encounters examined in one study, the great majority of prognostically relevant remarks were short, tangential, and casual, typically reflecting optimistic reassurance by the doctor that the patient would respond to the proposed treatment. They were routine. Examples include the following actual remarks:

- A muscle relaxant should help. I bet by Monday you're recovered.
- Use one suppository a day for a week. Sometimes there is a little bit of irritation left after a week, and you can take a second week. There is a refill on there but I think one week should do it.
- The reason your knee is uneven and distorted like that is that we took a big chunk out of it. Then we pulled everything together. But that will smooth out just fine.
- If a new breast lump ever shows up, we should be able to find it.

In most cases, remarks such as these are the *only* prognostically relevant remarks made during a clinical encounter between a doctor and patient in an outpatient setting.[72] Usually, such remarks are embedded in the routine business of the visit, not presented as a distinct part of the clinical encounter, and neither the patient nor the physician elaborates on them. Both doctor and patient seem to gloss over prognostic statements with little or no analysis, especially in comparison to diagnosis or therapy. Cases where patients inquire or doctors volunteer what would happen if things did not go as the doctor had predicted—for example, if a prescription did not work—are quite rare in routine settings.

Although a majority of the encounters in the study of outpatient practice from which these examples are drawn (58 percent) contain at least some prognostic information, only 14 percent contain a substantial or deliberate discussion of prognosis. Moreover, the median amount of time devoted to prognosis is only three seconds (out of an average encounter length of 14.6 minutes). The overriding impression from this study is that explicit prognostication is only a peripheral part of everyday outpatient medical practice.

When one thinks of prognosis, however, one tends to think of a more serious type of prediction, one involving more formality or higher stakes. Medical care often involves especially meaningful and serious concerns, such as reproduction, fetal development, physical incapacitation, cognitive impairment, and, especially, terminal illness. Predictions regarding these topics tend to be ritualized, somber, and anxiety-provoking. Although physicians realize that most clinical encounters do not involve serious prognostication, they nevertheless tend to associate prognosis with life-or-death issues. Other, less important criteria, including attributes of the patient and of the social situation, may also influence physicians' views regarding this distinction; predictions in young patients, in important persons, in those with dependents, or in those whose illness is iatrogenic may also be deemed "serious" rather than "routine."[73] In all of these situations, the stakes in the outcome are high, and bad outcomes are regarded as particularly meaningful, deplorable, or sad. Predictions that are particularly uncertain or in which dramatic reversals are possible can also be serious. Finally, predictions involving outcomes with moral overtones (e.g., about a fetus, about a person's genes, or about the likelihood of death after withdrawal of life support) are serious. It is in serious prognostication that the starkest examples of how physicians generate and use prognostic information are found, and in which the most prophetic aspects of prognosis are apparent.

Modern American Death

The most important objects of prognostication are generally whether a patient will die and, if so, when and how. Physicians have a substantial impact on such matters; therefore, prognostication about the results of their actions can play an important role in the management of death and dying in contemporary society. The impetus to foretell death is both fundamental and ancient (reflected, for example, in stylized depictions of deathbed scenes in which the dying person has time for confession or last rites because the death is anticipated). However, the notion that death can and should be accurately predicted is especially consistent with broader contemporary beliefs about the possibility of *managing* death.

To understand the centrality of death in medical prognostication, it is helpful to begin with some features of dying in contemporary America: more then 80 percent of American adults die in health care institutions rather than at home;[74] 25 to 35 percent receive intensive care or other high-tech treatment prior to their deaths;[75] 70 to 75 percent die after a prolonged chronic illness, with the time from diagnosis to death usually exceeding two years;[76] 40 to 70 percent unnecessarily suffer significant pain;[77] 50 to 60 percent are short of breath;[78] 10 to 30 percent express preferences about end-of-life care that are disregarded by their health care providers;[79] and 25 to 35 percent impose significant personal and financial burdens on their families.[80] Over 75 percent of adults are hospitalized at some point during the year before they die, and almost 60 percent see a physician at least five times during the last year of their life.[81] Thus, patients tend to be ill for quite a while before death, tend to have significant involvement with the medical profession and with medical technology in the period leading up to death, and yet tend to have dying experiences that are suboptimal in fundamental ways.[82] That is, physicians have ample opportunity to make and act on prognoses regarding the timing and manner of death, and to optimize care at the end of life in accord with these prognoses, yet patients and their families complain of being neglected near death, of not being made as comfortable as possible, and of not being given enough information to make appropriate end-of-life arrangements.

As a result of both the proliferation of medical technology and the ever-greater contact of dying patients with physicians and hospitals, contemporary American physicians, more so than ever before, influence the timing, rapidity, and nature of patients' deaths. Life-threatening illness and death are routine parts of most physicians' professional life.[83] Physicians have control over the treatments instituted to forestall death; the degree of symptom relief;[84] the withholding or withdrawal of medical interventions;[85] the information patients have about their terminal illnesses;[86] the location where patients die; their state of consciousness at their death; and the policies regarding resuscitation. Indeed, in our society, one is not even legally dead until a physician so pronounces.

The role of medical technology and of physicians in the management of death suggest that death, like prognostication, is not only a physiological but also a social phenomenon. Attributes of death and how they are perceived are not fixed and immutable: they are socially constructed.

This proposition finds support in the substantially varied perceptions of death across time and place.[87] Sociologist David Sudnow's classic book *Passing On*, for example, shows that the recognition that someone is dying, the recognition of death itself, the specification of permissible causes of death, and, finally, the occupational rituals of the professionals who tend to the dying are all culturally constituted.[88] Patients are socialized to the dying role.[89] Indeed, the "trajectories" that patients experience while seriously ill—in the sense of their biological, psychological, and interpersonal experiences—are largely socially defined.[90] These trajectories in turn dictate the professional and personal responses by the patient, family, and medical staff.

The explosive growth in both the amount and sophistication of technology deployed by physicians to combat disease has given physicians unrealistic expectations about their own abilities. Indeed, physicians tend to regard death as a personal failure.[91] Powerful emotional and intellectual (and not just fiduciary) elements of their professional culture cause physicians to feel this way: optimistic, activistic, melioristic attitudes are endemic in American physicians. Indeed, when physicians speak of the death of their patients, they often use expressions that suggest either rectifiability ("we lost the patient") or a failing on the part of the patient ("that patient died on me"). Physicians' rituals (such as false reassurance of the dying or "heroic" efforts on their behalf) and institutional practices (such as rapid sequestration of dead bodies in hospitals) serve to protect physicians from being identified with a betrayal of confidence or a failure to fulfill their duty to eliminate disease.

Nonetheless, the material and psychological costs of this technology have also gradually come to light; patients and physicians are addressing the suffering and waste that the unblinking application of technology to prolong life may entail, as well as the dehumanizing transformation that dying has undergone. Describing physicians' attitudes toward death in America and the change they are undergoing, sociologist Renée Fox has observed that

> the Judeo-Christian tradition emphasizes that, because human life is divinely given, it is inherently sacred and important, has absolute, inestimable worth and meaning, and should be protected and sustained. . . . [But] in recent years, the unqualified commandment to support and sustain life has become increasingly problematic in American society, particularly in the medical sector. The sanctity of life ethic has helped to push physicians, nurses, and other medical professionals into a pugilistic tendency to combat death at any cost, and to define its occurrence as a personal and professional defeat.

This heroically aggressive, "courage to fail" stance has been reinforced by the development of more powerfully effective forms of
medical technology that increase the medical team's ability to save
and maintain life. However, some of the consequences of doing
everything possible to keep all chronically afflicted and terminally
ill patients alive have come to be questioned.[92]

Patients have expressed deep sadness, frustration, and anger with modern medical care of the dying, especially in ICUs. A fundamental shift
seems to be occurring in our society with respect to perceptions of medical technology; modern medical care at the end of life, especially that
involving high technology, is often equated with "excruciating pain,"
"imprisonment," and "torture."[93] In a sense, greater technology, which
initially led to greater control over death, now leads to less control.
Such technical and invasive therapy is viewed as causing meaningless
suffering. Dying in modern American society has been characterized
as highly professionalized, institutionalized, mechanized, secularized,
and dehumanized. Americans appear to be so dissatisfied with these
developments that they are even expressing interest in euthanasia as an
alternative.[94]

Professional and public attitudes have thus been shifting to a notion
that death should be better managed if it cannot be averted. This shift
is reflected in numerous developments. The newfound tolerance for
voluntary euthanasia, the examination and limitation of life-support
technology, the assertion of a "right to die" (as if death itself were
optional and volitional), the increasing interest in hospice care and
palliative medicine, and the proliferation of advance instructions by
patients about how to care for them when they are terminally ill, along
with the ongoing public discussion of the limits of medical technology
and even the definition of death itself (with a confusing array of possibilities including "brain death," "whole body death," "irreversible death,"
and the like): these are all ways in which patients and physicians seek
to specify the timing and circumstances of death—as if, in so doing,
they can specify whether death will occur at all. Paradoxically, within
the context of modern medical practice, control over life is seemingly
achieved only through control over death.

There is thus a prevalent idea, if not ideology, in contemporary
medicine and society that death can and should be managed. This
management is often achieved through the withdrawal or withholding
of medical treatment and sometimes even the administration of lethal
drugs—acts that represent the highest possible degree of control over the
timing of death and thus the greatest foreknowledge.[95] An unavoidable

part of such decisions is making predictions about what would happen if life support were not withheld or withdrawn, what would happen if it were, and when death would occur in either case.

In contemporary American society, despite the actual way that most deaths transpire, death is ideally seen as a private, individual, and personal event.[96] Moreover, dying in modern contexts engenders fear of a loss of control, a loss that is antithetical to a core American value. There has been a change lately in a key element in the perception of what constitutes a good death, from a sudden and unconscious death (typified by dying in one's sleep) to an aware death that is individual-specific, that is subject to individual control, and that allows the patient to finish business (dying "my way"). The idealized perception of a good death is one that is painless, at home, and surrounded by loved ones, and also one that is in some ways anticipated. Such a death is managed, and thus must be predicted. Indeed, nowadays, death can often be anticipated long before it happens. This is partly a result of the fact that people are ill and interacting with medical professionals for longer periods before their deaths, but also partly a result of medical technology that can provide sophisticated diagnostic information.

Prognostication and Death

Prognostication is therefore another way for both physicians and patients to try to exercise some control over death. Predicting death is a way to counterbalance the sense of failure that arises when, despite the deployment of powerful technology in the care of the seriously ill, death cannot be prevented. If one cannot control whether death occurs, one can at least control, and thus anticipate, how and when it occurs. Patients and physicians alike believe that patients should have some general—albeit carefully circumscribed—awareness of death and its impending occurrence.

It is therefore not surprising that the technological forces arrayed to treat serious illness, in an effort to control death by postponing it, have in recent years come to be focused on controlling death by managing and predicting it. This development finds expression in the increasing technicalization of euthanasia (with attention, for example, to the pharmacology of inducing death as well as to protocols for the withdrawal of life support). It also finds expression in recent efforts to develop prognostic models of considerable sophistication, models themselves requiring technologies such as computers, statistical algorithms, and complex data acquisition system.[97] In other words, technological developments in therapy are beginning to be mimicked by technological developments in prognostication, in part to justify the therapeutic technology that is being used in the first place.

Physicians use prognosis to manage death in another sense as well: they use it as a means to avoid being held responsible for the patient's death. Unanticipated or sudden death has always been problematic for those responsible for attending to the dying.[98] By configuring the patient's situation as one that leads inexorably to death—whether it is called a "terminal illness" or "dying state" or "fatal process"—the physician can avoid being held responsible for the death and can, simultaneously, get credit for having discerned the nature of the situation. As David Sudnow has observed:

> The least comfortable circumstance of death, from the doctor's perspective, is when it occurs where there has been no predictive statement of its possibility in advance. Here the physician is in the situation of having possibly to confront accusations of his own incompetence. These accusations, in turn, may establish the conditions under which he, rather than a disease's inevitable, natural operation, can potentially be considered as material in the occurrence of the death.[99]

Death must be made to be a consequence of *dying* (which itself is seen as an inevitably transitory status).[100] Without such an orderly transition and trajectory, death might be seen as unnatural or wrongly caused. From a professional point of view, sudden death is abhorred even if, from the patient's point of view, it has both advantages and disadvantages.[101] Sudden death is deplored so much that unexpected deaths sometimes evoke historicizing by physicians, as when they are at pains to note that the patient "must have been ill for some time" or that "their body was too weak to fight this new disease"; histories may be retrospectively constructed to cast the death as more anticipated (or anticipatable) than it really was.

To predict death is a way to control it. Yet to engage in the business of predicting death is to further associate with it (and, as we shall see, possibly to be held responsible for causing it)—and this runs against several powerful forces within medical culture. Although the impetus to predict death is strong, equally strong are numerous reasons *not* to predict it, or to predict it in only the vaguest or most general ways. Nevertheless, death and prognosis are intertwined: each often involves the other.

A clinical situation involving prognostication about death is apt to be filled with unpleasant and intense emotions. These emotions arise as a result of both the obligation to prognosticate and the underlying situation itself. Such a situation, moreover, highlights the limitations of medical knowledge in general and, perhaps worse, the limitations in the physician's knowledge and ability in particular. Physicians ideally would like to employ techniques to decrease the uncertainty of the future and the anxiety that it engenders. But paradoxically, as we shall see, foretelling the future is not necessarily more certain or reassuring than the future itself.

The act of foretelling the future represents in medicine—as it does elsewhere—an attempt to grasp an elusive future. In general terms, prognostication—whether implicit (usually) or explicit (rarely), and whether routine or serious—permits clinical work to take place. It motivates action because it obviates an epistemological and therapeutic paralysis that might arise from the great variability in a patient's expected subjective and objective experience of a disease. It forms the basis for the clinician to treat and for the patient to respond. It frames the illness episode by specifying its severity and its ordinary, permissible course. And, for the patient as well as the physician, prognostication is often a way to express (and partially to fulfill) fervent wishes for a favorable outcome and for a victory over death.

Two

MAKING USE OF PROGNOSIS

A man came in to see me after having been fired from his job as a stockbroker. He had been working in that job—and had quite a brilliant career—for about twenty years at the same place. He was in his early 70s but he had been doing fine until about five months before, when his decisions became erratic and he began to lose a lot of money. But beyond just losing money, the people who worked with him saw immediately that there was a major change in his analytic ability. And they just fired him. They gave him a going-away party and they gave him a watch, and he was gone. So he came in to me kind of depressed. But I suspected that underlying the depression was a serious cognitive disorder, like Alzheimer's disease, that had actually not yet manifested itself with his family or his day-to-day interactions. I ordered some cognitive testing by our neuropsychologists, and they agreed.

So there I was with this man who was depressed, who knew he had been fired, and who was feeling ashamed. And I said to him: "I don't know how much time you've got, whether it's six months or a year or two years, but in the time that's left that your brain is working reasonably well, I want you to stop brooding over getting fired. That's behind you. I want you now to apply yourself to your family, to your hobbies (he liked to dance), to all the things you enjoy doing—because I don't know how much longer you've got to function."

That was an instance where I used prognostication. I thought that was, in retrospect, the right thing to do. He actually had a little under a year of reasonably good functioning before his dementia became rapidly progressive. At this point he's still living at home with his wife, but he requires caretakers around the clock and it's not clear whether there's much communication or how much longer he'll live. That was a time when I used an estimate of the progression of the disease to influence my care of a patient.

— EXPERIENCED GENERAL INTERNIST

Effective prognostication serves many functions, but perhaps the most poignant is to empower patients to manage their lives more effectively. "How much longer do I have to live, doctor?" has become a cliché in popular depictions of doctor-patient relations precisely because the question reflects such a central concern of patients. Having some sense of what to expect allows patients to make the most effective use of their emotional, fiscal, and temporal resources and to regain some sense of control over lives thrown into disarray by serious illness. The desire for accurate information on which to base personal decisions is pronounced in people who suffer from terminal illness. Indeed, one of the central attributes of a good death in contemporary society is a death in which the patient has had a chance to put his affairs in order and otherwise organize aspects of his terminal care.[1] Patients need prognostic information.

Physicians do as well. Most of the time, physicians' use of prognosis is latent and incidental. Sometimes, however, it is manifest and deliberate. Indeed, even though prognosis tends to be neglected and inexplicit, it is still a critical part of clinical care. Prognosis can inform a great deal of physicians' behavior, from therapeutic and diagnostic decision making to communication with patients. In general, physicians too like to have some sense of where they are heading.

Patients' Need for Prognostic Information

Circumstances where patients require prognostic information are common. Patients with Alzheimer's disease and their families want to know the likely course of cognitive decline and when to expect that specialized services might be needed; patients with rheumatoid arthritis want to know whether and when they might become severely disabled; patients with hypertension want to know their risk of having a stroke or a heart attack and whether treatment might be expected to modify that risk; patients with prostate cancer want to know what they might expect with watchful waiting as compared with surgery; patients about to undergo hip replacement want to know their likely postoperative course; patients with colon cancer want to know their chances of survival to a certain point in time; patients with diabetes want to know the likely interval of time until they go blind or require renal dialysis; patients with a genetic test suggestive of an increased risk of breast cancer want to know what to expect; and patients with terminal illness want to know when they should be referred for hospice care.

Getting prognostic information is often the highest priority for seriously ill patients, out of a desire both to know what is in store (to decrease uncertainty and its attendant anxiety) and to make practical decisions better. Indeed, getting prognostic information can eclipse interest in treatment options or diagnostic details, and it is the principal motivation of patients undergoing testing for numerous conditions.[2] Prognostic information, moreover, is a key determinant of patient decision making, especially with respect to end-of-life care,[3] and the inadequacy of this information is often the greatest complaint patients and their families have about the terminal care they receive.[4] Physicians are aware that patients usually want prognostic information, and the great majority have experience with situations that are likely to require formulation, if not communication, of a serious prognosis—making decisions, for example, about withdrawing life support, admitting patients to intensive care units, or referring patients for hospice care. In an average year, general internists address the question "How long do I have to live?" a median of six times, intensive-care specialists twenty-five times, and oncologists one hundred times.[5]

Physicians identify a number of reasons that patients want prognostic information. One pediatrician noted:

> Parents always want to know what the prognosis is. They obviously want you to tell them something good, but I think that they just want to know what to be prepared for. Is the mother going to need to quit her job and stay home and take care of the child full-time? Because that's going to affect their income. That's going to impact their life profoundly. I think that they want to see these things coming. I can't think of any families that *don't* want to know.

Another physician explained why he makes predictions in his practice:

> If you deal with diabetes—which I do a lot—you see that for people who have the disease when it is newly diagnosed, prognosis is an extraordinarily important area to discuss. And I often will discuss this before I even do a physical examination! They want to know, for example, what's the potential outlook for their vision, their circulation, or their kidneys, because they know based on public knowledge that diabetes has a dramatic impact in terms of all these issues. So the future and its predictability is a thing that comes up very early and in considerable "density" in the care of a patient.

Still another remarked:

> I think that is one of the things that patients like to hear and know: something about the outcome of their disease processes. But I don't think that doctors communicate prognostic information to their patients. I think a large majority of physicians do not—in part because I don't think they communicate well with patients in general. I think a great number of them just go ahead and treat patients, and don't discuss what the future will bring or don't, for example, try to allay

their fears by assuring them that this is going to be a short-term
incident in their life as opposed to a long-term incident in their life.

These physicians express many of the commonsensical reasons that
patients want prognostic information, including their desire to plan
their practical and financial affairs and their desire to know what will
happen to them physically. They also imply, but do not explicitly state,
that knowing the future is a way for patients to understand the meaning
of their condition, a way to decrease their uncertainty, their anxiety, and
their fear about the impact of the illness on their lives and their families.
Patients usually want their condition to be given a name and a cause,
want to know what can be done to ameliorate it, and want to know its
outcome. They want to know the past, present, and future, and they
want to know that they are scrutable to the doctor. Not surprisingly,
when physicians give prognostic information to patients, patients are
more satisfied with their care.[6]

Uses of Prognosis in Patient Care

Physicians use prognostication in their practice in a number of ways
beyond answering patients' questions. Physicians use prognosis to serve
clinical objectives (to affect their therapeutic or diagnostic management
of the patient's condition), interactional objectives (to affect their relationship with the patient), and symbolic objectives (to imbue certain
actions or events with meaning).

Clinical Uses of Prognosis

Prognosis is instrumental to decisions about whether and how to treat
patients. Decisions about treatment depend upon (typically implicit)
prognostic assessments regarding the likely outcome of the condition if
it is left untreated or the outcome of the condition if it is treated with
various alternative means. When a physician chooses to treat a patient at
all, the physician implicitly presumes that the prognosis for the treated
condition is more favorable than that for the untreated condition.

Similarly, a major determinant in choosing one form of therapy
over another is the likelihood of its resulting in a preferable outcome.
Implicitly, if not explicitly, a physician uses prognosis in making such
decisions. This can occur at several levels. The most straightforward
is when one treatment is predicted to yield a better outcome than
another. However, prognosis can also inform therapeutic choice when a
prediction serves to clarify what therapy a patient can actually receive.

For example, in oncologic practice, it is not uncommon for a patient to be "too sick" for certain kinds of chemotherapy but not too sick for others, or a patient might be considered too sick for one surgical procedure but not another. Finally, prognosis can inform decisions about the details of how a patient is treated, even down to the level of choosing between drugs with very subtle differences. As one physician described:

> You make predictions to help you make therapeutic decisions. For example, we have a young patient in the ICU right now with lung failure due to an acute lung injury, and the patient had to be paralyzed for a particular mode of ventilation. And what we had to do was predict, or give a prognosis, about how long we thought the patient was going to be on this type of ventilator. Our estimate was that the patient would be on it for longer than two weeks (because of the severity of his lung injury) and this was important to deciding which sedative we were going to choose, whether it was going to be a long-acting agent or short-acting agent—because there are significant cost differences and metabolic concerns and all sorts of things that made us think that this was an important decision. So this prognostic assessment changed a therapeutic decision for us in a very concrete way. We used a long-acting benzodiazepine, whereas the patient had been getting a short-acting benzodiazepine.

Most of the time, however, physicians do not consciously or explicitly prognosticate in making such decisions.

Prognostic expectations can also affect the very *goals* of therapy. As one physician observed:

> Prognosis informs your treatment choices. If you predict that an illness has a very poor outcome regardless of your treatment, that will inform how many steps you take in the treatment. If I predict that a certain illness will not respond well to any treatment, I may be less likely to have cure as a goal in my interaction with the patient. My goal might be more maintenance or comfort for the patient.

A prognosis can radically reshape the physician's and the patient's therapeutic management of a condition, resulting, for example, in a shift from a curative to a palliative approach to care. In short, if various treatments are available, prognosis may be a means to an end: foretelling the future under alternative kinds of therapy can be a prominent part of choosing the therapy. On the other hand, if therapy is unavailable, prognostication can be an end in itself.

The relationship between prognosis and therapy is thus extensive and complex and occurs on many levels. These levels may be evident simultaneously and may influence each other, as the following exchange, between a surgeon and a patient with a knee injury, illustrates:

> *Doctor:* I am convinced by examining you today that your problem is a torn anterior cruciate ligament. I think that surgery is likely to be the best approach for you. You don't absolutely have to do it; this isn't the only approach. But I think if somebody stuck my feet in the fire and said, "Tell me which way this guy is going to wind up in the long run," I would say that sooner or later you are going to want an operation because this knee is just not going to be acceptable to you, even in your daily life.
>
> Now, even if we operate, we do want to wait some. Your knee is still swollen and it does not move fully normally. That will come in the next few weeks. I suspect bending is probably limited some, and it is still sore and hurting you, so we want to get all of that out of the knee before you have an operation. . . . I would estimate two to three weeks minimum before we would want to put you on the surgical schedule. You could even wait months, as long as you don't tear the knee up any more and you don't go out and do extreme things.
>
> *Patient:* Mmm. Well, can I walk without crutches between now and then?
>
> *Doctor:* Yes, definitely. Though that is going to take a while yet, probably two or three weeks. As soon as you get strong and your swelling and soreness go away, you will be able to walk without the crutches, even though the knee is loose. We can schedule it as soon as then and as long from now as you want. But no sooner than two or three weeks from now. Three would be the safest thing.
>
> *Patient:* Yeah.
>
> *Doctor:* The surgery itself will keep you in the hospital overnight with two hours of surgery to make a new ligament called a graft. Then most people need a week or ten days of primarily home stuff, although a couple of hours at the office after a week or so is not a big deal. But we want you to be able to lie down a lot and keep ice on this thing. If you do that for the first week to ten days, then anything after that is a piece of cake. Usually you are off the crutches by ten days or two weeks after the surgery. Sometimes you need a brace for a little bit just to be comfortable walking. But generally, you will be crutch- and brace-free by two weeks, maybe three weeks after the surgery. And if you can stand down that first week to two weeks, it really helps you to recover quicker. It takes about six weeks to get a good normal limb underneath you walking around. It then takes about four to six weeks of rehabilitation therapy, and then you are back to service. Things like biking, even running straight ahead,

swimming, all that kind of stuff, we can get you to fairly soon after surgery, within six to eight weeks. But hard, cutting sports where you are changing directions suddenly—we don't like people to do that any sooner than four to six months. Okay, that gives you some idea of the time frame of this whole process.

Patient: Mmm. With what you have seen without surgery, what could I expect?

Doctor: In terms of?

Patient: Mobility.

Doctor: Without surgery? Well, I will bet you will walk around just fine. However, as loose as the knee feels to you and to me on exam, I would predict that if you step off a curb and miss a step, this is the kind of knee that is apt to buckle. In terms of sports, this is almost certainly the kind of knee that is going to buckle.

Discussions such as this between a patient and a doctor are filled with prognostic detail. The surgeon predicts the patient's course in the near future, predicts the outcome if the condition is not treated, predicts the appropriate time to treat the patient, predicts the outcome of the treatment, and predicts the course after (and as a consequence of) the proposed treatment. The surgeon also uses prognostication as a means to encourage the patient's adherence to his recommendations; a favorable outcome (and a more rapid recovery) is predicted if the patient complies. Finally, the prediction is used to encourage the patient to undergo the treatment to begin with. Surgery is presented as the option that yields the best future.

The surgeon provides a meticulous trajectory of the disease after future treatment, along with a week-by-week, month-by-month time frame. He lays out a course for the patient to follow. This kind of prognostication is more typical of surgery than internal medicine. A fracture presents a different, and typically easier, prognostic challenge than a cancer; diseases differ in their prognostic tractability. Generally, this kind of prognostication is more common when physicians prognosticate about the treatment of, and recovery from, acute injuries (whether surgical problems, such as trauma, or internal medicine problems, such as heart attacks) than for chronic ailments (such as inflammatory bowel disease or diabetes). Because of this disease-specific variation in the kind of prognosis that physicians can offer, it is much more difficult to provide such time frames (with all their detail and implied certainty) in some medical specialties than in others.

It is worth noting in the preceding example that it is the patient who asks what would happen *without* the surgery. It seems the need for surgery is obvious to the surgeon, and that he would not present the prognosis if the procedure were not done—unless asked. This pattern of the doctor discussing the prognosis with treatment, followed by the patient asking about the course without treatment is not uncommon. In some cases, the discussion of the prognosis is a key component in a kind of negotiation between the physician and the patient about what to do therapeutically. Discussion centers not so much on the therapeutic options themselves—their nature, side effects, costs, risks, and so forth— as on the prognosis to be expected with each.[7]

The extensive relationship between prognosis and therapy is also illustrated by an altogether different case involving an internist and an elderly patient with a much more serious problem, an aneurysm of the abdominal aorta that could rupture and kill the patient at any time.

> *Doctor:* I notice in your chart that you have an aortic aneurysm.
> *Patient:* Yes, I think they said it is 4 centimeters in size.
> *Doctor:* It is 4.5 centimeters. If it got any bigger, would you consider having surgery for it?
> *Patient:* I don't care for surgery, to tell you the truth. Unless it is really, really necessary.
> *Doctor:* OK, let's talk about this. An aneurysm is when the blood vessel starts to balloon out. Like a bubble almost. When these break, often times they burst and . . .
> *Patient:* That's it, you're dead!
> *Doctor:* Exactly. The whole point in getting an ultrasound of the belly is to measure the size of it to see if it is getting larger. What we are trying to do is find out what the best time to operate is if we are going to try to fix that, because the bigger these things get, the more chance they have of breaking. So you are at the point where it is not so big that we would decide to operate right away, but it is in that sort of gray area where we would like to follow it. We are really not sure whether or not it is worth it to operate.
> *Patient:* What causes it? Age or what?
> *Doctor:* Well, it is a combination of things. As you get older, the blood vessel deteriorates and gets weaker.
> *Patient:* I know a couple of guys who had this. The one is doing all right but the other one died. Now, I don't know if he died from that because he went through the operation and he didn't die for a couple of months. He might have had something else wrong with him.
> *Doctor:* Right, some complications. Well, as I said, the surgery is significant.
> *Patient:* That is a pretty dangerous operation.

Doctor: They do everything they can to make it as safe as possible.

Patient: Well, but that is almost like heart surgery.

Doctor: Yeah, it puts a big stress on you. I just wanted to make sure you had all the information you needed. Right now, you seem to be suggesting that you are not interested in having an operation.

Patient: No.

Doctor: If a doctor were to come to you and say that we think it is very, very important that it be operated on, would you reconsider that?

Patient: [*Pause.*] If you convinced me it was dangerous the way it is, I might.

Doctor: Yes.

Patient: But, I don't know. That is a pretty tough decision. There is a woman who lives near me, she has a heart aneurysm. They give her a 10 percent chance.

Doctor: Of living or dying?

Patient: Of pulling through the operation, of making it through.

Doctor: Yeah.

Patient: 10 percent—that is pretty low.

Doctor: 90 percent chance of dying.

Patient: Yeah, she turned them down.

Doctor: What if they told you there was a 20 percent chance of dying from the operation?

Patient: [*Laughs.*] Twenty percent chance, I don't know. It is pretty hard. There is always a chance every time they put you under for the operation, always a chance of not coming out of it, right?

Doctor: Oh, sure. All surgeries have risks. Anytime you go for surgery, the ideal situation should be that we are saying that your chances of dying from that aneurysm are greater than your chances of dying from the operation.

Patient: Yeah.

Doctor: Otherwise only a fool would go ahead.

Patient: Yeah.

This case again illustrates the use of prognosis to guide the decision to treat the condition or not. This patient is in a "gray area," diagnostically, therapeutically, and prognostically. How big is the aneurysm? Will it rupture? If they operate, what are the patient's chances of survival? At what level of probability would an operation be indicated? It all seems very unclear, yet prognosis is central to the therapeutic and diagnostic management of this patient's condition. The physician proposes to use a diagnostic test (ultrasound) to help guide the decision-making process by quantifying the risk of the aneurysm rupturing. If the ultrasound showed that the aneurysm was likely to rupture and kill the patient, then surgery would be indicated. On the other hand, if the aneurysm was still relatively small, then no surgery would be needed. Diagnosis, therapy, and prognosis are all interconnected.

Prognosis is particularly important in helping to decide what treatment to use in extreme cases where there is no "gray area" and where prognosis may indeed help the physician determine whether to provide any therapy at all. When the prognosis is very favorable, as with a patient expected to recover quickly from a simple, "self-limiting" condition, therapy might be deemed unnecessary. Conversely, when the prognosis is very unfavorable, as with a critically ill ICU patient facing imminent death, therapy might also be deemed unnecessary. At both extremes, the prognosis is sufficiently instrumental as to obviate therapy.

Thus, prognostic assessment in seriously ill patients can result in decisions *not* to use treatments even when they are available. For this to happen, generally speaking, the available treatment must be expected to be of no material benefit to the particular patient. The patient might be deemed "incurable" and the therapy "futile."[8] A determination by physicians that a patient will die regardless of treatment can thus, either explicitly or implicitly, lead them to stop trying to save the patient. Life support may be withdrawn, or the patient or family may be encouraged to prepare for the end.[9] A physician's prognostic assessment that a patient is terminally ill is indeed a required and essential element in the withdrawal or withholding of life support from critically ill patients.[10] Similarly, a prediction that treatment is likely simply to diminish the quality of whatever period of life is predicted to remain may also justify withdrawing treatment. As one intensive care physician observed:

> If I feel that the person has a chance of making any type of recovery, back to anything, of improving at all, then we proceed full guns. But if a person is clearly dying, then I think that life support should be withdrawn. There really are only two factors (taking the patient's preferences out of the equation for the time being): the physician's intrinsic desire to continue to treat the patient, and the physician's conception of whether he thinks the patient can get any better.
>
> So I go to the family and say, "By everything I can measure, see, believe in, have seen in the past, etc., etc., the patient is not going to get any better." And I say that I think that we should consider that life support should be withdrawn. I pretty much tell them point blank. They understand the issues, there is no reason to cloud them in proper, insulated language. You tell them what the story is: "He's

dying. And we tried for a week by these and these means to try to reverse the situation. He's not getting any better, he's getting worse. Really, I see no hope for his improvement, and I think that at this point we should consider—you should consider—letting go." That's what I say to them.

It is typical for physicians to use a rendered prognosis to justify stopping therapy, especially when a very unfavorable prognosis is used to justify withdrawing life support, as we shall see in Chapter 7. This use of prognosis helps to insulate physicians from the perception, on the part of themselves or others, that they are shirking their obligation to treat patients. But this use of prognosis also creates a new obligation, namely to develop the prognosis accurately and communicate it sensitively.

Prognosis may also be used to deny intensive care in the first place. Triage, after all, is a classic use of prognosis. Speaking of such admission decisions, one physician noted:

You try—with very little information, usually—to predict whether or not a patient could benefit from the ICU. Sometimes, patients are too sick. For example, there is actually something known as a "burn index." If a patient's age plus the percentage [of their body surface with] third-degree burns is over 100, then their chance of survival is minuscule. So we essentially wouldn't take those patients, because we don't think that they would benefit from intensive care. Virtually all of those patients die. I think that physicians do this stuff all the time. I don't know if they think about it enough to articulate it, but I think that people do this relatively routinely. Every day the critical care doctors are making predictions and changing their decisions based on what their estimate of the probability is.[11]

Prognosis may influence decision making in the allocation of scarce resources, such as ICU beds, blood products, or physician time and effort. This physician's observation also illustrates the at once fundamental and latent role of prognosis in therapeutic decision making. Physicians prognosticate without thinking about it.

Not only the valence of the prognosis (whether the expected outcome is favorable or unfavorable), but also the relative certainty with which the prognosis is held, may influence the choice of extraordinary versus ordinary treatments. In general, substantial prognostic uncertainty leads to one of two extremes in the formulation of prognoses (pessimism or optimism) and one of two extremes in therapeutic decision making ("paralysis" or "aggressiveness").[12] When the prognosis in critically ill patients is uncertain, doctors may make choices that leave survival uncertain; that is, they may moderate the level of therapy, thus letting survival depend on the innate prognosis—they "let nature take its course."[13] For example, they may withhold surgery or hemodialysis but offer antibiotics or intravenous fluids.[14] Other temporizing behaviors may also serve as mechanisms for coping with uncertainty—for example, physicians may order more tests or ask for consultations.[15] Conversely, physicians may confront unpredictability with maximal intervention and systematically err on the side of treatment.[16] This is particularly likely when the prognostic uncertainty is felt to depend on diagnostic uncertainty.[17] Given uncertainty, they "overtreat" so as to avoid failing to treat a patient who might benefit from therapy.

The link between prognosis and treatment has in some cases been institutionalized and made quite explicit. For example, a "terminal" prognosis—specifically, a life expectancy of "less than six months"— is a criterion for access to such interventions as referral for hospice care.[18] A similar criterion was recently codified in proposals in Oregon regarding physician-assisted suicide; a physician there is supposed to render the prognosis that a patient has less than six months to live before engaging in the practice.[19] Yet physicians have been sharply critical of the assumption that they are able and willing to make such precise predictions. Critics have noted that physicians are frequently inaccurate and that they may be unwilling to have such patient-care decisions based on their estimates of survival.[20] Other examples of the bureaucratization of prognosis include the specification of Medicare benefits for "end-stage" renal disease patients and the "five-year survival" rates for cure that are the standard for so many cancer studies.[21]

Finally, prognosis can inform *diagnostic* strategy and testing. First, testing may be sought specifically to acquire prognostic information that may not have any therapeutic implications.[22] Here, prognosis influences diagnosis in that the diagnosis is made in order to determine the prognosis. Second, if a physician examines a patient and is unsure of the precise diagnosis but certain of the outcome (whether favorable or unfavorable), then diagnostic tests may be considered unnecessary. Here, prognosis influences diagnosis, but the prognosis is made in order to determine the diagnostic approach.

More generally, prognosis is an implicit basis for "differential diagnosis," the widespread, standard process by which physicians consider possible explanations for a patient's complaints. When physicians examine a patient, they develop a list of possible diagnoses. These diagnoses are then ordered from first to last in a way that satisfies two criteria: the most likely explanations for the patient's condition and the most unfavorable explanations for the patient's condition. The first diagnosis on the list, in other words, may not be the one that is most likely to be causing the patient's complaint: it may be—indeed, as a form of fail-safe mechanism, it often *should* be—the one with the worst prognosis, the one that the physicians should exclude before assigning the patient another, presumably more benign diagnosis. Thus, the choice of how vigorously to "work the patient up" is influenced by the nature of the prognoses implied by the list of diagnoses generated. Overall, however, the link between prognosis and diagnosis is less extensive than that between prognosis and therapy.

Interactional Uses of Prognosis

Prognostication finds use in clinical practice not solely through its influence on therapeutic and diagnostic decision making. It also is used by physicians, both advertently and inadvertently, to fulfill other objectives, such as fostering compliance, cultivating hope, managing expectations, relieving anxiety, and engendering confidence. The use of prognosis here resides in the interaction between the patient and physician, and the prognosis, especially if it is articulated, may be a way for the physician to influence the patient's outlook and conduct, as well as a way for physicians to enhance their relationship with the patient.

When physicians describe a prognosis to a patient, they are not merely describing the likely outcome of a given condition in general or for the patient in particular. They are affecting the subsequent actions, thoughts, and emotions of others and of themselves. The stated prognosis can be a means for the physician and patient to resolve conflicts about expectations and to integrate their actions. Prognostication may be used to manage patient expectations (especially by aligning them more closely with the anticipated or observed outcomes) and to increase patient hopefulness. By resolving discrepant views and fostering particular actions, stated prognoses are *effective*. This is more true with respect to prognosis than diagnosis because not much can be done about the diagnosis. While the diagnosis is a fait accompli, the realized prognosis is yet to be known and there may be the belief, if not the fact, that the physician and the patient may influence it.

Prognostication may thus be a way to persuade the patient to do what the physician recommends. Descriptions of what is likely to happen, whether favorable or unfavorable, are perceived as effective means of persuasion. Such remarks can span the spectrum from threat ("If you do not stop drinking, you will suffer a fatal hemorrhage") to reassurance

("Take this medicine and you will feel better"). More generally, however, prognosis and discussion of it can be a basis for doctor-patient communication and can serve as the basis for joint action. As one physician observed, "Estimation of approximate prognosis and its discussion creates better understanding and expectations between the doctor and the patient." The prognosis, in other words, gives the doctor and the patient something to cooperate about, especially because over 90 percent of physicians believe that patients "accept" the prognosis they offer.[23]

One physician characterized this use of prognosis in one of his patients as follows:

> There is one guy who comes in to my clinic. He's fifty years old and he's been to doctors for the last year. All he knows is that he wheezes whenever he goes anywhere. He's getting worse and worse and worse. He's spitting up green stuff right and left. They tell him he has asthma. He knows it's not asthma: he feels like crap. [*Laughs.*] So he leaves and comes to me. He won't even give me his old records because he doesn't want me to be biased by what other physicians have told him he has. I hear his story. The guy clearly has an obsessive-compulsive disorder. He took his own sputum and looked at it under his kid's microscope! [*Laughs.*]
>
> By history I think he has allergic bronchopulmonary aspergillosis. It's a weird thing. I've never seen it before, but he has it. It's a textbook case. The treatment is the same as the treatment for asthma, miraculously enough, which is steroids, which he's been taking from another physician anyway. Gets better but hates it; goes off of it and his illness recurs. So I do the diagnostic test to prove that he has aspergillosis, and I show it to him. I say this is what you have. And the treatment is steroids, at the same dose he is already on. He's very interested. He's already pulled the European literature that says that steroids aren't necessary to treat asthma. He doesn't want to be on steroids. So we have this huge discussion about who is the doctor [*laughs*] and what his illness is and the proper way to treat the illness. He is more than welcome to bring in any outside source he wants, and I will listen to him. But as far as I know, this is how you treat it the best way. And so I put him on steroids, and I tell him the complications and what is likely to happen: that he was going to improve. And that he could have recurrences. And that I would lower his steroids as I could. And he could have an exacerbation requiring an increase in the steroids. Steroids *are the treatment* and he *should* get better. And I tell him that if he doesn't take his steroids that it has been shown that you go on to fibrotic end-stage lung disease, so he has to take his steroids. I told him all of this stuff. I gave him all this information *because I wanted him to be compliant.*

In this case, the patient was predisposed to question both medical care in general and his physician in particular. However, the physician used his predictions about likely outcomes—both with and without treatment—to draw the patient in. After all, regardless of the patient's ability to double-check the diagnosis and therapy, he cannot as easily double-check the (not yet realized) prognosis, and so he must put his faith in the doctor's expertise—in this domain if not in the others.

In another lengthy example, a physician describes how, by prognosticating, he persuaded the patient to cooperate with a treatment the physician believed was life-saving.

> One way to use prognostication is as a battering ram, to persuade people to do what you want them to do. I had a patient in her late seventies who I had looked after for thirty years. She had high blood pressure, heart disease, and peripheral vascular disease, and she had an aortic aneurysm resected in the past. She developed chronic renal failure and her creatinines [a test of kidney function in which higher numbers are worse] were about 3.0. I took care of her and I anticipated six or seven years ago that her kidneys were going to fail at some point. And they did so very slowly, very slowly. The creatinine probably went from 3.0 to 5.0 over a five-year period. Once it got to 5.0 it began to move more quickly. Throughout this time I had been talking to her about end-stage renal disease and the availability of dialysis and the fact that, with dialysis, she could live for an indefinite period, but that without it she would die whenever the kidneys failed. She said she was in God's hands and she didn't want to talk about dialysis. She was feeling well and she wanted to live life to its fullest.
>
> I said, "We have to talk about it because what are we going to do if I'm not around when you come in and you need life-saving dialysis. What do you want?" She said, "Well, you know what I want, I know what I want: I don't want anything done." So we kept talking about it. I'd bring up the subject and she would just dismiss it out of hand and say, "We talked about that, you know my feelings."
>
> As her creatinine crept up to 9, 10, 11, she was getting nauseated, and not eating well and losing weight, just feeling quite terrible. I brought the subject up again. And she said, "No, I don't want to talk about this. We've gone through it. I don't want dialysis."
>
> I saw her in clinic on a Monday a few months ago when her creatinine was 14 [an extremely high level], and I said, "This may be our last visit together. I think you're probably going to die in the next week or two." I really thought she was going to die. She was in heart failure too, and she was not making any urine, and I couldn't treat the heart failure without dialyzing her. And she

had all kinds of electrolyte abnormalities. I said, "It's sad for me, because you and I have known each other for thirty years, and I honestly think that if you leave the office today having made up your mind not to be dialyzed, I'm not sure you're going to be around to come back and see me in a week or two weeks." She said, "Well, give me an appointment for a week." I said, "All right, I'll give you an appointment for a week, but I really am deeply worried." This was at the culmination of two years of discussion like this. But here I was using prognosis very directly to plead with her to change her mind. The prognosis I gave her was not unreasonable with the creatinine of 14 and potassium of 7.0 and some minor EKG changes. She left, and I really thought that I had seen the last of her.

The next day was a Tuesday, and in the late afternoon I got a call from the emergency room saying that they had a patient of mine down there who had come in asking to be dialyzed. And I said, who is it? And they gave me this lady's name! And I said, "I'm not sure that she's mentally competent"—though she was when I saw her the day before—"because this is quite the opposite of everything she's ever said to me up to yesterday at noon. Before you call the kidney people, I must come down and see her to make sure she's with it, because I have to defend the interest that she's repeated to me time and again that she does not want to consider dialysis."

So I went down and she was her old feisty self—feisty in a nice way, blunt, direct—and she made it very clear that she had changed her mind from Monday to Tuesday. And she actually said something to the effect of "The idea that I might not see you again was one of the things that I really began to think about." I said to her, "That's very nice of you to say, but what was it? What was it that led you to change your mind?" And she said, "To tell you the truth, up until that day that you told me I had a week or two to live, everything was in the future. I didn't have to make a decision. I was still there, I was still functioning, even though I wasn't feeling well. When you put it so bluntly, something that has been a question of theory became a real practical issue, and I knew that if I didn't decide soon I might not be able to, so I changed my mind."

This example illustrates, first, the discrepancy in how elements of the prognosis (predicted time to renal failure, projected experience of dialysis, benefits of dialysis, and so forth) are perceived by the physician and the patient, at least for the first few years of the patient's course. The patient does not contest that her kidneys will continue to fail or that she will die without dialysis; she simply does not regard these outcomes as negatively as her physician does. In other words, the valence of the prognosis was the contested domain ("So what if my kidneys fail?" she seemed to be asking). Second, this example illustrates the centrality of the prognosis to this physicians' interaction with the patient. The physician is mystified but respectful of the patient's refusal to consider renal dialysis. But he eventually wears her down by using his prognostic pronouncements like a "battering ram," especially by being blunt about impending death (when the situation got that far) and by personalizing the prediction (that he would not see her again). These elements of prognosis (the proximity of the outcome predicted, the precision in the information transmitted, and the personal touches in the communication) can be powerfully effective in getting patients to comply with physicians' therapeutic recommendations—and not just in life-or-death situations like this one.

Physicians use prognosis broadly to support their proposed therapeutic interventions, and not simply in the narrow sense of persuading patients to comply. Prognostically relevant remarks typically emerge during clinical encounters in connection with discussions of treatment. Even when they are short, prognostic remarks are usually subordinate to discussions about treatment and usually reflect physicians' opinions about how patients would respond to various therapies. For example, half of routine prognostic discussions in one study of outpatient practice were about the patient's response to treatment, more than about any other type of outcome.[24] The prognosis usually took the form of a statement that the proposed therapy would be successful. Thus, prognosis was used not so much to guide or choose therapy (the "clinical" use described earlier) as to support the physician's chosen therapy. For example, one primary care doctor used a favorable prediction about a drug's effectiveness to support his proposed therapy as follows:

> *Patient:* So, polymyalgia is something you never get over then?
> *Doctor:* No. The patients that have that are on some prednisone all their lives. OK? Now sometimes you can cut the prednisone back quite a bit, and then sometimes there are flare-ups and the disease gets worse. But it's not something that you are going to be cured of.
> *Patient:* There isn't any other treatment for it either, is there?
> *Doctor:* Prednisone is it. I've never heard of anything else that works. And prednisone works pretty well, actually.

Here the proposed treatment is problematic in that it is not curative. In this type of situation, the physician must try to maintain the patient's

confidence in the physician's ability, in the treatment the physician recommends, and in the patient's chances for response to the (suboptimal)
treatment that is indeed available. This is done through prognostication.

Equally commonly, the physician may use prognosis *after* an outcome has been observed, especially an outcome that is either unexpected
or unsatisfactory to the patient. This use is distinct from explaining
why things happened as they did. In such situations, physicians use
prognosis as a way to keep the patient hopeful, diverting the focus of
attention from the unsatisfactory present to a potentially more favorable
future. Oncologists, for example, often handle their patients' disappointment at relapsing by manipulating their prognostic pronouncements. They may take the opportunity to make a new prediction about
the chances of success of some new therapy, or they may attempt to
shift a patient's focus from one outcome to another, for example from
survival to tumor size ("The disease is still here, but the tumor has
shrunk, and that's a good thing."). Surgeons talking to patients with
a (so far) unsatisfactory outcome may encourage them to wait longer
for "healing to be complete." Physicians may also take the opportunity
to highlight adverse outcomes that *did not* occur, outcomes the patient
had not even considered. In general, physicians may direct patients to
focus on another course for their illness: the patient is not so much
experiencing a bad outcome as realizing an alternative prognostic trajectory, a trajectory that is "well described" and known to the doctor.
Recasting an apparent setback in terms of a standardized, familiar
pathway can help the patient maintain hope as well as confidence in
the physician. The doctor too may derive satisfaction and a sense of
control. Thus, the articulation of standardized (and, it is hoped, favorable) prognostic pathways may be especially significant after previous
therapeutic failure.

Prognostic statements are often used to enhance confidence in therapeutic success; they are not neutral or merely factual but encouraging and hopeful. The prognostic remarks are themselves part of the
treatment. In many cases, the doctor's optimism that a condition will
respond to the prescribed treatment is well founded clinically—that
is, the patient is likely to do well. This does not explain, however,
why doctors actually articulate the prediction; the mere fact that an
outcome might be favorable does not *necessitate* that this be articulated.
Doctors find ways to express optimism even when it does not seem
to be well founded clinically. Doctors believe their optimism serves
other important—virtually therapeutic—functions during the clinical
encounter.

At other times, although much less frequently, physicians' recommendations are not accepted by the patient, despite the physicians' predictions, as in the following interaction:

> *Doctor:* What did you decide about doing that colonoscopy?
> *Patient:* I frown on invasive procedures.
> *Doctor:* Yeah, but this is not terribly invasive.
> *Patient:* I will let them do an autopsy on me! How about that?
> *Doctor:* Well, *I* would just as soon they not do that for a while.
> *Patient:* Yes, that is going to be a few years off.
> *Doctor:* You know, I think we can get this thing [a colonic polyp] out of there before it turns into cancer.
> *Patient:* I don't think that it is going to.
> *Doctor:* There is a significant likelihood that it will, though.
> *Patient:* Yeah, I know. Doctors are statisticians now! They are quoting the odds on that.
> *Doctor:* Well, if something is one out of a million, then probably you don't worry about it a lot. If it is one out of ten, then—
> *Patient:* I still don't worry about it. I am convinced that at my age two-thirds of health is right up here in the brain box.
> *Doctor:* Well, there are some things that are really easy to take care of, and a polyp is one of them.

Here, the patient's discordant perception of the future (presuming that the polyp would not turn into a cancer) supports his choice of therapeutic plan over the physician's proposal (which hinged on a different prognostic outlook). What was contested was not so much the appropriateness or even the invasiveness of the procedure as the prognosis.

In addition to using prognosis to foster compliance and to support a proposed therapy, physicians also use it as a way to relieve the patient's anxiety. In speaking of the client-professional relationship in general, sociologist Robert Merton has argued:

> Motivated by anxiety, the client thus develops exaggerated hopes and exaggerated fears. Above all, he has a profound desire to know "how things really stand." He is peculiarly unable to tolerate that ambiguity that comes from uncertainty of outcome. He develops an insatiable desire for information, of the kind that would be supplied by a definite diagnosis of his situation and by a firm prognosis.[25]

Knowledge of the future can function to limit the patient's anxiety. Prognosis, especially if favorable, may be used to reassure patients. For example, one physician noted:

Prognosis is immensely important from the standpoint of the doctor knowing what to expect in the course of an illness, but it's also one of the most important things the doctor does for the patient. It often has a reassuring quality to be able to tell a worried person that "the symptoms you have are not those of any significant disease that I can see any sign of." This is one of the places where I think the primary care doctor can be so effective in stopping that patient's quest for medical activity right off the bat—especially if there is no sign that there is anything wrong.

In such a circumstance, the patient's "reassurance" comes both from the knowledge of the (favorable) future communicated by the physician and from the fact that the physician is capable of providing this knowledge.

The prognosis need not necessarily be favorable, however, in order to serve this anxiety-reducing function. Another physician observed:

One of the chief reasons that patients go to a physician is to say, "Tell me what's in store for me." And I think that physicians do very, very little to change the natural history of disease. We do a little bit—penicillin, a few things like that, have been really major triumphs—but disease generally plays itself out. So I think that prediction is extremely vital to a patient, and to really talk about it—I find very few physicians do so. But I sit down and say to patients, "You've got a fatal disease. I can't tell you when you're going to die, but I can tell you you've got it, and I can tell you how people go through that disease, and what the limits are on either side. What the average course of the disease is and where the standard deviations lie." And I find that is always very reassuring to patients. People don't mind being told they're going to die as much as they mind not knowing what's ahead for them.

Thus, an important function of prognostication is to reassure patients by decreasing uncertainty—regardless of whether the outcome is expected to be favorable or unfavorable. The reduction of uncertainty can lead to the reduction of anxiety. Not surprisingly, this is often a reason patients seek out clinical evaluations and diagnostic tests.[26]

Physicians may carefully control how they articulate a prognosis in order to maintain hope. One physician described how she gives information as follows:

I think a doctor can very easily foster a sense of hope just in how she frames the information she gives a patient. You can give the same information one way and have patients feeling upbeat and hopeful about their illness, versus framing it a different way and have them feeling negative, pessimistic, or sort of neutral about things.

   In the gastrointestinal malignancy clinic, we treat a lot of cancers that tend to be fairly chemo-resistant, such as pancreatic cancer and metastatic colon cancer. . . . We had a man who's been on drug therapy for locally advanced pancreatic cancer for three months, and he had a reevaluation scan, and his disease was stable. So, the way I framed it to him was, "You have this incredibly aggressive cancer and it's stable. So that's great. It's not growing." Now, it wasn't shrinking, and I could have said to him, "Oh gee, you know, this kind of looks the same after all this chemo that you've been through. Isn't that terrible?" But communicating this way is something that I definitely use in my practice to try to help people feel I'm upbeat about what they're going through. I look at things that way, rather than a more pessimistic way.

Indeed, prognostication may itself be changed into a form of therapy, as the following case description provided by a medical resident reveals:

   The patient was admitted with a diagnosis of GBS [Guillain-Barré Syndrome], an acute paralyzing neurologic condition. Shortly after admission, he underwent electromyography. The results, which confirmed the diagnosis, suggested that he was in a poor prognostic category. These results were not given to him by his attending since he was doing so poorly and was still in the acute phase of his illness. However, the attending said he would have told the patient the results if he had been in a good prognostic group—that is, if he had been doing well in the acute phase—in order to boost his spirits and accelerate his recovery. In the case of GBS, only certain patients receive the "therapy" of being told their prognosis.

Controlling revelation of information in order to influence patients' thoughts or behaviors is a key aspect of physicians' action with respect to prognosis. The fact that physicians feel the need to control the information they formulate or communicate at all suggests not only the power that they believe is inherent in prognosis, but also their considerable professional duty in this regard.

   Finally, the articulation of a prognosis may serve the critical function of aligning both the physician's and the patient's conduct with social norms. For example, an unfavorable prognosis may be used by a physician—explicitly or implicitly—to justify suspending the physician's traditional role of saving life and moving to withdraw life support. For a physician to abstain from treatment, the treatment must be deemed futile—that is, it must be *predicted* to be ineffective. Similarly, an unfavorable prognosis may be used by patients to excuse themselves from some social obligations (quitting a job, say, and taking a trip around the world) or to reinforce other social obligations (for example, repairing relations with estranged relatives). Adhering to a new set of obligations may in fact be the price paid for exemption from established ones. Indeed, patients with particular prognoses are expected to act in particular ways.[27] This trade-off between acquiring new obligations and suspending old ones, conditional on prognosis, is part of the more general behavior of sick patients.[28] In short, prognosis can imply both responsibilities and exemptions—for both the physician and the patient.

Symbolic Uses of Prognosis

Distinct from its clinical and interactional uses, prognosis may be used to provide a sense of meaning in the patient's illness. The offering of a prognosis may symbolize that the future is scrutable, that the disease is tractable, and that the doctor is sufficiently competent to both know and control the future. Paradoxically, however, the offering of a prognosis,whether favorable or unfavorable (but especially the latter), can symbolize that the disease, too, is powerful; it is intractable and neither the doctor nor the patient can, or should, be expected to change it.

Prognosis may be a way for the physician to allay the patient's feelings of responsibility regarding the outcome of his condition. There is an emphasis in American society on individual thought and personality as causes of human action. By stressing that disease entities indeed have probable or permissible outcomes, explicit prognostication reaffirms the importance of the biological cause of human illness, thereby reducing reliance on human action as an explanation. Prognosis reaffirms that there is a domain over which the patient and the physician have no control—and for which they are not responsible. This sentiment may be especially beneficial to patients and physicians when little can be done therapeutically. However, this is a double-edged sword, because it also curtails what physicians and patients feel they can do about the future.

The offering of a prognosis can also symbolize, or stand for, the assertion of efficacy on the part of the physician. The doctor "lays out the course" and the patient follows it. In this sense, prognostication can represent an effort to regain cognitive control over something that cannot be controlled operationally: the disease is at least predictable and therefore orderly. Prognostication, however, stands not merely for the scrutability of the future, but also for its malleability. The act of prognostication is almost a willful domination of a fundamentally unknowable future. When physicians make predictions, they are often expressing hopes.

Paradoxically, therefore, prognostication can be used both to avoid and to take responsibility for, to repudiate and to seek control of, the future. A prognosis, depending on the circumstances, can symbolize, and be used to symbolize, either the fact that the disease is more powerful than the physician *or* the reverse.

A prognosis, when a physician in fact develops and articulates one, outlines the types of events that the physician and the patient can expect to happen or not to happen. The patient's subsequent experience in the illness thus has a constant referent, and the patient—according to medical parlance—will either "fulfill" or "defy" the prognosis. These characterizations (fulfillment and defiance) summarize the patient's relation not only to a natural order, but also to the physician's professional knowledge, a man-made order. In either case, the prognosis provides a sense of meaning. Fulfilling a prognosis—whether favorable or unfavorable—confirms for patients that their condition is comprehensible and that the unknown is actually less unknown than previously supposed. In recognizing the fulfillment of the prognosis, patients may find order and meaning in their plight. Conversely, and paradoxically, to the extent that patients find themselves defying the prognosis—especially if it is an unfavorable one—the patients' belief in their own uniqueness is confirmed, and there is meaning in this as well. As for physicians, when things happen as expected, they feel that they understand disease and can influence it. And when things do not happen as expected, they may be reassured that there is a larger force of nature at play and conclude that they are not truly responsible for outcomes.

Uses of Prognosis in Professional Matters

Physicians use prognosis not just in caring for patients, but also in a number of areas that might strictly be considered professional. For example, a physician's ability to predict the future accurately is viewed by both colleagues and patients as a mark of clinical acumen, and physicians may evaluate other physicians for choosing to make predictions or for their errors in them. Colleagues might also use prognostic ability as an index of each other's cognitive performance.[29] Yet when physicians refer to another physician as a "clinical fox" or a "doctor's doctor"—two high forms of praise—they tend to have clever diagnostic or therapeutic, rather than specifically prognostic, maneuvers in mind.[30] Indeed, one of the most widespread showcases of clinical acumen in modern medicine, the occupational ritual known as the "clinico-pathologic conference" (wherein a physician tries to figure out what caused a patient's problem on the basis of a case presentation), is exclusively about diagnosis.[31] Similarly, another common showcase for clinical judgment known as "tumor board" meetings, where the optimal treatment of a patient's cancer is discussed by physicians from many specialties, is primarily about therapy.[32] Comparable institutionalized showcases specifically for prognostic ability simply do not exist. Nevertheless, although prognostic performance is not as highly valued as diagnostic performance, inaccuracy in prognostication can still lead to mild professional censure in the form of the unfavorable opinions of one's colleagues.

Prognostic information is also used—albeit typically implicitly—in evaluating the practical performance of other, nonprognostic clinical tasks by colleagues. One doctor described his judgments about the competence of his surgical colleagues as follows:

> I look at several things in order to assess whether a surgeon is good or not: (1) his technique when I watch him in the operating room; (2) his judgment about whether to operate on a patient and, if so, which operation to perform; (3) his complication rate; and (4) my assessment about whether the outcomes of his procedures differ from what I would have expected them to be, even allowing for his case mix.

Physicians thus use prognosis as a tool to assess the professional competence of their colleagues; in order to assess whether another doctor's care is inferior or superior, one must be able to predict what a patient's outcome should have been. Physicians try to discriminate the true prognosis from the observed outcome (which may be better or worse) brought about by the colleague's intervention. The role of prognosis in providing a basis for such evaluation of colleagues has not always been appreciated. Sociologist Eliot Freidson, in his analysis of social control among physicians in a group practice, considers how physicians might observe the results of other physicians as a means of forming an opinion about their competence.[33] But against what standard should these results be evaluated? Against textbook descriptions, average performance by physicians in general, or expectations and predictions about the cases in question?

Prognostication may also form the basis for self-assessment. Physicians will sometimes test their mettle by predicting outcomes and then intervening in order to avoid them.[34] Similarly, outcomes that occur unexpectedly—outcomes not in keeping with prior predictions—may provide the opportunity for self-evaluation. Physicians must determine whether they have made a mistake and, if so, try to avoid such mistakes in the future. Physicians may use prognosis as a way to learn about disease, in that it provides a test of their understanding of uncertain phenomena.

Prognosis thus plays a role in professional comportment by providing a basis for the evaluation of colleagues and oneself, and by helping physicians to cope with the stress associated with uncertainty. Prognostication, as we shall see, can help to limit the strain associated with physicians' obligation to cure disease by providing a mechanism to vouch for their technical expertise while at the same time protecting it from being undermined, especially when the outcome proves unexpectedly unfavorable.

Finally, whether and how physicians communicate prognoses may be affected by self-interest. Physicians may choose to offer a particular prognosis, whether favorable or unfavorable, if they feel that it will encourage a patient to remain under their care or otherwise comply with their recommendations, with the professional or financial advantages that might attach to this. For example, patients may be given unduly optimistic prognoses, which may encourage them to continue seeing the doctor.[35] Or they may be urged to enroll in trials of experimental chemotherapy; enrollment of patients in such trials, regardless of whether it benefits the patients, can advance a doctor's career. These behaviors are not usually as sinister as the doctor wanting to profit financially from a patient or frankly deceiving a patient: physicians themselves are often not consciously aware of these implications of the use of prognosis, patients themselves often have interests in particular kinds of prognoses being offered, and patients obviously expect to receive emotional support and treatment when they see a doctor.

Uses of Prognosis in Bioethical Decision Making

Prognostication is also a major underpinning for many bioethical decisions, a fact which is often unappreciated in the consideration given to such decisions. For example, bioethical reasoning about the withdrawal of life support often proceeds as follows: The patient is going to die. Life support is of no further benefit. Should we withdraw life support? This type of reasoning often neglects such questions as: How do we know the patient is going to die? How do we know life support is of no further benefit? What if there are errors? Who must make these predictions? What if they are wrong? How might these predictions vary across prognosticators, and what would this mean? Analogously, much of the current debate regarding the ethics of physician-assisted suicide has focused on the ethical and legal aspects of doctors' engaging in such behavior, taking for granted that doctors are willing and able to predict when a patient will die.[36] Prognostication is, indeed, the fundamental and essential basis for a determination of "futility," a relatively new doctrine whereby physicians are not obligated to provide care that they deem inevitably ineffective to critically ill patients.[37] This doctrine is being invoked increasingly often to justify the withholding or withdrawal of life support from patients who are being harmed by it; in rare cases, it is invoked to withdraw life support over family objections. Yet the key issues of how futility is determined and by whom are often neglected.

Prognostication is a core and nonignorable element not only in bioethical decisions at the end of life, but also in cases of caring for newborns with congenital anomalies, counseling parents about genetic disease, allocating organs for transplantation, informing patients about the risks and benefits of procedures, and respecting patients' autonomy. In organ transplantation, for example, a key (though not the only) component of allocation decisions is the "greatest benefit" criterion, whereby organs are allocated according to who stands to gain the most from the transplant and who has the least chance of rejecting it immunologically. Organ allocation, however, typifies a broader type of ethical concern, namely the allocation of scarce resources (ICU beds, blood products, and so forth); to the extent that allocation is premised on the likely success of the medical intervention, prognosis is an essential element of the ethical decision making. The notion of patient autonomy holds that patients should be respected as persons and thus allowed to determine their own care. The implications for such decision making of the accuracy and quality of the prognostic information given to patients and the means by which such information is developed are, however, rarely examined. Often the quality of prognostic information they are given is poor.[38]

Indeed, many ethical decisions, ranging from advance directives to informed consent, involve a sort of "hypothetical prognosis" in which physicians describe various scenarios that patients might experience in the future. These scenarios need not be ones the patients are actually expected to experience; this is type of prognosis that is merely illustrative. Consider, for example, the role of prognosis in advance directive documents, in which patients express their wishes with respect to life support should they become both critically ill and unable to speak for themselves.[39] Ideally, discussions about such documents are initiated and guided by physicians.[40] But in order to elicit the patient's preferences, the physician must first engage in hypothetical prognostication about various possible situations. Some of the outcomes predicted might be quite realistic and well grounded in the patient's medical condition; others might be more disconnected and *very* hypothetical (e.g., those that might arise in an advance directive discussion with an elderly but healthy patient).

In the following case, the physician uses hypothetical prognosis to elicit advance directive preferences from an elderly patient with a history of cancer, coronary artery disease, and two past stays in intensive care units (one for pneumonia, lasting thirty days, and involving successful cardiopulmonary resuscitation). The patient is therefore experienced in the kind of technology at issue and likely to need it again.

> *Doctor:* I know you've been really sick in the past and been in intensive care and everything like that. But I don't know that you and I have ever had a conversation about what your desires or wishes would be if you were real sick with a terminal illness—you know, if you had something that could not be cured and you started to get really, really sick.
>
> *Patient:* I haven't told any doctor, but I've told my children that if I come to that, I don't want to be kept alive.
>
> *Doctor:* Right. Because in your feelings, there would be no sense in that?
>
> *Patient:* I don't know why they did it [resuscitated me] when I was in the hospital. If I'd known anything about it when I had that pneumonia . . .
>
> *Doctor:* Yeah, your were very sick. Now, the thing is, doctors usually treat something like a pneumonia. You had pneumonia that you acquired in the community that anyone else could have gotten, and you just got extremely sick with it. But in retrospect, you seem to be saying, you were so sick you really wondered why they shocked your heart and did all those kinds of things. But what I'm talking about is if, in fact, you had a terminal illness like your cancer had spread through your body, and it was affecting your mind, and there was no cure, and you started to die. You're saying what? That you couldn't see the use of machinery, right?
>
> *Patient:* No, I don't want that, no.
>
> *Doctor:* Because that's the kind of thing that, when we discuss it with people, they have strong feelings. And they often say, as you did, "Well, I've never told my doctor but I told my family." I am encouraged that you told your family, because I'm unlikely to be right there if you got that sick. But your family might be, and if they knew how you felt that would be really good. But certainly if you feel that way, you could sign a form saying, "If I got this sick and the

doctors agreed that my outlook was terrible, that I wasn't going to get better from this illness and that it was very likely to kill me, then I wouldn't want machinery to prolong this whole thing for week or a day or ever how long it would be."

Patient: That's right. I feel that way, yeah.

Doctor: Mm-hmm. Mm-hmm.

Patient: And I'm going to tell my oncologist about it next time I have an appointment.

Doctor: Well, you need to, because we all have this paperwork that we have people fill out. What it says is just what I've said, that "If in the decision of the doctors, my condition is fatal or terminal" or something like that. And it's not just the one doctor that comes running to your bedside. I mean, it's when more than one doctor agrees that you have a terrible condition and that we don't have a cure for it. Then we would not shock the heart and do what I call heroics to keep you alive. An oncologist has paperwork that he could put on his chart, so that if you went to the regional hospital in the middle of the night and he was out of town, then any doctor could see that if your condition was that fatal, that you wouldn't want to be put through all that.

This discussion hinges almost entirely on prognosis. It involves life-threatening possibilities that might arise in the future and that are described by the doctor. Moreover, not only do the patient and doctor peer into the future to imagine various clinical scenarios, they also foresee the actions they would and would not take.[41]

The role of hypothetical prognostication is also critical in the broad class of bioethical concerns known as "informed consent." Informed consent is the expressed, uncoerced willingness of patients or research subjects to undergo a medical intervention about which they have adequate information, predominantly through a disclosure of risks and consequences. Informed consent is ordinarily taken to involve five elements: disclosure, comprehension, voluntariness, competence, and actual consent.[42] During the informed consent process, the physician characterizes the proposed intervention by describing possible outcomes of both the intervention and any alternatives, along with possible side effects of each. By its very essence, informed consent takes place before conducting the intervention, so such statements are a type of hypothetical prognostication. Every time doctors or researchers get consent from a patient to administer a drug or procedure, they are using prognosis. The extent to which the doctor is willing and able to make accurate predictions is therefore an important factor in the patient's decision.

Consideration of the role of prognosis therefore ought to be an important factor in the strictly ethical analysis of such decisions.

What might a greater attention to the role of prognostication in such bioethical decisions entail, and how might it be used? The analysis of ethical dilemmas cannot be separated from the social context in which both the theory and the reality of these dilemmas emerge.[43] This suggests that the various factors that influence prognoses and physicians' responses to them need to be accounted for both in making and in analyzing such ethical decisions. What if doctors are systemically overoptimistic in their predictions of benefit from life-support technology, for reasons I will explore at length later, and are therefore unwilling to withdraw it, or overestimate its utility? What if doctors refuse to make predictions or regard predictions as fundamentally immoral? What if accurate prediction is not possible? Such questions cannot be ignored when considering the right thing to do in many bioethical decisions.

The Advantages and Disadvantages of Prognostic Uncertainty for Physicians

Prognosis may be both a source of uncertainty and a way of coping with uncertainty. Uncertainty in medicine has been classically described as having three principal sources:

> The first results from incomplete or imperfect mastery of available knowledge. No one can have at his command all skills and all knowledge of the lore of medicine. The second depends upon limitations in current medical knowledge. There are innumerable questions to which no physicians, however well trained, can as yet provide answers. A third source of uncertainty derives from the first two. This consists of difficulty in distinguishing between personal ignorance or ineptitude and the limitations of present medical knowledge.[44]

Predicting the future, however, involves a singular type of uncertainty that transcends these three types. A fundamental uncertainty arises in prognostication from the mere fact that *knowledge of the future is irremediably provisional;* the future cannot be empirically observed in the present. Uncertainty about the future results both from a personal ignorance that is unavoidable and from a limitation in medical knowledge that can never be fully remedied. This inability to predict future events and their timing is a particularly thorny form of uncertainty, especially since, paradoxically, situations in medicine with high unpredictability both demand and subvert efforts by physicians to render prognoses.

Nevertheless, formulating prognoses may be a way for physicians to cope with the uncertainty in medicine. Making predictions can make physicians feel as if they have some rational understanding, and therefore control, over a patient's disease. One physician described this function of prognosis as follows:

> Leukemia is a disease where I was taught that if you're a girl and your white blood cell count is between this and this and your age is between three and five, then you have a much better chance. I think that is really important and really interesting information because, when you meet a child who meets those criteria, it makes you feel better. It is the same way with Hemolytic Uremic Syndrome: if you know that they meet all the criteria for a really good prognosis, it is much more rewarding and you're more motivated to try hard. Whereas with oncology patients, sometimes you walk out of their room and you have *no* idea—no idea about their prospects! You find yourself, after taking care of a child for two weeks, asking, "Does this child have a prayer?" No idea! "Is this child doing well or not?" You wish you had a better sense of the prognosis.

The uncertainty associated with such serious, life-threatening disease is both unsettling and threatening to physicians, and they thus welcome situations where they can cope with it through prognostication. The ability to prognosticate can provide reassurance.

Prognostic *certainty* can, paradoxically, also be problematic for physicians. Certain knowledge of an unfavorable future can be perceived as a burden. One physician recounted the case of a patient with pneumonia and cardiac disease whom she had to care for over the course of a month, despite her certainty that the patient would not benefit:

> It was really horrible. I actually became really depressed that month. Because of this patient. I went in there everyday, and I had to do something that I so strongly didn't believe in. I was so against treating this patient. I was against it I felt it was mean and cruel toward him and his family. And I had this huge psychic conflict about it: "You're an intern, and you don't know what you're doing and you're supposed to do what people say because you don't have enough experience." But I had these very powerful emotional and philosophical beliefs and they wouldn't go away. I actually had a very disturbing dream about this patient. He basically came to me in my dream and said, "Get out of here, you are not supposed to participate in my death. You're not supposed to be here. This is not your job, get the hell out of here." And the most powerful thing about this dream was the feeling I had that I was in violation. It was like I broke some cardinal law. It was a very powerfully disturbing experience for me.

Although perfect knowledge and clinical acumen can be gratifying, acting against a certain prognosis can seem a violation, an unnatural act. Consequently, it can be disturbing. In a sense, then, uncertainty can be a source of relief. Uncertainty is a prerequisite for hope: in situations where the future looks grim, it is comforting if uncertainty permits patient and doctor alike to entertain the possibility of a favorable outcome.

Medical uncertainty itself may be seen to be a socially constructed and manipulated phenomenon. Physicians may exaggerate the amount of uncertainty in a given situation and use it to avoid having to discuss their true beliefs about the clinical reality with patients, as in the case of polio described by sociologist Fred Davis.[45] More generally, uncertainty may be manipulated by the medical profession in order to gain control over particular domains of human experience. For example, physicians may exaggerate the level of uncertainty regarding the outcome of pregnancy so as to encourage women to believe that childbirth is properly the domain of obstetricians, or, conversely, they may mask the level of uncertainty associated with the outcome of serious illness so as to encourage seriously ill patients to accept high-technology care provided by intensive care specialists.[46]

Less problematically, uncertainty can provide a vehicle for a bond between the patient and the doctor. One physician characterized it this way:

> I have found that letting patients know that I don't know for sure what will happen to them can be a great thing. I think it's very relieving to them sometimes. Because when they realize that *no one* knows, they feel "OK, I don't have to worry about knowing now." Or they can see that I can relate to their experience as a human being. I often tell people, "I really wish I could tell you exactly what's going to happen. I really wish I could tell you when this is going to end, but I can't." It's kind of like acknowledging that you know what situation they're in, but you're just as vulnerable and human as they are. You're in the situation with them. So I don't feel uncomfortable with that.

Indeed, this aspect of prognosis is very unusual in medical practice. This is one area where physicians' revealing their ignorance, uncertainty, fallibility, and vulnerability to patients may have positive effects, helping to build relationships with patients and to humanize physicians in their eyes. But its impact can go beyond this; as we shall see, physicians can find prognostic uncertainty reassuring and evocative of exculpatory religious sentiments.

In general, however, physicians rarely explicitly express any uncertainty when they make predictions. For example, in one study of routine clinical encounters, physicians acknowledged the fallibility of their predicted outcomes less than 10 percent of the time.[47] In more serious prognostication, they acknowledge prognostic uncertainty somewhat more commonly; one study found that 31 percent of physicians reported acknowledging uncertainty when communicating prognoses to terminally ill patients.[48] Nevertheless, when physicians express uncertainty, they typically express it in an offhand and tangential manner. For example, doctors might simply say it is "hard" to predict something. In other cases, they might discuss the source of the prognostic uncertainty: it might be related to therapeutic uncertainty (will the patient respond to this treatment?) or diagnostic uncertainty (what is the cause of the patient's illness?). It is striking that physicians seldom explicitly acknowledge uncertainty and fallibility in prognostication in the context of actual prognoses they do make. This partly reflects the fact that the prognosis is often construed as being connected to the treatment and so is standardized and uncontested: the treatment is obvious and certain to have known effects, so the prognosis is ipso facto favorable.[49] Physicians very rarely attribute uncertainty to their own ignorance, and we do not find physicians saying that the reason they do not know what will happen in a patient's case is that they have inadequate training, experience, or knowledge. That is, the uncertainty in prognosis is seen as being caused by the disease rather than by the doctor.

Expectation and Outcome

Patients with a serious illness under the care of a physician are in a vulnerable state that makes them want to know what the future will bring. Will the illness end and, if so, when? What should they plan for? How much certainty is there? Patients want answers to these and related questions, and physicians are supposed to provide them. Physicians too find good reasons to make predictions, to serve not only the patients' objectives but their own. Of course, making predictions is fraught with error and stress, and formulating, much less communicating, prognostic information is difficult.

Physicians feel that they are judged not only by the outcome of their efforts, but also by the difference between the outcome and expectations. As a consequence, they have two means to be effective in their work. The first is to deploy the science of medicine to manage outcomes: for example, they intervene therapeutically in order to change an outcome

from death to survival. They attend to the outcome regardless of expectations because people deplore bad results. The second means, however,
is to manage expectations. The two means are not mutually exclusive, of
course, and physicians often do both, simultaneously attending to the
outcome of their efforts and to the difference between the actual and the
predicted outcome.

Knowledge of the future—even if it is unattainable, or incorrect, or
idealized, or "false" knowledge—structures the experiences and actions
of both the patient and doctor. Doctors choose what to say and do
for their patients on the basis of what they expect to happen, whether
their expectation is explicit or implicit (though it is usually the latter).
Their use of prognosis is broad, deep, and influential: among other
things, prognoses influence whether and how doctors treat patients,
what kind of diagnostic evaluations they subject them to, whether they
encourage hopeful expectations, and whether they stop efforts to save
a patient's life.

Prognostication in clinical practice serves two important overarching purposes. The first is that prognosis, even more so than diagnosis,
can serve to cultivate a common vision; the sharing of a prognosis
is a fundamental predicate for the coordination of collective action.
Motivated by an implicit or explicit understanding, and possibly by
their agreement or even by their disagreement about what the future
holds, patients and physicians take action. Even in the extreme (and
typical) case when the prognosis is not actually discussed, the patient
accepts the doctor's prescriptions with the tacit understanding that
they will lead to a better outcome. Prognostication, even if implicit
or incorrect, is *effective* precisely for this reason. It effects changes in
patients' and physicians' behavior and it effects changes in the eventual outcome.

This is especially true when seen from a phenomenological perspective that allows for an indeterminate future. Compared to the patient's
diagnosis, which is generally seen as immutable, the prognosis is typically seen as more open to change. It is the fact that, in addition, the
future is not known that is so important to understanding prognosis
in clinical practice. Whereas diagnosis is generally perceived as the
province of the physician (the patient *has* a diagnosis definitively *made* by
the doctor), prognosis is much more open to patient modification (the
patient *experiences* the prognosis that the physician tentatively *offers*).
Although patients can reject a physician's diagnosis, they are certainly
much freer, in general, to reject a prognosis. Moreover, whereas patients
already have the diagnosis when they meet the physician, they do not

yet have the prognosis, and there is the hope, if not the expectation, that both actors can and should do something about the latter.

These considerations lead to the second overarching purpose of prognosis in clinical practice. The development and communication of prognostic information is in some sense about power and professional control. On the one hand, the future course of an illness is actually for the patient to experience, and this experience indeed often takes place outside of the professional domain—removed from the doctor spatially, temporally, and psychologically. In other words, although prognostication results from the application of professional knowledge to biological reality, it nevertheless has its origins and realization in social interaction and personal experience: the physician gleans information about the patient from the patient and then communicates information back to the patient, after which the patient experiences the prognosis. The patient is in control of the future. On the other hand, the patient clearly occupies the subordinate position in the dyadic, socially structured relationship between physician and patient, a relationship that likens them to prophet and supplicant respectively. Through its impact on patients, prognostication is used, directly or indirectly, deliberately or incidentally, to buttress professional authority. By supporting the physician's claim to special knowledge (here, of the future), by lending credence to the physician's proposed therapeutic interventions, and by enhancing patient confidence in the physician's abilities, prognostication in clinical practice strengthens the physician's position with respect to the patient. The physician is supposed to transform the patient's symptoms and complaints into an official, legitimate, professional diagnosis, after which the physician also uses professional knowledge and power to transform (both metaphorically and literally) the patient's course into some unseen future experience. The patient awaits the prognosis that the physician offers, and both the patient and the future are thus controlled.

Three

ERROR AND ACCOUNTABILITY
IN PROGNOSTICATION

*I just get so damn nervous when I have to make a prediction. I feel
as if there is no way that I can be right and that if I make a mistake
my patients will be angry or hurt. My colleagues would think I
was foolish to hazard a prediction in the first place. The way I see
it, the only thing I can say for sure about prognosis is that you are
bound to be wrong—unless you are so vague that the prediction is
meaningless. And people will blame the doctor no matter what: if he
predicts a good outcome and a bad one occurs or if he predicts a bad
outcome and a good one occurs. You just can't win.*

— GENERAL INTERNAL MEDICINE FELLOW

Error is unavoidable in prognostication. And it is quite common, often
sizable, and usually consequential. For patients, error means that they
are misinformed about their illness, that they may take foolish actions
as a result, and that they may be given inappropriate or needlessly
painful treatments or denied appropriate ones. For physicians, error
may result in adverse judgments by their patients or colleagues. The
fear that physicians have about being judged adversely as a result
of prognostic error is a major restraint on their willingness to offer
prognoses. Physicians cope in a number of ways with the fact that error
is both inescapable and consequential: they may avoid prognostication
altogether, they may adopt certain behaviors with respect to how they
prognosticate, or they may adopt certain philosophical, even religious,
attitudes about the meaning of prognostic error.

The possibility and reality of error is critical in understanding physicians' attitudes and behaviors with respect to prognosis. Indeed, it is
hard to think about prognosis without immediately thinking about error.
Although prognostication would occupy a problematic space in clinical
practice even if it were not subject to error, the existence of error adds
substantial complications and engenders meaningful compensatory attitudes and behaviors in its own right. Moreover, when the stakes are
the life or death of a patient, physicians find the problem of prognostic
error particularly acute.

Physicians' attitudes toward prognostic error are complex, however, and are not simply restricted to aversion. On the one hand, any

prediction entails the possibility of error, and a prediction which is unduly favorable or unfavorable may be perceived as a professional failing. On the other hand, developing and communicating a prognosis can be a way for physicians to avoid errors in their clinical practice, because if they can make correct predictions, they can avoid *unexpected* occurrences, especially bad ones. Through prognostication, physicians may try to configure the future as being *expected*; prognostication may thus paradoxically serve as a way to cope with uncertainty. Prognostication, in other words, not only can cause professional problems but also can prevent them. Moreover, physicians regard the very possibility of prognostic error as *both* harmful and helpful. It is harmful because in particular, realized situations, it can result in difficult clinical management problems. It is helpful because, when seen as a general, inherent, and unavoidable attribute of prediction, the possibility of error can function to exculpate physicians.

There are several ways to think about the nature of error in prognosis and to break it down into different elements or aspects. One way is simply to examine what percentage of patients in a given group have accurate predictions made about them—for example, by determining the percentage of patients for whom predictions of life or death proved correct out of the total for whom such predictions were made. Of course, a standard for accuracy must be chosen, or a time horizon over which the accuracy of the prediction is to be evaluated must be specified. The extent to which there is such "correct classification" of patients is only one possible measure, however, of the magnitude of the error. Another aspect of error in prognosis is whether errors in prediction occur at random or whether they have a particular bias—whether physicians making predictions for an entire group of patients are more likely, for example, to predict survival in patients who die rather than death in patients who survive. Depending on the circumstance, biases toward optimism or toward pessimism will be valued differently; in some cases, erroneous predictions of survival may be seen as more consequential than erroneous predictions of death, and in other cases, erroneous predictions of death may be seen as more consequential than erroneous predictions of survival. Thus, "prognostic error" is not a unitary concept.[1] Physicians are sensitive to different aspects of it, including the direction and size of the error and the particular clinical circumstance in which it occurs.

In the everyday experience of patients and physicians, the key aspects of prognostic accuracy are whether errors are common and, if so, what shape they take. For instance, do physicians commonly misestimate the duration of survival? If so, do they tend to overestimate it or underestimate it, and by how much? In what circumstances do they make such errors? What explains such errors? What are the consequences of such errors? And finally, how do physicians respond to the anticipated possibility or the observed reality of such errors?

The Direction and Magnitude of Prognostic Error

There have been extremely few evaluations of the accuracy of physicians' predictions.[2] Such evaluations take the form of comparing physicians' predictions about the outcome of an illness with the outcome that is eventually observed. The extant evaluations have tended to assess physicians' ability to predict survival in either terminally ill cancer patients (typically those referred for hospice care) or critically ill patients with diverse diseases in intensive care.[3] Virtually all of these studies have documented frequent and large errors in prediction, though the standard for accuracy has varied across studies. No study has concluded that physicians are, overall, very accurate (in the sense of being able to correctly classify patients) when they make predictions. Unfortunately, these studies have, as a group, neglected the causes or sources of prognostic error.

Studies evaluating physicians' ability to predict survival in cancer patients have generally shown not only that doctors err but also that they substantially overestimate survival. In this type of clinical situation, that is, physicians are prone to an optimistic bias. The classic study, conducted by psychiatrist C. Murray Parkes at Saint Christopher's Hospice in London, was published in 1972. Parkes showed that, for a number of physicians making predictions about duration of survival in 168 cancer patients, 53 percent of the predictions were in error (even using a very liberal standard for prognostic accuracy), and that 80 to 90 percent of the errors were optimistic.[4] In general, the physicians overestimated survival by a factor of two, with the median predicted survival being about six weeks and the median observed survival about three weeks. No variation among physician types (at least in terms of the one measured attribute, their specialty) was noted. A followup study conducted by different investigators and published fifteen years later found that for fifty patients with "terminal cancer," survival was overestimated in 88 percent of the cases, by a factor of almost three overall; the average predicted survival was 9.5 weeks, and the observed survival about 3.5 weeks.[5] Several other studies, typically involving fewer than four physician prognosticators, have confirmed these findings.[6]

My own work with 365 physicians predicting survival in 504 patients (65 percent of whom had cancer and all of whom were being admitted to outpatient hospice care) found that only 20 percent of predictions were "accurate," meaning that the predicted survival was within 33 percent of the observed survival (a standard that, for example, deemed a prediction of eight days to live accurate if the patient lived six days, and a prediction of four months to live accurate if the patient lived three months).[7] Of the remaining 80 percent of predictions, most (63 percent of the total) were overestimates of survival, while only 17 percent were underestimates. Overall, the patients had a median survival of twenty-four days, and physicians overestimated survival by a factor of about five. Close examination of the sources of prognostic error revealed that attributes of the patients (such as their age, sex, race, diagnosis, functional status, and illness duration) and attributes of the physicians (such as their age, sex, specialty, and dispositional optimism) were *not* associated with optimistic prognostic error. However, in general, the better the doctor knew the patient—as measured, for example, by the length and intensity of their contact—the more likely the doctor was to err in the prognosis, most frequently by overestimating survival.[8] Physicians explain this finding by noting that they do not want to believe that a patient they know well is going to do poorly.

Three studies have evaluated physicians' prognostic accuracy in cancer patients with a longer observed survival than the three to four weeks of the preceding studies. One study of the predictions made by nine physicians of various specialties for 196 patients with lung cancer found that the patients had a median survival of about five months; of the predictions made for these patients, 36 percent underestimated their survival time, 54 percent overestimated, and 10 percent were "correct," that is, within one month.[9] On average, the physicians appear to have overestimated survival by about a month. Again, no variation in accuracy across physician specialty was noted. Another study of the predictions made by an unspecified number of doctors for 319 patients with cancer (most of whom were outpatients) revealed that doctors were reasonably good at discriminating patients likely to live longer than a year from those likely to live less than a year. Of those patients estimated to live more than a year, 17 percent died before that time, and of those estimated to live less than a year, 31 percent lived longer. Nevertheless, since more patients were estimated to live more than a year, pessimistic and optimistic errors were nearly equivalent in frequency, though pessimistic errors were slightly more common.[10] Finally, a well conducted study of predictions by oncologists of the likelihood of "cure" for 98 cancer patients and of the length of survival for 39 "incurable" cancer patients revealed a similar pattern.[11] In the incurable patients, actual survival was about ten months; in 30 percent of the cases, the physician was "accurate" (within 33 percent of the observed survival); of the remaining cases, the physicians overestimated survival in 30 percent and underestimated survival in 40 percent.

The pattern that emerges from these studies of cancer patients is that physicians are "accurate" in their predictions only 10 to 30 percent of the time. Moreover, they tend to overestimate survival—depending on how long the patient actually has to live—by a factor of two to five.[12] Most of the studies did not investigate how attributes of the patients or of the physicians affected the prognostic error; however, when this issue was addressed, significant correlations were generally not detected. Overall, prognostic error and optimistic bias are common and are relatively uniformly distributed across patients and physicians when the patient is seriously ill with cancer and the object of prediction is how long the patient has to live.

Studies of physicians' prognostic accuracy and error rates in intensive care unit cases reveal a somewhat more complicated picture than the one seen in the studies of cancer patients. In general, errors are again rife, but here there is a tendency toward pessimistic bias. ICU patients have a high risk of immediate death, but the majority (70 to 90 percent) do indeed survive ICU admission (which typically lasts less than a week), and, depending on the population, overall survival can be quite long. One of the classic ICU studies was published by physician Allan Detsky and colleagues in 1985.[13] For 1,831 admissions, the investigators elicited estimates for "survival to discharge from the ICU" from the resident physicians caring for these patients. When predicted survival was compared to observed survival, the physicians were found to be somewhat pessimistic; for example, 63 percent of those patients estimated to have a 21 to 40 percent chance of survival actually survived. This study was particularly concerned with the effects of prognostic error on cost. It found that among those patients who *did not* survive, the highest costs were incurred in caring for those who had the *most favorable* estimated prognosis on admission. Conversely, among patients who *did* survive, the highest costs were incurred in caring for those who had the *least favorable* estimated prognosis. In other words, patients with unexpected outcomes incurred the greatest expenditures.

Another classic paper, published by health services researchers William Knaus, Douglas Wagner, and Joanne Lynn in 1991, reported preliminary results from a study of thousands of patients admitted to several representative medical centers around the country.[14] Reporting on 850 patient admissions, for which a total of thirteen experienced ICU physicians made predictions of survival, the authors found that the prognoses were in general somewhat pessimistic, with 25.5 percent of patients predicted to die before hospital discharge and 20.7 percent actually dying. For example, the forty-five patients whom the clinicians identified as having not more than a 10 percent chance of survival actually had a 48 percent survival rate. And, similar to the Detsky study, approximately 68 percent of those estimated to have a 30 percent chance of survival survived. Thus, there was significant pessimism in doctors' prognostic estimates in this setting.[15] These authors noted that objective, statistical estimates of survival can perform better, according to some measures, than physicians' subjective estimates, and that objective estimates offer a way to compensate for decision making by individual doctors, which varies in response to their personal clinical experience or preferences. Nevertheless, the authors noted that physicians resist the use of objective prognostic estimates for a number of reasons: physicians always have more information available to them about a particular case than can be incorporated into a generic statistical algorithm; they may be concerned that their particular patient's case is not comparable to those in which the algorithm was developed; or they may fear that deferring to objective estimates will diminish their authority and prestige.[16]

Several other studies of ICU patients conducted by other investigators (assessing patients' prospects for survival either to hospital discharge or to 180 days) have presaged or confirmed the results of the foregoing studies. Although the precise degree of prognostic accuracy has varied, these studies have tended to find meaningful inaccuracy in prediction, usually in the pessimistic direction,[17] though optimistic bias has also occasionally been found.[18]

As with the studies of cancer patients who were less acutely ill, most published studies of prognostication for ICU patients have not examined the role of physician or patient factors in explaining prognostic errors. The few that have done so have concluded that physicians' accuracy in predicting survival was not related to their age, level of training, experience with dying patients, or the number of times they had to prognosticate.[19] However, accuracy was related to physicians' self-rated confidence in their prognostic estimates in one study[20] and to their familiarity with the patient in another.[21] As in the studies involving cancer patients, greater familiarity with the patient was associated with greater (and misplaced) prognostic optimism.

What might explain the varying types of bias in studies involving cancer patients and those involving ICU patients? One explanation is that the background expectations in the two populations differ. Physicians may tend to overestimate survival for patients who are not critically or acutely ill or not in need of life support, and they may tend to underestimate survival for patients who are critically and acutely ill or in need of life support. Another possible explanation for the tendency to be optimistic about chronically ill patients and pessimistic about ICU patients is the strength of the personal relationship between the patient and the physician. ICU physicians usually do not know their patients before admission; conversely, physicians may know chronically ill patients quite well and have an interest in being optimistic or in overlooking ominous information. It is also possible that the specialty training and clinical background of the prognosticators accounts for the difference; the doctors caring for, and predicting the survival of, patients with cancer are primarily oncologists and general internists, who may be more optimistic by disposition and training than intensivists. Yet another possible explanation is the different contexts in which such predictions are made, a fact aptly illustrated by the rationales motivating the research. Most studies of physicians' accuracy in intensive care are conducted with an eye to rationalizing the use of scarce ICU resources. On the one hand, there is a wish to avoid needless expenditure (or needless suffering) in those patients who are "certain" to die; on the other hand, there is a wish to avoid needlessly expensive intensive care for patients who would do well even without it. In contrast, the studies of cancer patients reviewed above were conducted in a context where there is a desire to find ways to enhance the accuracy of information that is communicated to patients and to colleagues. In other words, whereas in the intensive care studies the impetus to prognosticate is somewhat impersonal (i.e., to avoid wasting resources), in the cancer patient studies the impetus to prognosticate is personal (i.e., to provide information to patients about their prospects). It is therefore not surprising that errors, while substantial in both situations, tend to be pessimistic in the former and optimistic in the latter.

Indeed, the relatively pessimistic errors seen in the studies of ICU patients run counter to much of the data on how physicians prognosticate in general, as we shall see. That is, overall, physicians are quite optimistic in how they both formulate and communicate prognoses. Several additional factors account for the relative pessimism seen in

ICU settings. First, the ICU setting is a special case in which physicians may indeed see a role for pessimism, at least in certain circumstances, such as when their intention is to limit the use of medical technology.[22] Second, ICU patients are a minority of all patients who doctors care for at the end of their lives. The great majority of medical care takes place outside of ICUs, and we may expect that the patterns of behavior seen in these other settings will predominate over practices seen in the ICU. And third, the foregoing studies have exclusively involved the foreseeing of the future by physicians rather than the foretelling; that is, they have examined how physicians formulate but not how they communicate prognoses. There is a difference in physicians' behavior in these two activities, however; even if they are pessimistic in the prognostic esti-mates they formulate, they may still be optimistic in the estimates they communicate—and, indeed, as we shall see in chapter 5, they often are.

These studies of prognostic accuracy also draw attention to the issue of the time horizon over which prognoses are made. The patients in the foregoing studies, whether outpatients with cancer or inpatients in intensive care, have generally survived six months or less. The ex-perience of practicing clinicians suggests that, if anything, physicians' survival estimates would be even less reliable over longer time horizons, such as five to ten years.[23] In general, however, when patients and physicians are concerned with prognosis, it is typically in a setting where a serious illness has been diagnosed and death is possible in the relatively short term.[24] Temporally specific prognostication usually takes place—and patients appropriately expect it to take place—over time horizons of less than two years, and we rarely see or expect physi-cians to predict whether a patient will live, say, for precisely eight or ten years. Of course, physicians are expected to say whether a patient will recover from a disease or not (e.g., be "cured" of their cancer), and such recoveries may indeed mean that the patient will live for many decades.

Error and Accountability

Physicians are aware that their predictions are often mistaken, and they realize that it is hard for them to predict outcomes accurately. How do they think that other physicians, and patients themselves, feel about such errors? Do they worry that they will be held accountable?

Physicians believe that prognostic error can indeed pose a signifi-cant threat to their professional standing, as reflected in the judgments of patients and colleagues. For example, 50 percent of surveyed internists believe that an error in prognosis might cause their patients to "lose confidence in them."[25] They believe, however, that their colleagues are more forgiving than their patients and that both groups are more forgiving of prognostic errors than they are of diagnostic errors. That is, 88 percent of surveyed internists believed that an error in diagnosis might cause their patients to "lose confidence" in them. Similarly, a majority of physicians, 81 percent, believed that if they made an error in diagnosis their colleagues might lose confidence in them, as compared to 29 percent who believed colleagues would lose confidence after a prognostic error. Moreover, physicians believe that they are more forgiving of their colleagues than their colleagues are of them; only 17 percent acknowledged that they would lose some confidence in a colleague who made an error in prognostication.[26]

The pattern of responses to these questions suggests two general observations about physicians' attitudes. First, physicians believe that both patients and colleagues recognize that prognosis is more difficult and uncertain than diagnosis and therefore regard diagnostic errors as more serious indicators of incompetence and threats to confidence than prognostic errors. Second, physicians differ in the extent to which they believe that colleagues would lose confidence in them compared with the extent to which they believe patients would. With respect to prognosis, the percentage of physicians who believe that other physicians might lose confidence in them in response to an error (29 percent) is lower than the percentage who believe that patients might lose confidence (50 percent). With respect to diagnosis, the percentage of physicians who believe other physicians might lose confidence in them in response to an error (81 percent) is also lower than the percentage who believe patients might lose confidence (88 percent), albeit to a lesser extent. Apparently physicians believe that colleagues are *relatively* more forgiving of prognostic errors. This pattern illuminates a "colleague-centered appreciation" of what constitutes a professional error—and a special recognition of the inherent fallibility of prognosis.[27] Physicians believe that mistakes in prognosis—much more so than in diagnosis—are inevitable and that criticism regarding such errors should be withheld. As with other types of professional errors, they feel that colleagues are more forgiving than patients.

Patients' and Colleagues' Judgments

The claim that physicians feel accountable for prognostic errors is strongly supported by certain experiments incorporated into a survey of a random sample of practicing internists in the United States. In these experiments, the physician subjects received identically worded, hypothetical clinical vignettes describing seriously ill patients being cared for by hypothetical doctors; the clinical details were carefully chosen so that the patients might have had a favorable or unfavorable outcome. Subjects were randomized into one of six groups representing one of three different prediction behaviors by the hypothetical doctor (no prediction, prediction of unfavorable outcome, or prediction of favorable outcome) combined with one of the two possible outcomes for the hypothetical patient (unfavorable or favorable). All subjects were then asked a series of identically worded questions about the vignettes, and comparisons were made of their responses.[28]

The experiments show that physicians realize that the prospect of error can affect how they are perceived by patients and other physicians in complicated ways. To begin with, physicians have ideas about whether they should make a prediction at all. Regardless of whether the clinical situation is one of acute or chronic illness, and regardless of whether the prediction is favorable or unfavorable, physicians believe that patients' confidence would indeed be enhanced if they chose to make a prediction rather than not make one. However, they believe that other physicians consider the making of a prediction (again, whether favorable or unfavorable) as damaging to their reputation as good clinicians—at least in chronic disease situations. In acute disease situations, prognostication is somewhat more acceptable and is not regarded as inappropriate; however, it is not considered better than avoiding prediction, at least with respect to standing among one's colleagues. This pattern of gaining standing among one's peers for *not* articulating prognoses occurs even though the results also indicate that physicians realize that making accurate predictions does indeed reflect significant technical proficiency. Overall, physicians believe that, although patients might want predictions, other doctors consider it best to keep quiet.

However, these experiments show that, if physicians make a prediction, they feel differently about different kinds of error. Errors in prediction, regardless of whether the disease is acute or chronic, damage patients' confidence and result in colleagues feeling that clinical ability and prognostic acumen are in question. However, attitudes vary depending on the type of error. In the case of chronic illness, physicians believe that it is better, in terms of maintaining patients' confidence, to make an optimistic prediction than a pessimistic one. Physicians typically remark that physicians look foolish to patients when they are pessimistic and underestimate survival. Physicians believe that patients are more likely to forgive them for an overly optimistic prognosis than for a symmetrically pessimistic prognosis. In the case of acute illness, again with respect to patients' confidence, physicians disapprove of optimistic and pessimistic errors equally, though there may be a slight bias towards pessimism. A similar pattern holds with respect to how doctors judge their colleagues. In the case of chronic illness, an optimistic prognosis is less of a threat to clinical reputation than a pessimistic one. In the case of acute illness, on the other hand, neither optimistic nor pessimistic errors are preferred.

Different combinations of predictions and outcomes thus have different kinds of consequences for different aspects of how physicians are perceived. When making predictions for real patients, physicians appear to weigh these consequences (e.g., they balance patients' likely perceptions against those of colleagues, or their desire to be accurate prognosticators against their desire to have a reputation as a good clinician). Sometimes they prefer unduly favorable predictions, sometimes unduly unfavorable predictions.[29] Overall, the experimental results suggest that if a prediction is essential and unavoidable, and if an error is to be made, it seems best to be optimistic, especially in chronic illness, and it may be better to be pessimistic in acute illness.

The parallels between these experimental results regarding physicians' attitudes about prognostic error and the observations of their actual performance outlined earlier are striking. Physicians' ideas about the consequences of prognostic error correspond to the types of errors they make in real-life situations, for, as we saw, physicians tend in actuality to make optimistic errors in chronically ill patients and pessimistic or equivocal errors in acutely ill ones. Concerns about error are only one factor determining physicians' relative propensity to be optimistic or pessimistic, however; as we shall see, there are several other factors that tend to make physicians optimistic in their prognoses in general, whether the patient is acutely or chronically ill.

Responding to Prognostic Error

Physicians' responses to the possibility and reality of prognostic error—both in general and in their care of particular patients—may usefully be divided into those that are manifested *before* an outcome that reveals a previous prediction to have been in error and those that are manifested *after* an outcome.

Behavior before Errors

The behaviors that are manifested before outcomes are observed, and the attitudes that undergird these behaviors, include both broad traits that characterize the profession and specific ones that characterize individual cases. In the first instance, physicians try to avoid errors by not making predictions at all. Physicians cope with the problem of prognostication in general by using various other conscious and subconscious techniques to reduce the role of and need for prognosis. These techniques are generic—meaning that they are widespread practices with respect to prognosis in general—and they include a pattern of delay or avoidance of prognostication, a pattern of offering optimistically or pessimistically biased predictions, and an emergence of nonrational (magical and religious) beliefs about prognostication. We will examine all of these in detail.

The foregoing behaviors arise in response not only to error, but also to other aspects of the task of prognostication, including, for example, the fact that it is stressful to give patients bad news, even if it is accurate and error-free. It is important to emphasize that even if predictions were perfect, physicians still might show some of these responses. Prediction is fraught with emotional and social overlay, substantially beyond its propensity to error. Behaviors and attitudes regarding prognosis are overdetermined, and error is only one of the factors contributing to them.

For example, one technique physicians employ to mitigate the propensity to and consequences of error is to share prognostic decision making with patients and with other doctors. This practice serves at least two purposes. One is to increase accuracy. There is evidence that consensus prognoses are more accurate than those of individuals.[30] Physicians might cooperate and consult with each other in order to optimize prognosis, just as they do for diagnosis and therapy. Another purpose of this practice, however, is to diffuse responsibility. Physicians may choose to engage patients and colleagues in discussions in order to discover whether they agree with their prognostic pronouncements.[31] In the case of sharing prognostic decision making with patients, such behavior diffuses responsibility both for formulating the prognosis and for the outcome that is ultimately observed.

Behavior after Errors

After an unexpected outcome is observed, and particularly if an explicit and wrong prediction has previously been made, doctors usually feel obliged to offer an explanation. Indeed, physicians feel that both unduly favorable and unduly unfavorable predictions call for an explanation to the patient: 96 percent of internists indicated that when they "predict an outcome to a patient and things turn out unexpectedly poorly, [they] feel obligated to explain this to the patient," and 67 percent indicated that even when they "predict an outcome to a patient and things turn out unexpectedly well, [they] feel obligated to explain."[32]

Physicians' belief that it is necessary to explain unexpected outcomes and erroneous predictions, regardless of whether the outcome is favorable or unfavorable, is confirmed by the vignette experiments discussed above. Physicians generally feel that an explanation of an outcome is indicated after it has occurred, even if no prognosis was previously given to the patient. However, an erroneous prediction is even more likely to call for an explanation. Physicians clearly believe that they would have to explain an outcome when a favorable prediction is made and an unfavorable outcome is observed. However, physicians even believe that they have to explain outcomes that prove *better* than predicted. On the other hand, although error in prediction calls for explanation, expected outcomes following a prediction (that is, correct predictions) are no more likely to require an explanation than outcomes occurring in situations were no prognosis was made. It is the inaccuracy of the prediction, rather than the valence of the outcome, that causes the need for explanation.

The compunction to provide an explanation for unexpected events originates partly in the general obligation physicians feel to explain to patients what is happening with their bodies—regardless of whether they predict the events correctly. Physicians believe that both their profession and their patients demand such explanations, as indicated by the following physician's observation:

> Physicians are trained that we need to give explanations, and they need to be clear and foolproof: "This is what happened and this is why." "You have a rash, this is why." "Your mother died, this is why." "Your brother got better—well, I knew he was going to get better, and this is why." I think we're trained to do that because we think people expect that—expect us to say exactly what happened and why.

Explanations of outcomes originate in the desire of patients and doctors alike to understand what has happened and to find meaning in medical events. There is a special desire, however, to find meaning in unexpected outcomes. When expectations of success or failure are disturbed, patients and doctors alike wish to know why. This desire is so fundamental that it can arise even when something unexpectedly good happens.

Then, an explanation can be instrumental in framing the experience for the patient, as the following physician's observations illustrate:

> A patient I remember, a priest, had a brain cancer. It was partially resected and he also had radiotherapy. He was told that this is a cancer where death in a year is a coin toss. It's a very horrible disease to have, with a very poor survival rate and many clinical problems. He had two or three operations, several treatments of radiation, and the tumor went into remission. He was in his second year of life when it recurred. He lived still another year. And when he had had his disease for three years, he ultimately went to see a specialist in neurologic oncology. The specialist came into the room, and he said, "There's no reason when I look at your records that you should be alive now. I have nothing to offer you, and you probably knew this when you came here. There are no more treatments." The patient had even had gamma-gun treatment [sophisticated radiotherapy], so he had really maxed out all the therapies. And he knew this fact; he was a priest, he was educated. But he was just looking for one more answer from a specialist. And the answer the specialist gave him was really almost metaphysical: "You're a miracle, and to be with you is a privilege because no one would have ever thought that someone like you would have lived this long. You've taught me a lot. God must really love you. People must really care about you. You must be really valued. Because there's no way you could have lived this long just from what we, the doctors, did." And the patient felt elated. He felt like his existence was justified. He was so happy. And he got nothing, nothing substantial, from the doctor. No additional therapy. No secret chemical. But he was elated nonetheless.

This case demonstrates the powerful capacity of physicians to reframe patients' experiences, even in such a complex situation as this, where the patient has a lethal illness and a better-than-expected course. Here, the doctor and the patient both ascribe meaning to the unexpected outcome: that the patient must be very loved—by his friends and by God—to have lived so long. His unexpected survival was thus "justified." The case illustrates the satisfaction that both patient and doctor often derive from the notion that the outcome in medical situations can be disconnected from the actions of doctors.

An additional point illustrated by this case is the role of specialist knowledge in prognosis. What this patient was seeking from this consultant was not a diagnosis (for he already knew this) or even treatment (which he knew he had exhausted); what he was seeking was a prognosis. He wanted, in a significant sense, to know the meaning of his condition, and this meaning was discussed with reference to his having outlived his prognosis. This is particularly ironic because physicians often speak of sending their patients to a specialist for a "blessing," by which they mean a review of the patient's case and a confirmation that the actions being taken are correct. Here the blessing is prognostic and occurs in more than this narrow sense.

Although physicians in general feel some obligation to explain events that are unexpected or counter to prior predictions, this is not always the case. Physicians realize that they do not always need to explain events. As one noted:

> I'm not convinced that patients always expect us to be able to explain what happened. I don't think that there always is an explanation for why things happen. And I think people are a lot more spiritual than we realize or than we give them credit for being. And they just accept the fact that this is what *happened.*

This physician invokes a spiritual sensibility on the part of the patient to explain why explanations are not, in fact, always necessary. Such invocations of spirituality and religion in discussions of the occurrence and meaning of unexpected events and of prognostic error are not uncommon, as we shall see.

Sometimes, physicians simply do not have an explanation, as described by one physician:

> When I don't know what is happening and when I am not able to give an explanation, that bothers me. And it bothers the patient too because I'm told that you have to give people an explanation. I don't like to make up things to appease people. I see other doctors do that, rather than say, "I don't know what happened." I think doctors are very scared. For example, we recently had a woman who died unexpectedly in the middle of the night, and the husband looked at us funny. You have to give him a reason that makes sense about why she died, so that he doesn't say, "You don't even know why she died. She came in the hospital, you told me she was fine, then she died. And you don't know why." Our cynical view is that this guy is going to sue. I think that might be one reason why doctors feel they have to have a logical explanation for everything, so that it makes sense and people don't think twice about it. But I'm impressed when people can be honest enough to say we don't know what happened.

The fear of being judged adversely by patients and their families, or of being sued, are given as reasons compelling physicians to explain the unexpected. When death and failure upend the patient's expectation, if not the physician's prognosis, of therapeutic success, the physician must say something.

Another way physicians cope with unexpected events and prognostic errors after the fact is to see them as an opportunity for learning. One physician characterized this as follows:

> I feel really bad when something unexpectedly bad happens. Because I feel like if we had been more aggressive or recognized the problem earlier, then maybe something could've been done. A patient comes in and then eight hours later he rapidly deteriorates: you feel bad when something like that happens. But in general, you learn from everything that goes wrong. You learn to recognize the pattern. If I ever find someone similar to this, I'll be thinking along these lines: Is that something we need to work up really quickly? I think from everything like that you learn, it's part of your medical information that you can apply to the next patient.

Viewing unexpected events as an opportunity for learning allows them to be reframed positively, in this case, for the benefit of the doctor. After an unexpectedly bad outcome, physicians may also employ retrospective justification, such as concluding that the patient would have died anyway, regardless of the therapy instituted or the prognosis pronounced. The error is rationalized as innocent or unavoidable.[33]

An unexpected outcome is an occasion for considering whether an error in prognostication did in fact occur, whether it could have been avoided, whether it was a result of a professional error, and if so, whether that error is excusable. Mistakes in prognosis can be fateful for both the patient and the doctor.[34] Nevertheless, mistakes in prognosis are the doctor's to make; society delegates to physicians the right and responsibility of making legitimate prognoses.[35] However, when mistakes do occur, physicians must find ways to cope with them, as they must with other types of medical errors. Physicians must cope with the fact that any maloccurrence might be seen (and often is seen) as a failure to anticipate events adequately, that is, as a failure to prognosticate competently and to take action accordingly.[36]

The Paradoxically Reassuring Nature of Prognostic Uncertainty and Error

Error in medicine is not limited to prognosis, of course, and diagnostic and therapeutic errors also occur.[37] While prognostic error is problematic for physicians, they are definitely more likely to believe that patients and colleagues will judge them adversely for diagnostic errors. Indeed, some physicians feel that the fact that prognostication is recognized to be more difficult than diagnosis insulates them from the stress and responsibility associated with making predictions.

Prognostic errors differ from other types of medical error in certain other important respects. Whereas diagnostic and therapeutic error typically cause physicians to question their knowledge and power in self-critical ways, prognostic error can cause them to question their knowledge and power in self-forgiving ways. Although making mistakes in prognosis is a problem for physicians, such mistakes—especially an unexpectedly good outcome—can paradoxically be *reassuring* to physicians.[38] One physician described two such cases:

> There was a fifty-year-old guy who came in from another hospital with Wegener's disease [a serious immunological disorder], and when he came in he was having frank lung hemorrhage and renal failure and was critically ill. We put him on appropriate medicines and started mechanical ventilation. But he progressed not only to have lung hemorrhage but lung failure and pneumonia. By all rights, his mortality now approached 100 percent. And after three weeks on the ventilator, progressing to jet ventilation and bilateral bronchopleural fistulas [holes in the lung], and four chest tubes [drainage tubes placed in the thoracic cavity], it seemed rather hopeless. And we told the family that, and we were entirely ready to start withdrawing support. Then, for whatever reason, in one day, we noticed that all of his chest tubes stopped having air leaks. The very next day, his oxygen requirements turned around and he was requiring much less mechanical ventilation. And within an amazing ten days, he was off the ventilator. And he left the hospital! If I saw that case a hundred times, a hundred times I would say that person has *no chance* of recovering, and I wouldn't push on any further. If it was my own family member, I wouldn't push on any further. But he lived.
>
> I had this other patient, a young man in his twenties or thirties: his girlfriend had left him, he became suicidal, drove his car off into the woods, and put a hose running from his tailpipe into his car. By sheer coincidence, he was found by hunters! He was helicoptered into our ICU, where he got hyperbaric oxygen therapy. He was in a coma! In a coma for three weeks or something like that. He was going to go to some horrible coma rehabilitation center. And he opened his eyes! And over the course of time, he came back to be an incredibly functional person. With absolutely no memory of this event or his girlfriend. By every measure that we have to evaluate people, his chances of recovering were not even minimal, they were *nonexistent*. And he came back to being very close to what he was before.
>
> I was wrong in both cases. But again, in both situations, by every right, neither of those patients should have turned out the way they did.

Asked how he felt about the way the cases turned out, this physician replied, "I was ecstatic! It was a minor miracle!" He summed up his response to having been so dramatically wrong as follows:

> Well, I still don't think that I would have predicted anything else, given the same situation again a hundred times. I think that the only thing that it makes you think is that in a situation like that there is a God. I find actually that this type of error is *hopeful*. I find it hopeful that there are these cases.

Another internist put it as follows:

> How did I feel when there was an unexpectedly good outcome in this woman with metastatic breast cancer? Well, I think that I was probably affirmed by the fact that there is a whole aspect of medicine we don't know about, and that makes me feel happy because I think therefore that there is *always* hope. I mean I don't think there is hope for cure in that type of situation, but I think there is hope for a prolonged survival with good quality of life.

The fact that there are limits to how much they can know of the future may thus be both a source of stress *and* a source of relief for physicians. There may indeed be a positive relationship between uncertainty, error, and medical limits, on the one hand, and hope and the possibility of a felicitous outcome, on the other. Physicians welcome unexpected outcomes (especially but not only if they are favorable) because they vindicate the belief that physicians are not, in fact, omniscient or omnipotent, attributes that confer considerable responsibility and stress.

Prognostic inaccuracy and the very lack of prognostic information offer hope not just to doctors but also to patients, doctors believe. For example, speaking of the development of kidney failure in children, one pediatrician observed:

> In a way, I think that not being able to make a prediction is kind of nice because it offers hope. I mean to some of the parents of the patients. You can say "He may develop renal failure but he may not. Right now we'll just try to use optimal nutrition and follow his growth and follow all his parameters and hope that we can get a lot of good growth before we need to start dealing with dialysis and transplant." It's kind of nice that you can offer them hope that the child will make it, but it's hard when they want an idea about when the kidneys will fail and you can't say whether it's going to be when they're a young adult or a young child. And you just can't tell them when they're going to become end-stage.

Rather than undermining their confidence in their own abilities or their devotion to the practice of medicine, the existence of prognostic error may ennoble physicians and relieve them of feelings of responsibility—as if certain things are beyond their control and are "God's responsibility."

Prognostication and Religious Sensibilities

The "God" that physicians sometimes invoke when discussing prognosis is not just a metaphor for the limits of physicians' ability, something akin to saying that the patient's prognosis is in the hands of "nature" or simply reflects the "natural history." It is a religious concept of God, a belief in a power that is beyond physicians' understanding. For example, one physician noted:

> We're not spiritual enough. Sometimes things happen and we just can't explain them, we just don't know why. I'm not a very spiritual person, but when I think about medical outcomes that I'm not sure I know 100 percent why they occur, I think about God.

Under ordinary circumstances, physicians do not openly discuss religion. They certainly do not spontaneously acknowledge its relevance to their work in general or to technical aspects of their practice in particular. It is not that physicians lack religious inklings or affiliations; rather, there are normative constraints within the profession against discussing religion.[39] Yet prognostication, especially about death, often spontaneously evokes this kind of talk and brings a latent religiosity to the surface. Prognosis evokes religion in a way that diagnosis and therapy, which are seen as much more under human control, do not.

Religious feelings about prognosis appear in two ways. First, physicians often defend the avoidance of prognostication on the grounds that it is too "God-like" to offer prognoses, especially if the prognoses are stated with any degree of certainty, and especially if they are about survival. Physicians often liken making predictions to "playing God" and say such things as "I leave the future in God's hands, that's not my job" or "Sometimes we're wrong; we can prognosticate, but we're not God." They regard it as arrogant and intemperate and even blasphemous to make predictions.

The reference to, and importance of, God with respect to prognostication, however, goes beyond physicians' opposition to prognostication on the grounds that it is hubristic. Religious sentiments about prognosis are also evident in a second, more remarkable way. When discussing prognosis, physicians sometimes see a truly religious God at work in medicine. Physicians liken making predictions to playing God in part because God is seen as being responsible for outcomes. The existence of dramatic turnabouts, especially favorable ones, evokes a recognition of the "miraculous" nature of medical practice. The knowledge that such events indeed occur lightens the enormous burden physicians feel they must shoulder in caring for patients. Miracles suggest to them that there is a God that is, after all, responsible for the patient's progress and prognosis. Indeed, physicians not only believe in the possibility of miracles, they sometimes wish for them. These miracles are deemed to be attributable to a higher power.[40]

The emergence of religious sentiments in this aspect of medical practice should not be too surprising, since religion is a fundamental way of coping with the strain posed by the limits of human ability and by the threat of death. Nevertheless, it is remarkable that physicians break through taboos about talking about religion when discussing prognostication, which might at first glance appear to be a purely professional function in medical care. For physicians, however, prognostication is not some kind of simple science, and this is not merely because it is difficult. Rather, prognostication touches on deep concerns. As one physician elaborated:

> My experience caring for the terminally ill has convinced me that there has to be a God. Even though I can't explain this, I find it reassuring. I cannot, in the end, really be the one who is responsible for whether the patient lives or dies, or even for knowing whether these things will happen. How arrogant! Not everything can be explained. It reminds me of that passage from Shakespeare, something like, There is more in heaven and earth than can be explained by philosophy.[41]

In its application to prognosis, religion gives meaning both to the patient's suffering and to the physician's limitations. It represents the victory of hope and sentiment over precision and science.

Such references to God in discussions of prognostication also suggest that physicians believe that predicting the future has both a forecasting function, which simply states what is in store, and a prophetic function, which frames, gives meaning to, and creates the future. Indeed, as we shall see, physicians believe in the effectiveness of prediction and in the self-fulfilling potentialities of prophecy. The emergence of religious sentiments reflects the extent to which physicians, in prognostication, cannot escape the prophetic role, a role that seeks to find grace in suffering, order in disorder, and meaning in disease.

PROFESSIONAL NORMS
REGARDING PROGNOSTICATION

Prognostication and good medical care are like acrimonious in-laws: they meet occasionally, but only when it is unavoidable and only at the risk of great stress. I refuse to make predictions in my practice unless I have absolutely no choice.

— GENERAL INTERNIST

The practice of medicine is like wine, and prognosis is the dregs.

— INTENSIVIST

Despite its usefulness, physicians regard prognosis with anxiety and disdain, and they avoid it if possible. If patients do not insist on being told, physicians generally will forswear making a prediction or will be as vague as the situation permits. Several professional norms restrict whether and how prognoses are offered to patients. These norms insulate physicians from both the need for and the consequences of prognostication—decreasing the strain associated with offering prognoses and mitigating physicians' concern that prognostication is arrogant, hubristic, or harmful.

The Stress of Prediction

There are several reasons physicians find it stressful to make predictions about the course of a patient's illness. First is the complex nature of prognostication. Most internists, even experienced ones, believe that prognosis is the most difficult matter in their practice. The difficulty in making prognoses is first of all technical, in the sense that it is complicated to formulate them. A great majority of physicians, 91 percent, report that making an accurate prognosis about the course of a patient's disease is harder than making an accurate diagnosis.[1] As one physician observed:

> You have much harder facts to pin a diagnosis on a patient. There are material things, there are X rays, there are laboratory studies, there is your physical diagnosis, your history, which is a lot of information that leads one to have a degree of certainty about what the diagnosis is. On the other hand, the course of illnesses is much more difficult to pin down—you're talking about what's going to happen in the

future. Once you've made the diagnosis, what you have to think about is what the course of the disease is most likely to be. And, you know, there is a certain degree of uncertainty as to what that course can be.

Moreover, although therapy does not change the underlying diagnosis, it can indeed change the prognosis, making alternative courses possible, depending on whether and how the patient is treated.

Physicians believe that there is inherently more uncertainty associated with predicting the future than with determining the patient's present state. Physicians in general do not enjoy the uncertainty associated with their practice, and they try to minimize it by avoiding prognostication. Moreover, in prognosis, as compared with diagnosis and therapy, physicians find it impossible—if not dangerous, as we shall see—to "act like a savant" and to adopt a "manner of certitude," key mechanisms for coping with uncertainty.[2] The great majority of physicians, 92 percent, are "reluctant to make predictions about a patient's illness when the clinical situation is uncertain." This reluctance is compounded by the fact that most internists, 80 percent, believe that their patients "expect too much certainty" in their predictions.[3]

But even when the prognosis is considered certain, it may still be difficult and stressful to prognosticate. This is especially true if the prognosis is unfavorable. As one physician observed:

> Seeing my patient with multiple sclerosis deteriorate slowly, and knowing with certainty what the future held for her: it was so depressing for me. Bladder problems, wheelchair bound, blindness. It was terrible.

While just knowing the future can be taxing, having to communicate an unfavorable prognosis may be even more unpleasant. The manifold nature of the difficulty of prognosticating is illuminated in the following physician's remarks:

> I had a patient with metastatic lung cancer. And she had a big, big hemorrhagic cerebellar metastasis that was compressing her aqueduct [a fluid passage in the brain]. She asked me how long she had to live. And, I was very honest with her. I told her that I didn't really know, but that from my experience I knew that she probably wouldn't live more than a year, and that we should think more about months than years. And I told her that since she had this lesion in her brain, that actually in her case she could die any time, and the lesion could hemorrhage further. But I also told her that it was very difficult for me to make this prediction.

The prediction was difficult to make in more than one way. It was technically demanding to make an accurate prediction (indeed, it was ostensibly impossible), it was emotionally draining and painful, and it was professionally frustrating (in that it forced the physician to acknowledge impotence).

Prognostication is likely to be especially painful for physicians who have known their patients for a long time and whose contact with the patient involves substantial, ongoing responsibility. Many general internists noted that it typically was more stressful for them to discuss prognoses with their patients than it was for consultant oncologists, for precisely this reason. For generalist physicians, the stress was compounded by what they feel to be their own relative ignorance about prognosis and by the allegedly crude handling of their patients by specialists. For example, one general internist observed:

> Prognosis is a difficult situation. As a primary care physician, I'm the one who is trusted since I know the patient, but I know less about the disease per se than the oncologist. When patients have cancer, they always seem to ask me "How long?" My answers are vague, and I give averages for the disease, and I reinforce that they are different for an individual.

Another general internist observed:

> Any physician who makes an official prognosis must first make sure he is in a position to do so. Being "the specialist" does not automatically qualify him or her. Moreover, the specialist must make sure the primary physician knows about it *before* he prognosticates. Nothing is more disastrous than a prognosis by a "professor" versus that of a longtime friend and doc.

The closeness of the relationship between the patient and the doctor can lead, however, not only to greater difficulty in making predictions, but also, as we saw in chapter 3, to greater errors.

On the other hand, physicians who have long-standing relationships with their patients also claim that it may be *easier* for them to communicate prognoses, compared to consultants—regardless and independent of whether it is easier for them to make the prognoses. One experienced physician noted:

> If in your mind the prognosis is absolutely zero, by anyone's accounting, then how do you impart this fact to the patient or the family members? In that arena, I'm quite straightforward. Now, the times I've done it, I must confess, I have been extraordinarily fortunate—if one could ever see it in that light—to have known the

families, so that I can sit down and review what the patient went through. I never would say, "You know, we're going to pull the plug tonight at six o'clock." I'd say, "You know, here is your mother, father, whatever; this is what's happened; this is where we stand; here are the resources that this institution has deployed for X days. By my view and by everyone else's view who has seen the patient, there is absolutely no way this . . ." And knowing the family makes a huge, huge difference. I feel very sad that the people who work in ICUs rarely know the patients' families, and it's really too bad, because they have to confront this kind of decision making and explanation to someone they don't know, and I think that's very unfair to them in some ways and certainly very far from ideal from the perspective of the patients' families.

Having a relationship with a patient can thus, with respect to the difficulty of prognostication, be both disadvantageous and advantageous. Despite the discomfort generalist physicians experience in prognostication, they would rather make and, especially, communicate the prognosis than have a specialist do it. They believe that specialists do not communicate well and do not "know the patient," both of which they consider essential for accurate and compassionate prognostication.

Many specialists, however, believe that generalists "dump" patients on them to avoid communicating bad news themselves. As one oncologist noted:

> My experience is that most physicians stress the positive and have difficulty giving bad news. Of patients I see in consultation, most describe a positive referral from the general physician. Most of my oncology colleagues, however, believe that they have given the straight facts and outlook to the patient and family.

There is thus a difference in perspective between specialists, who stress knowledge and accuracy in prognosis, and generalists, who stress empathy and individuality. This difference underlies a division of labor with respect to prognosis within the group of physicians caring for a patient.[4] Perhaps ideally specialists, with relatively less knowledge of the patient, would develop the prognosis, and generalists, with relatively more knowledge of the patient, would communicate it. It is clear, however, that knowledge, whether of the disease or of the patient, is considered essential for optimal prognostication.

An additional reason that physicians find prognostication stressful, beyond its technical and interpersonal difficulty, is that they believe they have not been adequately prepared. With regard to diagnosis only 7 percent of physicians believe their training was inadequate; with regard to therapy, only 6 percent. But fully 57 percent report that they had inadequate training in prognostication.[5] One young internist observed:

> In clinical practice, I find that patients will routinely request that we make prognoses regarding conditions which remain highly variable from patient to patient. I find this aspect of medicine the most difficult. This, in fact, may be the "art of medicine." Unfortunately, medical schools and residencies do little to guide us through this very difficult process.

The perception of the inadequacy of the training is widely and homogeneously distributed among physicians and does not vary according to their specialty or level of training, for example. Physicians reporting inadequate training in prognosis are significantly more likely to find prognostication stressful than those reporting adequate training.[6]

Prognosis is also stressful because, more than diagnosis or therapy, it is based on probabilistic reasoning, which physicians often regard as problematic and for which they are typically also poorly trained. Physicians see a tension between aggregate, population-based probability statistics on the one hand and the application of such data to identified, individual patients on the other. This reflects a more general attitude in the medical profession: although physicians see themselves as scientists, they disdain one of science's most prominent epistemologies, namely, probabilistic reasoning. For example, one physician noted: "Prognosis— unlike diagnosis and treatment—is a silly statistical endpoint." Another observed:

> Prognostication is inherently difficult at best, since is it based on statistics. It is great for large populations but very unreliable in individual patients (whose outcomes are *always* 0 or 100—a situation extraordinarily rare in statistics). When asked to make a prognosis, this uncertainty has to be related to the inquirer, and prognoses made reluctantly, if at all!

On the other hand, when they are obliged to communicate prognoses to patients, physicians often will use statistical expressions. Although the dependence of prognosis on statistics discourages doctors from developing or communicating prognoses, the dependence is nevertheless deliberately emphasized when prognostication is unavoidable.

Physicians find prognostication more stressful than other clinical tasks because they believe it reveals their professional limitations. Although making a prognosis increases the physician's appearance of omnipotence, and although this illusion of power is seductive, physicians fear that they may be expected to deliver on their predictions. Ironically, prognostication shows physicians the imperfect fit between what they do for the patient and what the outcome might be.

Unexpected events, especially unfavorable ones, can be humiliating, disheartening, and saddening, not just professionally threatening. One physician described such a situation as follows:

> There was a graphic case of a 40-year-old woman who was in a minor motor vehicle accident and who had to have fairly elective surgery done and who ended up having a pulmonary embolism. I told her and her family that this was a common event after such surgery and that we would put her on this medicine, and that she could only get better. And it wouldn't happen again. I said: "You won't have to stay on this medicine for more than three or four months. The cast on your leg is going to come off soon. You won't be sedentary any longer. And there is no residual damage in the leg from where the clot came from that we can see. Your lung isn't damaged and its function is preserved. We'll check a couple of things in a month or so once you're out of the hospital, but this shouldn't set you back at all. It's really not a problem."
>
> Only to have her have, four days later, another pulmonary embolus and go on to have heart failure and die! So, you know, those are the times . . . that's one case in a million that that happens. *(Almost tearful.)* It's totally unpredictable. You can say that it happens . . . it's "reported." But so what? Should I have told the family, "You know you have a 0.5 percent chance of having a recurrent pulmonary embolism and you have a one in a hundred chance of that pulmonary embolism causing heart failure." There is no reason I should tell them that kind of information. Because it's really not relevant. It's actually never relevant. I never would tell a patient that kind of a story. Though it happens.[7]

Prognostication can painfully confront physicians with the limits of their ability to help patients because sudden and unexpected reversals of previously articulated prognoses simultaneously prove the prognosis to be wrong and the therapy to be ineffective. Unexpectedly bad outcomes reveal both prognostic and therapeutic limitations. Moreover, in the above case and in others like it, there is an element of iatrogenesis, which compounds the physicians' perceptions of their limitations and increases the physicians' sadness and embarrassment at the erroneously favorable prediction. After all, the doctor both predicted a favorable outcome and was responsible for the therapy that undid the prediction. In such cases, where there is a sudden turn for the worse—especially when the patient is otherwise young and healthy—it is as if the patient is being punished for the doctor's arrogance in predicting recovery. For physicians, favorable predictions sometimes seem almost to invite the failure of therapy.

Finally, prognostication is stressful because physicians believe that prediction can sometimes harm patients. One physician described this as follows:

> I find prognosticating puts patients and families into more turmoil than the better alternative of simply telling them to take one outcome or stage of an illness at a time. The latter approach is less likely to create either false images of doom and gloom or false images of good outcome. The approach of keeping the family's "emotional balance" over their "emotional feet" produces less needless hysteria than might result from an assumed bad outcome that has, in fact, not yet occurred.

Moreover, as we shall see, physicians fear that unfavorable predictions might actually cause corresponding unfavorable outcomes, in a type of self-fulfilling prophecy.

Thus, the extent to which physicians find prognostication difficult, the extent to which patients expect prognostic certainty, and the extent to which physicians lack training in prognostication are all positively associated with physicians' considering prognostication to be stressful. In addition, physicians find prognosis stressful insofar as they believe that their patients, if not their colleagues, would judge them adversely for prognostic errors and insofar as it might harm their patients.[8]

"Maintaining Hope," "Being Honest,' and "Being Accurate"

Strain in the physician's role, as in other social roles, can arise from difficulties in fulfilling role obligations, for example, from the conflict between the imperative to do everything possible for the patient and the possibly intractable situation of a particular sick person.[9] Strain can also result, in particular cases, from conflicts between ordinarily unrelated role expectations. Physicians caring for an acutely ill patient, for example, are expected to act with both dispatch and prudence; moreover, they are enjoined to cultivate an attitude toward the patient that is both detached and concerned, and to treat the patient both respectfully and beneficently.[10] With respect to prognosis, strain emerges because physicians are expected to be honest and to be accurate on the one hand and to maintain hope on the other.

Physicians find prognostication, particularly about the end of life, to be troubling and stressful precisely because they must balance such conflicting expectations. One general internist expressed the problem as follows:

> I think that if a patient with an incurable disease asks in a direct question how long he has to live, a doctor needs to try to give a ballpark idea so the person knows what to do for himself in terms of getting his affairs in order. But I think this needs to be done in a way that takes into account the uncertainty of statistical probability and the uncertainty in life, and I never pin it down to a definite or exact time limit. I hate to destroy all hope, because I think that hope is very important. But I try hard to be realistic also.

For this physician, as for most physicians, being "definite" about the expected survival time "destroys hope." This is a paradigmatic tension that prognosis poses for the physician. Again and again, using very similar language, physicians explained their quandary: "Patients will not improve if all hope is denied, yet it is important to be realistic." "When patients are terminal, I tell them so in general, nonthreatening terms, and I always leave a ray of hope; but we should not mislead patients." "Prognosis should be done cautiously but with optimism." "It is helpful to be optimistic, but one should also be realistic to help patients and families prepare for death or life with substantial disability." "I believe we should be as optimistic as possible without being misleading." "Always exude optimism—tempered with reality. And be humble." This is truly an impossible combination of demands: optimism, honesty, accuracy, realism, hopefulness, humility, and foresight all at once.

With respect to prognostication, physicians thus find themselves in a situation fraught with what Robert K. Merton terms "sociological ambivalence." Merton argues that "sociological ambivalence puts contradictory demands upon the occupants of a status in a particular social relation. And since these norms cannot be simultaneously expressed in behavior, they come to be expressed in an oscillation of behaviors."[11] This social-structural ambivalence can in turn result in an intrapersonal, psychological ambivalence. Often, however, people cope not so much through an "oscillation" in behavior as through an avoidance of the problematic domain, a submersion of one extreme of the ambivalent dichotomy, or a syncretic melding of the extremes such as the establishment of a dynamic equilibrium between them.[12] Indeed, physicians use several approaches to cope with the sociologically ambivalent demands of prognostication. Clinicians may simply avoid prognostication altogether. They may cultivate ambiguity about the future, thus attempting to convey accuracy, honesty, and hope simultaneously. Or they may adopt one of two complementary predictive and communicative strategies: the "ritualization of optimism" or the "ritualization of pessimism." Here, I will consider especially the ways in which physicians avoid prognostication.[13]

The Avoidance of Prognosis

The strain induced by the conflicting obligations to maintain hope and to be both honest and accurate contributes to several norms regarding the avoidance of prognosis in the medical profession, an avoidance reinforced by the numerous other stresses associated with prognostication and by the feeling that prognostication can sometimes harm patients. By *norms* I mean shared ideals about behavior within the profession that are both formally and informally enforced. Norms are beliefs about what individuals in certain social roles ought to do, and they become part of individuals' patterns of behavior as a consequence of a socialization process.[14] Norms are more than merely typical or habitual behaviors and more than patterns of action: they reflect responses to distinctive stresses of the profession, codify underlying values of the profession, and symbolically represent these values.

The norms regarding prognosis may be arranged hierarchically in the order in which they are typically invoked: (1) do not make predictions, (2) keep what predictions you do make to yourself, (3) do not communicate predictions to patients unless asked, (4) do not be specific, (5) do not be extreme, and (6) be optimistic. These norms tend to make prognostication less prominent and to mitigate its potentially deleterious effects. From the perspective of both the profession as a whole and the individual physician, they operate as a sort of sequential, fail-safe mechanism, progressing from the most comprehensive and restrictive to the least. It is important to stress that these norms are not hard and fast rules: physicians *do* offer prognoses, especially when the prognosis is relatively certain or favorable or both, when the illness is routine or minor, when the patient demands one, or when clinical management depends on formulating or communicating the prognosis (for instance, for referral to a hospice or withdrawal of life support). And physicians are not always optimistic either.

The general prohibition against prognostication is widely internalized and reflects the belief that it is hubristic and even unethical to formulate predictions, let alone communicate them to patients. Physicians state the norm that prohibits even the formulation of a prognosis again and again: "I think a readiness to prognosticate displays arrogance rather than wisdom." "Prognosis should be avoided if possible; above all one should not be emphatic." "Making hard predictions is bad practice for both physicians and patients." Physicians thus go beyond the suggestion that prognosis be avoided; they also express the belief that it is "arrogant" and "stupid" to make predictions, and they show a disdain for prognostication: "Prognosis is dirty business." "The only thing that is ever true about the prediction is that it is wrong." "Prognosis is often an ego trip by the physician that patients should not have to suffer or pay for."

In a thoughtful observation, one physician argues that prognostication should especially be avoided if it is *idle*. Indeed, he argues that it is unethical—and not merely arrogant or foolish—to make predictions, unless they serve a narrow and specific purpose.

> If the role of diagnosis is primarily pragmatic (that is, knowing what the condition is allows us to determine what to do), then the role of prognosis is even more so—if it has any place at all. Mere morbid or intellectual curiosity and/or speculation has absolutely no place in the concerns of an ethical and humble physician. If considerations regarding outcome can serve no specific purpose (eschatologically for the patient or clinically/therapeutically for the physician), then it is morally and medically incumbent not to entertain them at all. If they have significance for the patient's plans or the physician's choices, then, within the envelope of prognostic concern, *then* they become morally imperative considerations.

The choice of whether to make a prediction at all is seen as a moral question, and humility about uncertainty and about what the future holds is seen as an ethical duty.

Prognostication is often viewed as being hubristic to the point of representing a godlike presumption on the part of physicians. Prognosis in general and the rendering of *specific* prognoses in particular are often proscribed precisely for this reason. In a typical observation, one doctor suggested that, whereas therapy and diagnosis were rightly his province, prognosis was "God's alone." Another noted: "My family, religion, education, and upbringing *forbid* 'definitive' statements of prognosis as a false god." Still another physician, an experienced general internist, observed:

> Being positive and optimistic really helps even if the reality of the patient's condition is poor or critical. Being premature in saying the situation is hopeless is playing God. Physicians are just human beings in whom patients put their trust and hopes. Physicians should not play God and make decisions about when a patient will die. We all die some day. I feel the God that is watching over us (regardless of

one's religion) will make the final decision. Patients and their family
will usually make their peace with dying much better this way.

These statements reflect a religiosity that is not commonly so explicit
among physicians, as noted in chapter 3. The expression of religious feelings in discussions about prognosis is yet another indication, however,
of the strain it imposes. Physicians liken rendering prognoses to making
God-like "decisions about when a patient will die." As we shall see in
chapter 6, this association arises partly because many physicians believe
in the self-fulfilling prophecy and partly because they do not want to
feel responsible for a patient's death. But they also liken the rendering
of a prognosis to playing God because it suggest an omniscience they
feel is superhuman.

In contrast to the foregoing, many physicians justify avoiding prognostication by comparing it to gambling. For example, one general
internist observed: "If physicians were that good at prognosis, then
we would spend more time at the track." Noting the "arrogance" of
prognostication, an experienced physician observed:

> It amazes me how colleagues who don't gamble at dice or poker, or
> buy stocks on margin, are nevertheless sometimes so explicit about
> prognoses. I think only those who are ignorant of the fundamentals
> of statistics can be so bold. When patients or families press me, I try
> to point out to them that knowing a coin will turn up heads in 50
> percent of tosses doesn't give us an ability to predict the outcome of
> a *single* toss. But I do try to be more specific in predictions when a
> patient or a family member informs me that certain decisions (about
> family or financial affairs of some weight) will hinge on the patient's
> prospects. In such situations, I think a physician has an obligation to
> be more forthcoming. In most other circumstances, I think a readiness
> to prognosticate displays arrogance rather than wisdom.

The analogy to gambling at once refers to the elements of chance and
uncertainty inherent (and deplored) in prognosis and suggests that
prognostication is vaguely illicit and perhaps outside the proper practice
of medicine. Physicians should not manage their patients as though they
were involved in games, let alone games of chance.

Although the reluctance to "play God" or "gamble at dice" helps to
explain physicians' unwillingness to formulate prognoses, it does not
explain why, when physicians do formulate a prognosis (for whatever
reason), they do not then communicate it to the patient. Apparently there
are restrictions not only on *foreseeing* the future, but also on *foretelling*
it. This is the second norm regarding prognostication: that, even if

physicians formulate a prognosis, they should not communicate it to a patient. Rather, they should keep it to themselves and use it to guide diagnostic and therapeutic maneuvers. Physicians typically say, when it comes to prognostication, the less said, the better. One pediatrician described her behavior in this respect:

> I can remember a case where I had to transport a child in from an outlying hospital. It ended up being child abuse; someone had whacked the kid upside the head. But this kid was basically obtunded and shocky in the ER and initially nobody knew why. I remember talking to the mother—who was not the perpetrator—and telling her that things were really bad, that the kid was not responsive and on pressors [drugs to support blood pressure] and really critical. I think I said that the child could die in the ambulance. I don't think I said, "I expect this child will die." I said, "She is very critical." But, yes, to myself I thought that the child would die. In fact, she was probably already brain dead at that point.

Physicians resist communicating prognosis even when it is obvious and material. They believe that communicating prognoses can harm patients, and, especially if the predictions prove to be wrong, can harm the physician as well.

The third norm regarding prognosis is not to *volunteer* predictions to patients. If prognoses are to be communicated at all, it should in general be in response to a patient's question; indeed, 44 percent of surveyed internists believe that they should "wait to be asked by a patient before offering a prediction about the course of a patient's illness."[15] One experienced physician observed: "It is very important to make prognoses only when asked, unless the patient and/or family are unrealistically pessimistic regarding the prognosis."[16] A young oncologist characterized the norm of not volunteering predictions, as well as the fact that certain circumstances may require violation of this norm, as follows:

> In oncology, we are strongly discouraged from offering prognostic information at all. I've seen it done maybe five times at most in the two years that I've been taking care of patients as an oncologist at an academic medical center. And when the prognosis *is* revealed, it's invariably only to people who just keep pushing the oncologist to say a date.
>
> Now the few times that I've seen prognoses be offered have been to people who have been incredibly ill with aggressive tumors such as lung cancer. It was fairly certain, that, without therapy, these people would be dead within a year, and that's essentially what the physicians said each time.

In such cases, in keeping with the interactional use of prognosis to modify patient behavior, physicians may make use of prognostication to encourage a patient to accept therapy. This appears to be especially true when the prognosis is relatively certain.

As one physician put it, doctors "feel that the number of unsolicited prognoses made varies inversely with knowledge and maturity."[17] Physicians believe that the wisdom borne of experience mandates circumspection and humility when it comes to making predictions. One very experienced physician described his beliefs as follows:

> When I was at this famous hospital, one of the senior surgeons was admitted to my ward with a shadow in his lung, and he hadn't had symptoms very long. He and his wife were neighbors of ours, and I looked at his X rays and went in to see him and I examined him and I talked to him. And, *for no reason at all,* I said as I was leaving: "One thing we don't seem to have to worry about is carcinoma of the lung. It doesn't look like that." He said, "Well, I'm glad to hear that because I was worried." But within a few days the sputum cytology came back, and it showed that I was wrong: it was carcinoma of the lung. I could have cut my tongue out for having *volunteered* that statement, when I didn't have to.
>
> I really don't think one should go out of his way to give a prognosis unless one is very *certain* in one's own mind that that's the way things are going to go. But then, I've told you why I think it is important for the patient and the family to know what to expect and to be able to communicate on the same level that the doctor and the patient are communicating. It is hard to balance these things.

Here, the physician expresses regret for having voluntarily offered a prognosis (about the test results and, implicitly, about the patient's condition), but he also affirms that there are important reasons to prognosticate. This is one of the paradoxes of prognosis: physicians find themselves in the ambivalent and difficult situation of wanting to simultaneously withhold and share information.

Sometimes the physician cannot avoid formulating and discussing a prognosis—for example, when a patient demands to know. Under such circumstances, several secondary norms come into play. The first of these is to avoid *specific* predictions about the timing or nature of events. Physicians consider general predictions to be better for both the patient and the physician, and to be better ethically. Being nonspecific avoids encouraging an idée fixe in the patient about a specific time, and it minimizes the possibility of error. In a typical observation, one oncologist remarked that, when asked to predict how long a patient will live, "At most, I will occasionally answer 'weeks to months' or 'months to years.' " This studiously nonspecific type of response is the most widespread and typical way physicians prognosticate about survival. Some authorities explicitly recommend this, stating that oncologists should "avoid giving a prognosis with a definite time scale, but, if possible [should] give the patient a broad, realistic time frame that will allow him/her to sort out personal affairs while still well enough."[18] Doctors are often also encouraged by numerous authorities to ask why the patient wants to know a specific time frame, as if such curiosity is misplaced![19]

One reason physicians avoid being specific is that they think it is detrimental to patients' efforts to remain hopeful. For example, one physician noted:

> I try to avoid predicting specific time intervals. I try to educate the patient and family about the uncertainties and I use qualitative terms like "soon," "not much longer," "you are in great danger," "you should have your affairs in order." I almost always try to leave some room for hope.

Another physician provided additional reasons to avoid specificity:

> I don't answer the question "How long do I have to live, doctor?" with a given, specific time. I phrase my response in a generic sense, in terms of my overall feeling, meaning that I say, "Things are not good, the outlook is guarded, and I would certainly talk to your family about making plans for, you know, 'beyond' so to speak." But if they come back and say, "Well, is it going to be two weeks, three weeks, four weeks? What's it going to be?" then I'd say, "At this stage I just can't tell you for sure," and I would make the prognosis in a generic time frame, but not a specific time frame.

Asked whether part of the reason for not giving a quantitative response was a belief that to do so was really impossible, this doctor continued:

> I'm certainly influenced by the variability in prognosis, which makes things hard to predict. But again I actually don't think it is critical for the patient to know whether it's three weeks, four weeks, or five weeks. I think they should know it's a short time. I feel that giving numbers like that does two things which, I think, have somewhat negative implications: the first is that it suggests that I know exactly what's going to happen in a given time, and the second is if they see that time [i.e., if they live that long], they might wonder if I would just give up on them, so to speak, and turn my back.

In sum, the reasons to avoid specificity include averting the possibility of hopelessness in the patient, avoiding a pretense to omniscience, and avoiding a fear of abandonment by the physician. As we shall see, a further reason is to minimize the possibility of a self-fulfilling prophecy.

A related secondary norm about prognostication is to avoid extremes. Physicians typically express this norm as follows:

> Patients with the same disease state and stage of illness still have variable longevity, which is unexplained. It is very important for clinicians to take a middle ground in discussions of prognosis but to always maintain some optimism. Unfortunately, there are some physicians who tend to extremes in prognosis—making excessively good or bad predictions.

Nonetheless, it is not appropriate, according to physicians, to stay purely in the middle either. It is important to maintain some optimism, to tilt at least somewhat to the optimistic end of the prognostic spectrum, depending on circumstances.

The final norm regarding prognostication is thus not phrased as an interdiction. When rendering a prognosis is unavoidable, physicians are expected to be relatively *optimistic*. As we shall see in chapters 5 and 7, there are a number of complex reasons that physicians are systematically optimistic in the prognoses they offer. Optimism is regarded as essential to fostering hope in patients as they confront the frightening prospects raised by illness. And it serves several other purposes as well.

Maintaining Prognostic Norms

Like social norms more generally, the norms regarding prognosis are associated with sanctions—albeit mild ones—that enhance both the effectiveness of the norms and the consistency of their expression. Specifically, these norms are supported by (1) the informal approval and disapproval of one's colleagues, (2) the relative absence of formal instruction regarding prognostication in medical training, and (3) a folkloric tradition in which physicians share stories about the problems with prognostication. The norms about prognosis, unlike certain norms about diagnosis (such as the practice of what is called "differential diagnosis") or treatment (such as the deliberate and explicit consideration of therapeutic alternatives), are generally not formally taught or enforced.

Professional Opprobrium

Professional opprobrium is one of the main ways in which the norms regarding prognosis are enforced. Physicians think less of their colleagues not so much for being inaccurate when making a prediction as for violating the interdictions regarding prediction to begin with. We have seen, for example, that physicians question the judgment of colleagues who communicate prognoses to their patients, even if a prediction proves accurate. Physicians think it is foolish to unnecessarily discuss prognosis with patients, and they judge their colleagues accordingly. Occasionally, though not generally, these adverse judgments have a more palpable effect; for example, some general practitioners reported that they would not refer patients to oncologists or surgeons who were "cruelly blunt."[20]

Structured Silence

An avoidance of prognostication is also cultivated and maintained through the nature of undergraduate and graduate medical training and the socialization process it entails. Relatively speaking, prognosis is missing from medical textbooks, neglected in journals, and overlooked in medical education.[21] And almost without fail, when physicians or others write about what doctors do, they refer to diagnosis and treatment and omit prognosis.

It is as if what the sociologist Renée Fox calls "structured silence" surrounds prognosis. The classic example offered by Fox occurs in the anatomy lab, where there is a collective understanding that students should not talk "too philosophically" about their cadavers. This understanding is present without anyone intending it or teaching it; certainly no instructor admonishes the students, "Do not talk about your feelings about the cadaver."[22] More generally in medical education, trainees learn not to talk about things that, like prognosis, arouse emotions or have metaphysical significance, including, for example, sexuality and death. Physicians have plenty of practice avoiding such topics, an avoidance that is not necessarily intended but that is nevertheless socially shaped and enforced.[23] The avoidance of such topics, including prognosis, is socially structured and is implicitly, if not explicitly, learned through the socialization process; moreover, it is reinforced through physicians' interactions with their colleagues. Physicians observe that their colleagues avoid prognosis and they come to feel uncomfortable when colleagues confess to having given a prognosis.

The Patient Who Outlived His Doctor and Other Cautionary Tales

An important reflection of the norms limiting prognostication in medical practice is a type of folkloric story sometimes shared among physicians. Such stories reflect many of the hopes, fears, and anxieties of the social group in which they arise and are told. In his engaging discussion of such stories, none having anything to do with medicine, folklorist J. H. Brunvand identifies their common characteristics: they (1) fit recurring, problematic social situations in which the teller and listener might find themselves; (2) are told as if the story were true; (3) are told as if the storyteller is not one of the principals; (4) have a foundation in actual behavior; (5) often carry specific local touches; (6) have a strong basic story appeal; (7) tend to concern deaths; (8) often involve poetic justice or irony; (9) often are embarrassing; (10) involve the "violation of an interdiction"; and (11) contain a moral. Such folktales "seem to convey true, worthwhile, and relevant information, albeit partly in a subconscious mode."[24]

Several anecdotes about prognosis recounted by physicians are remarkably consistent with this description. Typically, such a folk narrative consists of nothing more than a very short story about a humiliating prognostic error, often taking as its point of departure the facts of a particular case. Many physicians offered such stories about other physicians, yet virtually none of those whom I interviewed were willing to admit to having made such an error (involving the definitive pronouncement of a specific, terminal prognosis) themselves. It was always some other physician who made the error.

The cautionary tales typically take the following form: A physician describes the confident prediction made by another physician that a particular patient will die within some particular period of time (usually six months). However, the patient outlives this prediction by some large but variable amount of time, causing embarrassment to the original physician. The stories are often punctuated by the ironic observation that the patient outlived not only the prediction but the physician as well.

These stories thus suggest that prediction may be so hubristic as to invite retribution. They contain an implicitly supernatural element. The death of the physician belies the ordinary emphasis on the patient's illness, revealing the well-kept secret that the doctor is as frail and mortal as the patient—prone not only to error, like other humans, but to death as well. The humility that these stories encourage thus represents not just an implicit professional norm, but possibly a moral duty as well.

Here is a typical example:

During the oncology rotation of my residency, there was a seventy-one year old patient with metastatic adenocarcinoma of unknown source in the abdomen, possibly colon. This patient was given less than a year to live by her attending. But with an incredible determination, the patient proved the attending wrong. The attending died of a heart attack, and six years later this cancer patient would come into the office, smiling at the fact that she survived her doctor![25]

Another physician developed the same theme:

All of us have heard stories about patients who were told by the doctor, "You have six months to live," and then twenty years later the patient is going to the doctor's funeral. That is because we as physicians have been such idiots in prognosis.

The foregoing remarks hint at the punishment that awaits hubristic physicians, the ironic punishment of the patient's outliving the doctor.[26]

Another example of this type of story involves a similarly incorrect prediction, but with a different ironic ending:

I took over a case of a patient with metastatic prostate cancer from another doctor who had said, "Sell your business, you have six months to live." I said: "Keep the business, we haven't even started!" He lived fourteen years, riding horseback daily for thirteen of those years. But the business went to hell. Oh, well.

There is additional irony here in that business concerns are, after all, outside the physician's competence. Moreover, the story includes the implication that the business failure may have been the price for this unexpectedly good outcome.

Another way the prognosticating physician can be punished, other than by death, is by humiliation. The physician may be made a fool of, as reflected in this anecdote recounted by another physician:

A famous physician was making ward rounds with his team, and came by this bed. This old guy was in the bed, and he says to the doctor, "You saved my life!" And the doctor says, "How did I save your life? I don't remember." The patient says, "Oh, twenty years ago, I was in this hospital, and I was in a bed just like this. You came around with all the doctors, like you are now, and you talked about me and you looked at me and you said, 'Moribundus.'" And the patient said "From that time on, they [the other doctors] knew what was wrong with me and I just got well immediately."

By moribundus, of course, the physician in this anecdote meant quite the opposite of what the patient thought, namely that the patient was facing impending death. The physician who previously lacked humility endures humiliation, an occurrence made all the more poignant by the irony that the former and current circumstances are the same (the patient is in bed in the same hospital, and the physician is on rounds with junior colleagues). There is also the sense that the physician's use of a Latin term not easily understood by the patient, and thus ambiguous, could have had a felicitous impact on the patient's outcome precisely by virtue of the patient's misunderstanding. The story thus also reinforces the notion, explored in chapter 5, that physicians should discuss prognosis in ways that afford variable interpretation and that are obscure if not impenetrable.

These stories are analogous to the "horror stories" surgeons tell abut surgical error, which have been identified by sociologist Charles Bosk and which also serve as moral parables.[27] Like these stories, the cautionary tales about prognosis are sometimes told publicly. They also share the "integrative" function described by Bosk, serving to build professional solidarity and to reinforce the interdictions regarding prognosis. These stories are generally not told for the express purpose of enlisting the listener's support for a specific action. Rather, there is a sense that an essential and communal aspect of the condition of physicians is being illustrated: namely, the simultaneous need for, and danger of, making predictions, as well as the (professional and personal) vulnerability of the doctor himself. As such, these stories are part of a larger tradition of gallows humor in medicine. Such humor is often blasphemous and self-mocking, often involves bad events such as death, and often makes fun of patients, doctors, or medicine alike.[28] The humor is a sort of protective device physicians use to cope with the strain of making predictions in circumstances that are as inherently uncertain as the outcomes are inherently serious.

Even more common than the folk stories about prognosis are straightforward statements offered by many informants about the norm against making predictions in general—and against voluntarily offering specific predictions in particular. These admonitions emphasize unexpectedly favorable outcomes that are embarrassing for physicians and that may adversely affect the doctor-patient relationship. Such events, as a type of "crisis of good fortune," sometimes threaten social roles and cohesion as much as bad fortune does.[29] The following statement is typical:

> I learned long ago not to predict the time of death. You can hardly read the paper or watch TV without running into somebody who says, "The doctors gave me six months to live and look how well I am!" And this happens: we're very fallible. And I think if you're wrong once you will never forget it. I can't remember that I ever did

say to a patient, "You'll be dead within six months." But I certainly have had patients live longer than I expected them to.

Another physician observed:

> My general feeling is that physicians should almost never hazard a guess about a patient's expected date of death. They can almost never be right unless they phrase comments in the vaguest of terms ("soon," "probably not today," "weeks not months," etc.). I'd bet every general internist in this country has at least one patient (I think I have three) who was told, years ago, that they had only a short time to live. The implication here is, "Just look, here I am still going strong, and wasn't that doctor foolish to make such a prediction?" Yes, that doctor was!

Still another physician, again referring to *other* doctors, noted:

> Giving firm numbers about a patient's prognosis is a problem. I've had the experience of knowing doctors who have said to a patient with a putative illness, "Sir, you have only six months to live." And then, of course, the patient lives two, three, four years.
>
> In my role as a teacher, I've heard cases presented where people have had a disease, usually of an oncologic nature, where they were told by their physician that they had only a few months to live—and then the patient comes back a year and a half to two years later, still filled with disease, unfortunately, but by no means terminal in terms of what has happened. I think that's not a rare occurrence. And I think that can be very injurious to the doctor-patient relationship in terms of the patient; the patient then finds the physician's advice less than satisfactory. No surprise!

The theme of outliving a physician's prediction is thus a common one among physicians. Stories about such happenings reinforce the implicit and explicit professional norms of avoiding prognostication and avoiding specificity.

It is noteworthy that cautionary tales about unduly *favorable* predictions are very uncommon, if not nonexistent. I am not familiar with any. This absence is consistent with the systematic optimism in prognosis alluded to above and discussed in chapter 7. There is, it seems, little or no disapproval for being optimistic (though there may be other consequences). The absence of such stories is also consistent with the observation that unduly unfavorable predictions pose a greater threat to a physician's reputation than do unduly favorable ones; indeed, the medical profession applies harsher sanctions in response to unduly unfavorable predictions. In point of fact, it is best to avoid prognosis altogether.

Prognostic Norms and Physicians' Authority

Relieving and Causing Professional Strain

In his analysis of the social role of the physician, social theorist Talcott Parsons emphasizes the responsibility for the welfare of patients that lies at its core and the relationship of this responsibility to some of the stresses in the physician's role:

> [The] inherent frustrations of the technical expert acquire special significance because of the magnitude and character of the interests at stake. The patient and his family have the deepest emotional involvements in what the physician can and cannot do, and in the way his diagnosis and prognosis will define the situation for them. He himself, carrying as he does the responsibility for the outcome, cannot help but be exposed to important emotional strains by these facts.[30]

These strains are exacerbated by a number of factors, including the uncertainty in medicine, the vast extent of human ignorance, the intimate nature of medical practice, and the need sometimes to injure patients in order to cure them.

Physicians may indeed use prognosis as a tool to cope with the tension of their role, *decreasing* both the patient's anxiety and their own and increasing the confidence of both parties. When a patient accepts a prognosis that a physician has proposed, an interactional, social mechanism is called into play in order to deal with the strain. One of the purposes served by the articulation of a prognosis (particularly one that proves accurate) and by the solicitation of patient acquiescence with it, is to limit in advance the potential gap between outcome and expectation. This in turn limits the physician's obligation to explain should the outcome not fulfill the patient's expectations, and it limits inquiries regarding the physician's competence. Indeed, as we have seen, the majority of physicians feel that unexpected outcomes, whether favorable or unfavorable, require explanation. Prognostication is thus a type of anticipatory and preemptive account.[31] A related use of prognosis is to avoid—in a self-serving and potentially unprofessional way—patients who are likely to experience unfavorable outcomes in the first place. Thus, physicians may use prognosis to proactively limit their responsibility for unfavorable outcomes; this use has been recognized since ancient times.[32] Moreover, physicians may use prognosis retroactively by pointing to previously rendered prognoses that anticipated the outcome, thus defining the outcome as something that is perforce not the physician's fault.

One of the key paradoxes regarding prognostication is thus that although it is stressful, possibly harmful, and therefore to be avoided, it can also help to limit the stress of certain parts of the physician's role—by reducing the need to explain any disconsonance between the physician's efforts and the patient's outcome, by alleviating feelings of responsibility for the outcome, or by facilitating avoidance of patients prone to unfavorable outcomes altogether. In this respect, the act of prognostication itself, like the uncertainty in prediction, can have seemingly contradictory functions.

Physicians often believe that a patient is likely to be happy with an unexpectedly good outcome and that, by offering deliberately pessimistic prognoses, they will avoid both unpleasant surprises in patients and being held responsible for bad outcomes. On the other hand, pessimism may have adverse consequences. For patients, being sick requires an adjustment to a new social role; such an adjustment, which may be emotionally and otherwise taxing, might not be needed if one is actually not as sick as predicted. Similarly, in the opinion of physicians, an unfavorable prognosis may actually contribute to causing an unfavorable outcome, as we shall see in chapter 6. Moreover, pessimism can undermine a physician's appearance of effectiveness. Society accords physicians the mandate to cure disease, and bad outcomes suggest failure. The social pressure to fulfill this mandate (metaphorically if not literally), along with the ordinary human desire to avoid being the bearer of bad news, encourages the offering of optimistic prognoses.

These conflicting pressures to be pessimistic and optimistic raise two questions that I shall address in chapter 7: How do physicians navigate these extremes in practice? And in what circumstances does one pressure eclipse the other? Regardless of whether physicians in a given situation are pessimistic or optimistic, however, the rendered prognosis may indeed enhance their confidence in their own competence and effectiveness: a pessimistic prognosis enhances the physicians' belief that they are not morally or technically responsible for the outcome, and an optimistic one enhances their belief that they can help patients. Formulating prognoses may thus be seen as a tool with which physicians can distinguish things they might control from things they cannot, and this can help to exculpate them and to mitigate the stress associated with their role.

Physicians' Power

All but one of the norms about prognosis are expressed in "thou shalt not" form. Prognostication is surrounded with interdictions and cautionary statements. The presumption thus appears to be that physicians might find it tempting to violate the norms, that prognosis is to be avoided because, on some subconscious level, physicians might be seduced by the omniscience and omnipotence that prognosis, as a prophetic act, suggests. The cautionary tales, in particular, suggest that when physicians violate the norms, certain unpleasant consequences await them. Nevertheless, the norms serve more to foster humility and to avoid arrogance in those who are powerful than to punish those who transgress. In other words, in addition to privileging the power of prognostication itself, the norms privilege the power that prognostication gives to the physician. They function to restrain the physician's power to frame both the objective and the subjective experience of the patient—as this is a power that is recognized as real, and fearsome.

The norms regarding prognosis are, however, the physician's to violate. These are the norms of the powerful, privileging the physician at the expense of the patient. Although the norms assume that the prognosis is the patient's to request and experience, the norms make clear that the prognosis is the doctor's to formulate and articulate, on terms set by the profession. While these norms implicitly stand against the arrogance of the medical profession, they do so in a relatively self-serving and self-protective way. At every level, these norms serve to limit physicians' contact not only with prognosis but also, by extension, with death and adversity. Moreover, the complementarity between prognosis and therapy means that as prognosis is avoided, treatment is encouraged. As a consequence of this evasion of death and encouragement of treatment, the norms limit the appearance that the physician might be connected to unfavorable outcomes or to inaction. Thus, these norms serve simultaneously to decrease the strain in the physician's role and to bolster professional authority. We saw earlier how, when they actually do prognosticate, physicians can make use of prognosis to serve certain clinical, interactional, and symbolic objectives—some of which, in turn, serve their own needs, such as increasing the patient's dependence on, and obedience to, the doctor. Paradoxically, the existence of norms stressing the avoidance of prognosis can serve similar professional purposes. The attributes cultivated in patients by the application of these norms can help physicians to maintain their power and authority. Fostering ignorance, imprecision, or optimism about prognosis in a patient serves a useful purpose for the physician—even if such states truly are beneficial to patients or desired by them.

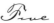

TELLING PATIENTS THEIR PROGNOSIS

*The thing that surprises me now with modern housestaff is they will
present a patient case to me and say that the patient has this or that
incurable disease. My first question after that is: "Now let's sit down
and decide how and when we're going to tell the patient about it."
And they say, "We've already told him." This has become a really
standard part of modern medical practice: to give patients bad news
quickly. We had a surgeon at [a prestigious medical school] who
couldn't get the bad news to the patient early enough. He would go in
to the recovery room when a patient was coming out of the anesthetic
and say, "I'm sorry, I've got to tell you that we found a cancer and
we couldn't remove it." I myself would do it by stages, and in the
immediate postoperative period I'd talk about how they were feeling
and relieving their pain and nausea and say, "Well, we'll let you
know in a day or two what the findings are after the pathologist has
had a chance to help us with it."*

— EXPERIENCED INFECTIOUS DISEASE SPECIALIST

Although some of the literature on physician-patient communication
has focused on the problem of how physicians *should* convey information about terminal illness,[1] there has been less attention to how
practicing physicians actually do so, or to what they themselves identify
as typical or ideal ways of discussing prognosis with patients, or to the
problems and meanings engendered by these ways of communicating
prognosis.[2] Physicians see prognostication as the stereotypical example
of giving bad news, and bad news is ordinarily seen as specifically
prognostic in nature. One authority defines bad news as "any news
that drastically and negatively alters the patient's view of her or his
future."[3] If you ask physicians what they think giving bad news means,
they are apt to respond, "telling patients they have a terminal illness."[4]
The association of bad news, prognosis, and death is well established.

Whereas in the preceding chapter I focused on norms governing
whether and to what extent prognoses should be developed and communicated, here I focus on the specific ways in which, when prognosticating is inescapable, physicians actually communicate prognoses.
Physicians describe as ideal a form of prognostic communication that in-

corporates truthfulness, accuracy, and empathy, but that also preserves hope in their patients. To achieve these objectives, they believe that communication should take place in stages, should be optimistic, and should involve reference to statistics about similar patients. They also believe strongly that the amount and type of prognostic information they communicate to patients should be influenced by what they think patients want to hear and by their understanding of patients' own predictions.

A "Warning Shot"

According to physicians, the communication of unfavorable prognoses should take place in stages. This admonition is one of several elements in a strategy that also involves other basic communication skills, such as allowing adequate time for discussion of a serious topic, being polite and respectful, clarifying patients' expectations, and showing empathy for patients and their families. Among other benefits, communication in stages allows physicians to evaluate how well patients have understood each element of the information being shared with them. One physician who is expert in communicating bad news advises:

> The cardinal rule, therefore, is to give the information in small chunks. One useful technique for starting this process is the "warning shot." If there is apparently a large gap between the patient's expectations and the reality of the situation, you can facilitate the patient's understanding by giving a warning that things are more serious than they appear to the patient (Well, the situation does appear to be more serious than that . . .) and then grading the information, gradually introducing the more serious prognostic points, and waiting for the patient to respond at each stage.[5]

Practicing physicians provide similar examples of how prognostic information typically should and should not be conveyed. For example, one clinician observed:

> The physician has to be willing to go back to a patient time and time again and make sure she understands her situation and her unique position and review her options with her. And as time goes on, you tell the person more about what they can expect and what the options are, if any, and lead them down the pathway. And then at that point, they've heard it enough times and are comfortable with it.

Another experienced clinician gave the following example:

> I had a secretary who had breast cancer. And her physician told her, just after she had a breast removed—while she was still recovering from the anesthesia and had just got back to her room—that she had six lymph nodes positive for cancer. I thought, "Hell, you don't need to discuss all those things that early. It's better to go slow." But there seems to be a real feeling on the part of physicians today that the more open they are the better. I don't think that's always true. We sometimes lack enough respect for our patients.

The unfortunate behavior described and deplored by this physician serves to highlight the correct way to communicate unfavorable prognoses—namely, in "small chunks," in a staged fashion over time.[6] Physicians advocate proceeding slowly, creating suspicion and preparing patients for the bad news to come.[7] More experienced physicians seem to endorse this strategy to a greater extent than younger physicians, suggesting that there may be a generational or experiential component to this strategy. Whereas older physicians see communication in stages as an appropriate and nondeceptive technique, younger physicians seem to believe that it is better to communicate information fast. Younger physicians appear, however, to confuse the speed with which information is given with its completeness or accuracy; experienced clinicians recognize that timing as well as the quality and quantity of information is important in communicating prognosis.

Although physicians sometimes violate the foregoing ideal characterization of how to give bad news, these violations nevertheless illustrate the general principle. Physicians call the practice of unduly rapid or excessively comprehensive prognostication "terminal candor" or "truth dumping," and they deplore it as irresponsible, though they recognize that it is not uncommon. Truth dumping amounts to an avoidance of responsibility, in several senses: physicians thereby avoid having to engage in a lengthier, more humane interaction, avoid having to face or discuss the limitations of their ability, and avoid having to address the implications of such bad new for patients. They can, however, conveniently claim that they have told the patient "the truth." Insofar as physicians believe that patients experience truth dumping as painful, it may be almost punitive in character—as if the patient were being punished for the temerity of having a serious illness, for putting the physician in a position of having to reveal this fact, and for undermining the physician's healing authority.

In describing the effect of truth dumping on patients, one physician noted:

> I don't believe it is appropriate to hit patients over the head with
> either diagnosis or prognosis. When the diagnosis is first made, it is
> inappropriate to give a prognosis of death at a certain time. We never
> really know in an individual case. I have seen people with advanced
> ovarian cancer have a cure from surgery and chemotherapy. I think
> that we should give the patient the benefit of the doubt and not take
> away hope.

The militaristic expressions used by physicians—such as "hitting,"
"dumping," "hammering," "bludgeoning," "crushing," "battering,"
"bombing," and even "oppressing," "imposing," or "dooming"—
capture physicians' belief that communicating prognoses in this way
may be injurious to patients' composure and optimism, and disrespectful as well.[8] Moreover, as we shall see in chapter 6, physicians believe
that receiving unfavorable prognostic information may be injurious by
worsening patients' outcomes through a sort of a self-fulfilling prophecy.

In giving the prognosis in stages, physicians also protect themselves. Communicating bad news gradually is a means of discouraging
"meltdowns" and extreme displays of emotion in patients, outbreaks
that might be unpleasant or time-consuming for the physician to cope
with. The patient's experience and expression of emotions are thus both
controlled.

Whereas being "blunt" regarding prognosis is disparaged within
medicine, being "frank" about diagnostic or therapeutic options typically is not. Physicians are expected to be specific and forthcoming
with respect to diagnosis and therapy but not with respect to prognosis.
Part of the reason is that physicians believe they should communicate
prognostic information in a way that preserves hope. To do so requires
ambiguity, whereas preserving hope while communicating diagnostic
or therapeutic information requires specificity and certainty. While confidence and certainty on the part of physicians are esteemed in diagnosis
and therapy, provisionality and ambiguity are seen as preferable in prognosis. But this dichotomous approach is also consistent with the notion
that prognostic information is much more dangerous than diagnostic
or therapeutic information. Information about the future—whether it
is uncertain or certain—is deemed more problematic than information
about the past or present, or about diagnosis or therapy.

Presenting the Bright Side

Physicians' descriptions of the ideal form of prognostication also emphasize putting the best light on the patient's situation.[9] Physicians
describe how they do this as follows:

A patient with newly diagnosed cancer might ask, "How long do I have?" Well, many of the diseases that I treat are curable, so I don't put it in those terms. I turn it around and say, "You've got an excellent chance of licking this disease." I don't usually like to give percentages of cure in diseases because what I like to do is really deal with the patient as an individual. And I like to say to them, "You know, for you it's either a hundred percent or zero percent, and I don't think knowing the statistics is really going to help you deal with this disease. But if you really want to know the cure rate in this disease, I'll be happy to share it with you."

Many times they actually come to me already knowing what the median survival of the disease is. And I always try to temper that with, "Again, that's lumping everyone together. That's not necessarily you." And I always try to say, "You know, you have a better chance than that." Although in reality, many patients have a worse chance than that.

This physician directs patients away from focusing on specific time frames or possibly unfavorable prognoses; if necessary, she takes advantages of the intrinsic uncertainty in prognosis to claim the patient has a better chance than she feels is true. This optimistic gloss on the patient's prospects, as well as the fact that the prognosis is configured as statistical, are typical of how physicians prognosticate.

Another oncologist described how she communicates prognoses:

You have to be honest with patients and tell them that there is this degree of uncertainty in their outcome. Normally what we do is start the chemotherapy and treat with two cycles of the therapy and then scan the patient to see how the tumor is responding. Then I'll say, "Great, it looks smaller. It looks like you're going to do well." Or, I'll say, "It does not look smaller," or "It looks bigger, and we need to change our therapy."

The physician matter-of-factly describes a remarkable asymmetry in how changes in tumor size would be handled. A shrinking tumor is evidence of success, but an enlarging tumor is not evidence of failure: it is merely an indication for a change in therapy. Physicians are thus able to remain optimistic about both prognosis and therapy regardless of the outcome that is observed.

Physicians, when they do give prognoses, believe that they should ideally be very careful in the words they use and the facts they focus on. This in itself is noteworthy because they tend not to be so self-conscious when the issue is diagnosis or therapy. Although physicians do not reveal all diagnostic or therapeutic possibilities to their patients any more than they divulge all prognostic possibilities, they are nevertheless less concerned about the specific ways they communicate about diagnosis and therapy. In a detailed explanation, one physician outlined his strategy for presenting prognostic information in a "cushioned" and "sanguine" fashion, and emphasized the importance of a careful choice of words and phrases when discussing prognosis. He draws a distinction between choosing words carefully and putting a positive light on things, on the one hand, and outright deception, on the other. It is a fine distinction that physicians make in both theory and practice.

> I'm basically candid and honest with patients when I discuss prognosis. But I think you have to cushion it from two perspectives: one is your interpretation of the data to begin with and the other is your interpretation of data that may well be modified in years to come by new developments.
>
> While I'm quick to recognize that many things can happen to patients with, for example, diabetes, the fact that they *can* happen does not necessarily guarantee that they *will* happen. And even if things do tend to go badly, the ability to intervene is better now than it was five years ago and hopefully will be better in ten or fifteen years than it is now. So in that sense I am not deceiving patients when I am optimistic, but I am sanguine in terms of care. And I use this foundation to suggest that follow-up care and ongoing evaluation is extremely important, so that any kind of deterioration in various areas of body function can be handled, and, hopefully, the course can be averted or at least delayed.
>
> You have to pay attention to how you impart the potential of bad news to anyone. You can be candid and truthful without being oppressive and blunt, though this is tough to do. I think there is a certain amount of choice of nouns and verbs that is very important in terms of how you communicate this kind of thing to patients and their families.
>
> For example, if the patient says "Well, doctor, am I going to be blind in twenty years?" and the answer is "Yes," you become more abstract and say: "Certain diabetic patients do become blind in twenty years, and they become blind because the diabetes takes its toll in terms of the eye. But there are newer modalities now that avert that for people and importantly there may well be dramatic changes in the next five or ten years that will change the disease course in terms of this outcome." That kind of cushioning is much more humane in general than to say, "You know, if you don't take care of yourself, you're going to be blind, or your foot is going to fall off," which I've seen some physicians do, in fact.

While I don't give any firm numbers when prognosticating, and while I don't say "You're going to be fine," I do think that one can speak in terms of "positive slope" and "sanguine outcome" without being misleading. I think one can at least give some cushioning phraseology that allows the patient to recognize that while something might well happen, in no way is it guaranteed. Nor is it in anyway suggested that if they don't do what you say something bad will happen.

This physician avoids both prognostic extremes ("Yes, you will be blind" and "You're going to be just fine"). But he does so in an explicitly optimistic way that takes advantage of the uncertainty inherent in the future to protect both himself and the patient. Physicians emphasize that unfavorable prognoses, even if certain, can and should be communicated in as sanguine, gentle, and optimistic a manner as possible. That prognoses are often uncertain only adds to the feasibility and importance of this approach.

As with other physicians engaged in prognosis, this physician's optimism is partly rooted in his belief in continuing scientific progress ("new developments"). This is one of the most frequent concrete justifications physicians give for optimism. When interviewed, however, physicians usually admit that the pace of medical innovation is not sufficient to justify a meaningful change in prognosis for most patients. Physicians and patients alike often have unrealistic hopes about the rapidity with which developments that might meaningfully affect the true prognosis can actually emerge, especially in conditions with survival horizons of only a few years. This varies across conditions, however. In chronic conditions that have a very long survival horizon, such as diabetes, this basis for optimism is both more credible and more frequently invoked. For example, the above physician continued:

Yes, I believe that holding out the prospect of new developments is truthful. I believe I'm being honest with myself as well as the patient. With diabetes, the outcome and complications often have a lag period of twenty years or so. So there may well be new developments in the treatment of this disease. Indeed, people who have the onset of their diabetes in their youth do have a very high likelihood of blindness at age thirty or forty. But those are data of the *past*; they may not be the data that are going to be relevant to the future, recognizing that research efforts in terms of treatment of diabetic eye disease are very intense.

The possible emergence of new technology thus not only affects how optimistic the physician can be when initially offering a prediction but may also modify the true prognosis. Moreover, such statements by the physician implicitly encourage patients to have ongoing contact with the medical profession, so as to avail themselves of these new developments as soon as they appear.

Overall, optimistic presentation appears more sensitive and respectful to patients and easier for physicians. It is also seen as more professional and proper. Physicians who are too exact when the prognosis is unfavorable are considered blunt and deemed to be less competent and less physicianly—in part because they are seen as acting in a fashion injurious to the patient. Favorable predictions are less strongly associated with the pretense to omniscience than are unfavorable predictions. Unfavorable predictions that are communicated to the patient, even if accurate in an objective sense, are seen as unduly definitive in a way that favorable predictions, even if inaccurate, are not.

"These Are the Numbers"

Another way that is considered legitimate for physicians to offer prognoses is "by the numbers," that is, by using statistics.[10] As we have seen, the fact that prognosis is often based on statistical data can be a source of strain and even derision for physicians; nevertheless, when prognostication is unavoidable, they will employ statistics. This manner of prognosticating is in keeping with the professional norm of not being specific; it involves the articulation by the physician of figures and percentages (whether precise or general) that are relevant to *groups* of patients, rather than the articulation of a prediction about a specific patient. In prognosticating thus, in a way analogous to their expedient use of prognostic uncertainty as a basis for optimism, physicians turn a problem to what is considered to be a good use: by communicating prognoses in terms of statistics, they distance themselves from what they are saying. Both they and the patient are meant to find hope in the indeterminacy of stochastic projections. One physician described this practice as follows:

> I *never* use time in years or months to answer the patient when questioned, "How long do I have?" I tell my patients that only God really knows, and next I refer to the seriousness of the illness. Many times I use statistics. For example, a patient with cancer of the lung with a pleural effusion *usually* does not live for more than six months. I tell the patient a ballpark figure, followed by saying that there are those patients with strong support (such as family, church, etc.) that do not follow statistics or rules.

Statistical prognostication is usually (and appealingly, from the point of view of both the patient and the physician) accompanied by the caveat that the prognosis might indeed *not* apply to the individual patient. However, it is extremely rare for the physician to mention that patients might do considerably *worse* than the statistical averages. Another physician elaborated on the benefits of such group data:

> The overall concept of prognostication is changing. Patients and families of patients often expect precise data regarding prognosis. Generally, I try to avoid individual-specific quotes but will give data for groups of patients studied with similar illnesses. Allowing the patient to have this data continues to foster hope even when the clinical situation is poor.

This statement captures the tension between using statistics as opposed to making the real predictions that patients "expect." The former practice is generally acceptable, the latter to be avoided. Like the techniques of communicating in stages and framing the prognosis in optimistic terms, statistical prognostication is sometimes justified by its beneficial effect of maintaining hope.

In addition, statistical prognostication implicitly situates the patient among fellow travelers on the road of serious illness.[11] It allows patients both the illusion that they might be spared the fate befalling their peers and the comfort—despite the coldness of the statistics—that others have been, and are in, their situation, and that the doctors have known about them. And for the doctor, statistical prognostication allows the illusion, and indeed often the reality, of accuracy, distance, control, and objectivity. Statistical prognostication is endorsed by physicians because it makes them feel more confident, as if they are on firmer ground. They feel more comfortable when they have "reference data." The existence of reference data, and their communication, allows physicians to prognosticate *safely* and to reduce the danger of prediction.

Indeed, statistical prognostication is a way to prognosticate to a patient without really prognosticating about a patient. Such predictions, while appearing to have scientific authority and significant content, are at the same time devoid of affect and of particularity. They are "sugar-coated," intended to seem less godlike and less threatening, to patients and physicians alike. But at the same time they are also less relevant. Statistical prognostication shifts attention from the particular patient to the disease entity or group of patients. As a consequence, statistical prognostication can be thin—devoid of humane, empathetic, meaningful relevance to the patients themselves.

There is nothing intrinsically wrong with placing patients' clinical experience within a context of hundreds of other patients like them. Indeed, statistical prognostication can be a concrete and productive way to provide prognostic information to a patient. The practice is problematic, however, when physicians use statistics to dodge meaningful discussion of temporality and of outcome with individual patients. The precision and honesty of statements such as "This chemotherapy has a 60 percent chance of reducing the tumor size" is largely illusory because the information is not linked to actual, important developments in the patient's illness (such as whether they would be cured) and when these might happen. Moreover, this information is not related to the feelings or hopes patients have about their future. Finally, it ignores the fact that patients are often less able than their doctors to make sense of statistical estimates.

Truth and Lies

In general, physicians see no conflict between delivering staged, optimistic, and statistically based prognoses and their desire to be honest and truthful. Such techniques are seen more as reflecting a considered *use* of information than as a deliberate *distortion* of information. As Japanese social scientist Naoko Miyaji has argued, "Few [American] physicians consciously categorize different modes of speech, such as sweetening, softening information, avoiding certain words, using euphemisms, giving hopeful information selectively, as 'lying.' [Such modes of speech] are rather seen as a necessary part of 'translating information.' "[12] More generally, it is important to realize that physicians often believe that prognostication is itself intrinsically and fundamentally a lie. Since, for a variety of reasons, they regard the future as stochastic and unknowable and indescribable, any statement about it—but especially one that might be construed as definitive—is seen as necessarily mendacious. Thus, failing to make such a statement is hardly considered to be a failure of truthfulness. Indeed, avoiding such statements is regarded as a virtue.

Physicians' "lies" about prognosis can take several forms. One of the most common is the "anything can happen" statement:

> I had a young patient who had pancreatic cancer. And he just kept pushing me, wanting me to acknowledge that he had some chance of a cure. But I've never heard of that, of anyone with pancreatic cancer who's not a surgical candidate being cured with chemotherapy. It was really strange, because he just kept pushing me and pushing me and pushing me, and I couldn't lie to him, so I said no. And then my attending went in, and he said that the patient also kept pushing

him, and the attending said to the patient, "Sure, it could happen. Anything can happen."

Another physician, an experienced obstetrician/gynecologist, put it poignantly:

> It's easy to criticize us physicians for being paternalistic, for not telling the truth, for sugar-coating reality. But try to imagine what it's like when a young woman with advanced ovarian cancer walks through your door. She is thirty-five years old and has two kids. More than anything in the world she wants not to die. You tell her the prognosis and that there is no good therapy for her, and she keeps saying, "But, doctor, are you telling me there is absolutely *no* chance I'm going to get better?" You feel yourself backsliding because you start thinking, "Gee, how can I speak with that kind of certainty about anything? And how can I deny her even a tiny shred of hope?" That's when a word like *truth* sort of loses its meaning.

For physicians, truth is not some monolithic concept that finds only one expression. When this physician responds to his thoughts and says to the patient that, after all, there is a chance she will get better, the truth he is communicating may be metaphoric or transcendent. What he may be saying is that he will do all that he can and that, after all, the future is in God's hands.

The intricate ways information is revealed and shaped, and also the different speeds with which the physician and patient acquire information, are also illustrated in the following example. At each step along the way, the physician is not being entirely truthful with the patient:

> I'm thinking of a woman who's just relapsed with acute leukemia. She is twenty-eight years old, and I've been taking care of her for just over a year. Typically such patients get a lot of chemotherapy within the first six months after diagnosis, and 40 percent of them or so will be cured. So we just follow their blood count and physical exam every month, and this patient had been doing very well.
>
> She came to see me on Tuesday. Her platelet count was low, suggesting a recurrence of her tumor. However, she and I both knew of another patient on a similar set of drugs who developed low platelets for a totally benign immunological reason. So, when her platelets were low she was very anxious. And I was very anxious that her tumor was coming back, and I thought it must have. But I suggested to her that it wasn't *necessarily* that her leukemia was coming back. There might be some other cause (like the immune mechanism) and she really shouldn't worry about it until we could get the rest of the information. We needed the rest of the blood exam

back. But if I had had to put money on it, I probably would have bet it was her leukemia coming back. Yet to give her that information in no uncertain terms isn't valuable. No good for her to go home and say, "Well, the doctor thinks that my leukemia might be coming back." Especially without a plan of action.

It turned out that it *was* her leukemia coming back. I looked at her blood smear after clinic and she clearly had leukemic cells in her blood. I felt really terrible. This is a young person who has three kids—they're all under five years old. It's terrible. She's not going to be cured now. And, she's a really upbeat person, and so, I mean, you just hope for the best.

Asked how the patient was given the bad news, the doctor continued:

Well, if you're careful about how you say stuff, you never have to come out and say it, to be honest with you. I called her on the phone and said, "There were some abnormal cells on your blood smear, and, with the platelets being low, I think we should check your bone marrow to see if the leukemia has come back or not. Come in tomorrow and we'll check." So she came in to the IV therapy suite to undergo the bone marrow procedure, and she told the nurses, "I've relapsed." So she knew. Without me ever saying, "You relapsed, your leukemia is back."

I have to call her today to tell her the final results of the bone marrow. But I think that delay is helpful for people's understanding. When I saw her in the clinic the first time, the *possibility* of a leukemic relapse was raised. It wasn't necessarily ranked higher than the immune problem. Then, when we talked on the phone, it was raised again, but it was a higher concern. So then this third time when I talk to her on the phone later today, it's going to be, you know, it's going to be it.

This doctor's account of how she slowly revealed information, in stages, contains several "lies." At each step, the doctor felt that the truth was in fact different from what she communicated. Yet neither the patient nor the doctor seemed to regard this behavior as lying. The reason is that the doctor's *intent* is beneficent. This perspective, which is often adopted by physicians, privileges a virtue-based rather than action-based ethic; in other words, this well-intentioned physician is perforce behaving ethically, regardless of her actions

When they think of lying, physicians tend to describe more extreme situations, often involving an ulterior motive on the part of the physician.[13] That is, twisting the facts for the patient's sake is one thing; misrepresenting them for self-interest is another: it is dishonest. One very experienced physician described his own personal experience with lying to a patient (decades earlier, at a time when lying was rife) and explained why communication in stages and optimistic presentation are much to be preferred as strategies for communicating prognoses:

> I think you've got to let the patient know the prognosis in almost every circumstance, almost every time. One of the things that we did so wrongly when I was in training was to lie to the patient. Usually, to protect himself, the doctor would indeed tell the patient's family. The family knows it, the doctor knows it, and the patient is left all alone.
>
> The good communication between a patient and his loved ones in the last few weeks of his life is lost because everybody is playing a game: the patient's family is coming in and saying, "Well, the doctor says this has to get worse before it gets better," and "We were counting on doing something next summer" and all these silly things. And the patient sees through that; the patient can tell that his or her symptoms are getting worse. And so this deserted individual is lying there, not able to talk frankly with anybody about plans for what's to be done after his or her death, whether the widow should sell the house, things of this kind that he would wish to be able to do. Moreover, if he were told the prognosis, he's not going to be so disappointed when he continues to lose weight and his symptoms are bad.
>
> I had one experience of this kind of lying when I was at [a prestigious university]. The patient was the wife of a professor. And the general internist called me up and said they'd like a second opinion and wondered if I could come over to the private floor and see her. And I said yes, and did. When I got there the doctor and the husband met me outside the patient's room, and they said, "We know she has a cancer and that her liver is full of it. She's jaundiced. But we have told her that she has hepatitis and that it may get worse before it gets better, and we would just like you to reinforce that."
>
> I went in and examined this woman. She had a great big hard liver and was deeply jaundiced, but she was an intelligent person, completely alert, and she looked me in the eye—and here I was saying, "Well, this certainly looks like a bad case of hepatitis, but they often get better." And then I finally got out of the room—I made a resolution right then and there that I'd never get tricked into the position of having to reinforce a lie. That woman and her husband could have had a meaningful relationship; instead of that, they were going to be playing a game as long as she lived. It's a terrible thing to do to a person who has a terminal illness.
>
> I know that's not the way to treat people. In most instances they have to be told. Often, the way to tell them is by degrees. If you tell them preoperatively, "There is a tumor that we want to operate on

you for," and postoperatively, "We're waiting for the pathologists to make a diagnosis of exactly what kind of tumor this was; there is a possibility of malignancy," and then a few days later, having got the patient warned, you tell him or her, "This is a malignant tumor and we may want to try to palliate it with chemotherapy or something, but the prognosis is pretty grim"—I think in the long run that this policy of honesty pays off.

Incidentally, one of the things that you say if you give them bad news is, "We're going through this together. I'll be with you as long as this goes on. You can count on me to keep on coming."

This passage illustrates many points about truthfulness. The physician specifically deplores the furtive collusion to hide the truth from the patient, in a way that seemed to him to serve the interests of the patient's husband and doctor more than those of the patient. In comparison to the previous example of the patient with leukemia, the case of the woman with liver cancer involves a lie of commission rather than of omission: in the previous case, accurate information was temporarily withheld from the patient; here, the patient was intentionally *misinformed*. Moreover, the physician in this case identifies the benefits of truthfulness: the ability it affords the patient to prepare; the potential enhancement in the patient's relationship with her spouse; the basis it would provide for a therapeutic alliance with the doctor. Yet the physician also endorses communication in stages and the use of softening language.

This physician's beneficent concern and good intentions are, furthermore, manifest in his explicit endorsement of a promise of nonabandonment: the patient can count on the doctor to be available "as long as this goes on." This action by the physician itself conveys other truths about the care the patient will receive in the future and the outcomes that are to be expected. Regardless of how and when the physician communicates the patient's prognosis, this promise assures the patient that the physician is committed to caring for the patient. This physician, in other words, does not dump the truth and will not dump the patient. There are different ways for physicians to be truthful, and different things for them to be truthful about; giving the patient prognostic information is only one way.

Another senior physician described the following case in which information was withheld:

When I started [in the 1940s], you didn't tell anybody that they were going to die unless they really pushed you. I think it is all wrong that today we operate in medicine the way we used to in the army, with a standard operating procedure [SOP], and that standard operating procedure seems nowadays to be that you tell people when they have a malignancy or, if they have a problem, you tell them just how big of a problem it is. I don't think that all patients can tolerate this. Medicine is something that just can't operate with an SOP. It is something that should be thought about and something where you treat the patient as an individual and involve the family as well as the patient. I don't think that every patient ought to know that they're going to die. That's just my feeling. But it's a whole new ethos that's developed during my time in medicine.

I think a physician always ought to let the *family* know, however. Long ago, my wife's father had angina and he came to Philadelphia, and I went over him, and there was nothing you could really do in those days. His electrocardiogram was all right, his chest x-ray was all right. It was clear that he had angina. And I guess I told him that he had a problem and that he did have heart disease, but I told my wife and his wife that he was probably going to die one of those days and die suddenly. But I didn't tell him that.

And what really happened was that sometime a year later, he was digging in the garden—he had always wanted to know whether he should stop digging in his garden, given his heart problem, and what he should do if he got pain while digging, and I said, "Well, stop when you get the pain"—but anyway, he was digging in the garden, which he loved to do, and he collapsed and died. Now, you know, I guess people today express various things to patients that this or that would happen to them. But anyway, my wife was very understanding about it and so was his wife. We just didn't tell patients in those days.

This lack of discussion by physicians was not always self-serving. Many physicians avoided discussion of death out of concern for the patient's well-being. This ethos of beneficent silence persists today among some physicians and in certain relatively traditional subcultures within American society.[14]

The distinction between lying and optimism, and their relationship to honesty, bears some resemblance to the distinction that social theorist Karl Mannheim draws between ideology and utopianism and their relationship to reality. Ideologies, according to Mannheim, are "more or less conscious disguises of the real nature of a situation, the true recognition of which would not be in accord with [the propounder's] interests."[15] As such, they are mental fictions, originating in the minds of people who seek to "stabilize a social order," and their function is to "veil the true nature of a given society." Conversely, utopias are wishes, inspiring action directed at effecting change. Utopian ideas may thus, in

Mannheim's view, "succeed through counteractivity in transforming the existing . . . reality into one more in accord with [people's] own conceptions."[16] Physicians seem to agree that utopian ideas (that is, optimistic predictions, especially consciously optimistic ones) are effective, and their way of prognosticating may be seen in a sense to be a striving, almost desperate way of attempting to change the situation of the patient. This mental process is consistent with physicians' professional role and duty: they are expected to be the repository and source of optimistic, against-the-odds ideas. At times, however, physicians' ways of prognosticating can border on being ideological. The way they prognosticate may be used, as we have seen, to protect their own interests. Moreover, optimism in prognostication may go beyond merely being a communication strategy and become so excessive and internalized that it shades into self-delusion. Indeed, physicians' intersubjective communication style may ultimately be correlated not only with their objective estimates of patients' prospects (as we saw in chapter 3) but also with their own beliefs and practices (as we shall see in chapter 7).

Discrepant Communication

Although withholding information from patients altogether is increasingly discouraged nowadays, certain traditional practices nevertheless persist. One is the optimistic bias in presenting prognoses to patients. Another is discrepant prognostication—wherein the physician communicates one prognosis to the patient and a different one to the patient's family or to professional colleagues. In the latter case, a difference may be discerned between the objective, impersonal prognosis communicated to professional colleagues and the subjective, personal prognosis communicated to patients.[17]

There is often a substantial difference between the prognoses communicated to patients and to colleagues or family members. For example, as part of a study of 504 patients referred for hospice care (discussed in chapter 3), the referring physicians were asked about the predictions they would make to patients and their families. In general, the physicians substantially overestimated survival in these patients. However, superimposed on this optimistic bias, two additional patterns were apparent. First, according to the physicians themselves, they would withhold prognostic information from 25 percent of patients, even though the patients were being referred to hospice for end-of-life care (indeed, the median survival was just twenty-four days). Second, in the remaining cases, when prognostic information would indeed be given, the physicians would give the patients their "objective" (albeit, as it turned out, inaccurate) estimate of survival only 45 percent of the time. In 35 percent of the cases they would communicate even more optimistic estimates to the patients, and in the remaining 20 percent, more pessimistic impressions. In other words, although in virtually all 504 cases physicians were willing to render an objective estimate for survival to the investigators, what they communicated to their patients varied: sometimes they offered no prediction, sometimes an especially optimistic or pessimistic one, but in only 34 percent of the 504 cases overall would they give the patient what they described as their best and most objective estimate.[18] This finding suggests that, at best, physicians have a special understanding of what truthfulness in prognostication means, an understanding many patients might not share. As a result, patients may be twice removed from the truth of their disease and its prognosis: first, because physicians themselves generally believe the prognosis to be more favorable than it is and, second, because they generally do not communicate their actual beliefs to patients.

Physicians find it more acceptable to communicate prognoses—in particular, those reflecting their true opinions—to colleagues than to patients. For example, one physician recounted the following experience:

> When I was a house officer, I was rounding one day with the team in the intensive care unit. And our attending, who was a world-famous intensivist, accompanied us into a patient's room. The patient was an elderly woman who was critically ill and comatose and had severe lung failure. The room was filled with her family and they asked my attending if their mother and grandmother would survive. My attending said it was "impossible to say" and that "only God knew." After we left the room, when we were further down the hall, I said to him: "You've been practicing intensive care for twenty years; you literally wrote the book in this field. Surely you must have some idea about whether that patient would live." And he said to me, "Oh yeah. She's not going to make it." And that was it! I was shocked at the discrepancy between how precise and definitive he was willing to be with us and how evasive he was with the family. Of course, he was right: the patient died twenty-four hours later.

When this attending physician was in a professional, objective domain, he was much more willing to communicate his best estimate of the patient's prospects, and he was much less optimistic than he had been with the patient's family. Experimental results with large samples of physicians support the generality of this phenomenon.[19] Such discrepant communication, however, is not limited to situations where the prognosis is unfavorable; physicians are also more willing to discuss favorable prognoses with colleagues than with patients.

Moreover, many physicians still seem to find it more acceptable to be frank and to communicate unfavorable prognoses when talking with families than when talking with patients. Some physicians describe their practice in this regard as follows:

> It is very important to give the patient some hope even when the prognosis is gloomy. I have found this to be very true. However, I will oftentimes be more painfully honest with the patient's family, oftentimes in confidence.

Physicians are conflicted about this behavior, however, and some physicians do not see it this way:

> If I have trouble with prognosis in my patients and their families, I simply tell them so quite straightforwardly, and we sit and take time and talk about it. I also always tell the patients themselves just whatever I tell the families, taking care not to deceive even with "harmless" lies—even if this means alienating a family member who wants to "protect" the sufferer.

Physicians invoke notions of "painfulness" and "harm" to support their positions, regardless of whether they endorse or reject discrepant communication to patients and their families. This is yet another reflection of the dangerous potential seen in prognosis.

Encouragement, Balance, and Reinforcement

Patients' own predictions about their disease also influence how physicians communicate prognoses—especially with respect to whether physicians communicate in an optimistic or pessimistic fashion. The relation between patients' and physicians' predictions is complex; generally, however, physicians respond to patients' assessments of their own prognoses in one of three ways, in order of descending frequency: (1) they may be generally encouraging and optimistic, reinforcing patients' optimism and correcting patients' pessimism; (2) they may balance both optimism and pessimism toward the center; or (3) they may reinforce optimism and (to a lesser extent) pessimism. (The fourth possibility—being generally pessimistic regardless of whether the patient was optimistic or pessimistic—was not observed.) These three responses may either typify a particular physician or be expressed at different times by the same physician.

Our survey of internists found that, overall, a majority of physicians, 64 percent, report that they reinforce patients' perceptions when patients are optimistic about their prognosis; only 5 percent report reinforcing patients' pessimistic perceptions. This pattern of asymmetric reinforcement reflects their own beliefs about the value of optimism, since 86 percent of physicians agree that it is "helpful to have an upbeat attitude when discussing possible outcomes with patients" and only 13 percent believe that a "downbeat attitude" can be helpful.[20] In general, then, physicians are optimistic when it comes to offering a prognosis, regardless of what the patient expects.

Sometimes, however, physicians adopt a communication strategy—in keeping with the norm of avoiding extremes in communicating prognoses—in which they try to *balance* patient expectations. One physician described his practice in this regard as follows:

> If I thought a patient was being too optimistic and if that was something that could compromise their health or could compromise what they might need to do, then I would talk to them. For instance, I had a patient with long-standing, life-threatening liver disease and neurological problems as a result. We hospitalized her with encephalopathy [mental clouding] and she recovered. And she said, "Wow, that was horrible and I'm so happy to be alive and things are going to go great." I said to her, "Yeah, but we've also learned a lesson from this, which is that there are certain things that I know you wanted to do before you die, and I don't know when something like this is going to happen again. So, even though it might be hard, I think we need to focus on that. You need to focus on things you wanted to accomplish before you die. I'm not saying that you're going to die this year or even in five years, I'm just saying you should think about those things now, in case something does happen this month. Because I can't honestly say."
>
> On the other hand, with pessimistic patients, I try to raise their hopes to some level, even if they have end-stage cancer and are dying. I would say, "Well, I completely empathize with you. I feel really depressed too, but you might think of it as if there are some things that this situation might open up for you. Like, are there things you want to do, or not do?" And the patient might say, "Well, I'm going to die and I'm not going to have time to do these things." So I might help them strategize on that. Or they might say, "I'm never going to feel well again." And I would say, "Well, maybe there are some things I can do to help you feel as well as we can make you feel," and then try to address that problem. So I also try to find out why they're feeling pessimistic and then try to address that in some way with them.

This strategy, in other words, involves gently correcting excesses.

In contrast, some physicians take a cue from patients and reinforce patient perceptions, whether they are optimistic or pessimistic. For example, one internist observed:

> My primary goal is to help the patient. If, according to the patient, the prognosis is good, then I am optimistic for the patient. If the prognosis, according to the patient, is poor, then my primary focus is on comfort and realistically preparing the patient for the inevitability of death. When prognosis is unknown or uncertain, I inform the patient of that. I often offer a "thread of hope" in my discussions, even in the more terminal situations. Depending on the patient, they may ignore this or use it. It helps me choose my course of action regarding the direction of the discussion. I try to make the patient understand how the prognosis is made so that he is appropriate in his expectations.

Physicians who respond to patients in this way basically reject responsibility for the prognosis they give, but they do so in a way that is different from truth dumping. Here, the patient, rather than the physician, is the source of the prognostic assessment.

Physicians do not always parallel patient optimism exactly, however. There are limits to how much they will reinforce patient expectations. For example, one physician noted:

> When a patient has an illness in which optimism favorably affects recovery, I have no problem being "overoptimistic." Even when a patient has an unreasonably optimistic perspective, if this helps him or her I do not challenge that perspective. But if the optimism means that he or she will not take precautions needed to recover or will not take care of his or her family's needs (such as business closeouts, wills, preparations for death), I may try to decrease that optimism. The bottom line is: What *effect* does the patient's perspective have on his or her outcome?

Though such physicians sometimes note a potential, adverse consequence of too much optimism in the patient, they nevertheless generally reinforce patient expectations, and they are guided by a concern for the patient's well-being. They are concerned with the effect of their actions on patients, and they use prognosis to serve specific clinical or interactional purposes.

To evaluate the extent to which the foregoing qualitative findings may be generalized, physicians' responses to patient perceptions about their own prognosis were further assessed by means of two experiments incorporated into a survey of practicing internists in the United States.[21]

In these experiments, physicians as a group were indeed found to be generally optimistic, correcting patients' pessimism and reinforcing their optimism.

In one experiment, for example, all of the physicians surveyed received a clinical vignette describing a hypothetical sixty-six-year-old man with chronic obstructive pulmonary disease and pneumonia necessitating ICU admission. At the end of the vignette, the patient, who has a substantial chance of dying, expresses an opinion about his "prognosis for being discharged from the hospital and returning to his previous baseline." Physician respondents received (at random) one of several different versions of the vignette in which the opinion expressed by the patient involved varying degrees of optimism, pessimism, or neither. They were then asked a series of identically worded questions about how much optimism or pessimism about the patient's prognosis they would communicate to the patient himself and to their professional colleagues. When their responses were compared, the patient's self-prognosis was found to be statistically significantly associated with what the physicians would have told the patient. The pattern, however, was such that, compared to situations where the patient expressed no opinion about the prognosis, physicians expressed optimism in response to both patient pessimism and optimism.

An additional finding was that physicians believed in the ability of optimism to materially improve the chances for a favorable outcome: not only did physicians express greater optimism to the patient when the patient was optimistic, but they also increased the degree of optimism about the prognosis that they communicated to hypothetical colleagues. In other words, patient optimism affects not only the articulated, but also the formulated, prognosis.[22]

Part of the explanation for why physicians tend to express more optimism to patients who themselves are optimistic is thus that physicians believe that optimism on the part of the patient actually does improve the prognosis. This does not, however, account for the observation that physicians also express more optimism to patients who are *pessimistic*.[23] Moreover, even after statistical adjustment for the physicians' objective prognosis (as measured by what they would say to colleagues), there is still a net effect of patient optimism on what physicians say to patients. Thus, physicians communicate prognoses to patients that are influenced by factors other than their assessment of the patients' prospects, employing optimism in a deliberate, strategic manner.

Finally, physicians were always substantially more optimistic when discussing prognoses with patients than they were with professional colleagues, which is consistent with the data regarding discrepant communication reviewed earlier. Whatever level of optimism respondents would have expressed about the patient's prognosis to a colleague (an indication of their "objective" assessment of the gravity of the patient's illness), they were likely to be substantially and significantly more optimistic when talking to patients.

In sum, these experimental results documented (1) the influence of patients' stated expectations on physicians' articulated prognoses, (2) the influence of patients' stated expectations on physicians' objective prognoses, and (3) the general presence of optimism in physicians' discussions of prognosis, out of proportion to their objective assessments. Overall, physicians correct patient pessimism and reinforce patient optimism. These behavior patterns manifested themselves even when the patient was quite sick, as was the case in the hypothetical situation described in this experimental vignette.

Negotiating the Prognosis

The interaction between patient and physician with regard to prognosis is not limited to the physician's use of a patient's perceptions to revise his estimates of the prognosis and to change what he says to the patient or to his colleagues. The interaction can also be more direct, in a sort of *negotiation* about the prognosis. Such negotiation is not usually deliberate and not particularly common, but it does occur, and it goes beyond the "bargaining" that sometimes takes place when patients try to persuade physicians to offer (or create) more favorable prognoses.[24] Negotiation regarding prognosis is broader and may focus on several aspects of the prognosis, including its valence, its object, its meaning, and its very articulation. This negotiation can be both a practical discussion (centered around instrumental objectives, such as the implications of alternative prognoses for treatment decisions) and a symbolic discussion (centered around the meaning of the prognosis for the patient, for instance, whether the predicted future is in keeping with the patient's hopes).

The ways in which prognosis is sometimes negotiated were described by one physician as follows:

> A patient of mine with breast cancer came to me after she had received primary treatment at [a prestigious center], then had received high-dose chemotherapy and bone marrow transplantation at another hospital, and then had been given another type of chemotherapy at the National Cancer Institute in Maryland. She ended up seeing

me because the two previous doctors who had cared for her had told her that her disease was incurable and that she had two to three years to live. She found that an unacceptable description. She said, "But I feel perfectly well, I'm healthy. I may still have cancer, but who's to say whether it's incurable and whether I'm going to live or die?" It was interesting: the reason she came to see me was precisely because several doctors had prognosticated, probably accurately (given the type of tumor she had and the fact it had spread), and the information was so troubling to her that she came asking me *not* to prognosticate. And I've never done so. I've now cared for her for about three years. She's doing reasonably well, although I still think her tumor is metastatic and probably incurable, although it's been stabilized on current treatments for the past six months. I don't think the prognosis is all that hot—it may be another year or two—but she's made it very clear to me that that's something she does not want to hear about.

This patient was unable to accept the prognosis that was offered, namely, that she would die. She and her doctor came to an agreement—almost explicitly—that they would uncouple the patient's serious diagnosis from the fatal prognosis that it ordinarily implies and not discuss the prognosis.

Sometimes the negotiation simply involves the patient and the physician trying to calibrate each other's predictions. For example, one patient who had had breast cancer surgery several years earlier observed at the end of a follow-up encounter with her doctor:

> *Patient:* Next September will be five years that I have been free of breast cancer.
> *Doctor:* Gosh, that'll be nice, huh?
> *Patient:* Yes, it will be.
> *Doctor:* OK. Bye-bye.
> *Patient:* Thanks.

The patient is seemingly inviting the physician to predict that she will *remain* free of cancer, but the physician dodges this implicit question by making a bland descriptive statement ("That'll be nice") rather than a predictive one ("You're likely to stay disease-free") or simply a more empathetic one ("It sounds like you are pleased—and you and I both think that you're likely cured"). This may be contrasted with another physician's handling of a similar situation:

> *Patient:* I just need to be reassured that if it is going . . . am I never . . . Can you just help me out a little bit with it?

Doctor: It is a benign-appearing breast cyst, both on the ultrasound and CT scan. It is not a tumor. It is not anything dangerous. In six months, we may want to repeat an ultrasound to make sure it is not getting bigger, but that is something you do not have to worry about.

Patient: OK, but could it duplicate?

Doctor: It is not likely to, but many people have these cysts and never even discover them. I mean it can sit in there dormant and not do a thing to you forever and that is probably what is going to happen.

Patient: OK.

In both cases, the prognosis is central to the patient's concerns. In the latter case, however, the physician's predictions specifically address the patient's anxieties about the future.

The notion of negotiation in prognosis, and also the fact that physicians respond to patients' prognostic expectations and "shade" the prognosis, sheds light on the fact that prognostication is, at times, a *dynamic* process. Prognostication is not always something the physician imposes on a patient. Patients, of course, can formulate their own ideas about what will happen to them. But beyond this, sometimes, the prognosis that the physician offers to patients (and perhaps even the one he formulates) is driven by patients' demands. This in turn suggests that physicians may specialize, in some sense, in the prognoses that they offer, allowing patients to shop for opinions in prognosis as they do in diagnosis or therapy. Certainly, physicians vary in their prognostic style, and some are blunter or more optimistic than others.

Ambiguity and the Preservation of Hope

The techniques of communication in stages, optimistic presentation, and statistical prognostication, as well as the practice of withholding information or adjusting predictions in response to patients' own assessments or wishes, can each be seen as reflecting an underlying commitment in medical practice to flexibility, indeterminism, and ambiguity in prognosis.[25] In turn, this ambiguity serves as a predicate for hope, in patients and physicians alike. That is, physicians do not regard the withholding of prognosis, much less the ways they communicate prognoses, as deceitful or self-interested; rather they consider them to be humane ways of preserving—or, even more actively, fostering—hope in their patients.

Ambiguity and vagueness also find expression in the most common and most typical way physicians communicate prognoses regarding survival, namely in stating that the patient has "days, not weeks" to live, "months rather than years," and so forth. These locutions do convey some information to patients, but because all of these temporal units can be transformed into each other, this verbal trick serves another purpose: it frames patient expectations while preserving the fluidity of time and the ambiguity of the future.

Medical sociologist Mary-Jo Good has argued that, in American oncology practice, hope is primarily conveyed by physicians' commitment to provide patients with diagnostic and therapeutic information and to employ a dazzling array of high-tech therapies; in contrast, physicians in Europe and Asia convey hope primarily by fostering ambiguity—not just with respect to their discussion of prognosis, but also with respect to their communication of diagnostic and treatment information.[26] Although this insightful characterization seems largely true, American physicians can also cultivate ambiguity, though they employ different means of doing so, especially in the case of prognosis. They too tend to avoid prognosticating, and when they cannot do so, they prognosticate in ways whose purpose is closely analogous to the rationales behind their foreign counterparts' avoidance of prognostication. American physicians are in the ambivalent position of being expected, when they communicate prognostic information, to do so honestly and accurately, but in a way that maximizes ambiguity and stresses the provisional nature of the information. This may be contrasted with the domains of diagnosis and therapy, where both doctors and patients tend to expect confident, specific, and certain information.

Moreover, many American doctors realize that there are different kinds of hope. There is, of course, the hope for cure. But particularly sensitive and practiced physicians also will sometimes deliberately reorient the patient's hopes toward other objectives, such as relief of symptoms, improvement in quality of life, resolution of interpersonal problems, or attention to spiritual growth.

How do the ways physicians prognosticate maintain or reflect ambiguity? The gradual, staged revelation of information to patients may be seen to mirror—and is sometimes said consciously to mirror—the gradual and tentative way that knowledge about patients and their illnesses becomes known to physicians themselves. In this sense, then, both the doctor's communication strategy and the patient's experience of prognostication reflect the epistemology of medical practice. In addi-

tion, communication in stages mirrors the way therapy is often imple-
mented; physicians will often employ gradually escalating therapeutic
interventions, which the patient also experiences in stages. The future is
thus neither revealed nor certain until it is experienced. Statistical prognostication, although it is cloaked in the seeming precision, objectivity,
and determinism of numerical expression, further fosters uncertainty
and ambiguity. Physicians feel comfortable using statistics because this
is a way of representing information about the future while allowing
for the possibility that the patient may deviate from the typical course.
The tendency to optimism, although not quite a source of ambiguity,
nevertheless takes advantage of it. All of these ways of communicating
prognoses in turn allow the physician the latitude to respond to patients'
own expectations regarding their prognoses.

Medical interactions are predicated on hope, on an optimistic vision
of the future, on the belief that physicians will be able in some way to help
patients, to relieve their suffering, to improve their condition. Patients
hope and doctors hope—they think about the future both consciously
and unconsciously—but they typically speak about this common (if
unshared) vision in coded, muted ways, if at all. The relative absence of
explicit or specific discussion about the future suggests that physicians
and patients fear that their most fervent wishes for success and cure will
not be met. It suggests a fear of disappointment.

Medical interactions are fundamentally triumphalist, based on the
optimistic conviction that things can be made better. Among patients,
this conviction manifests itself first and foremost in the fact of their
visit to the doctor, a visit made in the hope that the doctor will be able
to ameliorate their condition. Among doctors, this optimism manifests
itself in everything from the "courage to fail" ethos that drives their
attempts at therapy to their hubristic belief in their own power, from
their failure to acknowledge death to their avoidance of bad news, from
their belief in the benefits of an upbeat attitude to their minimization
of the possibly negative consequences of treatments. For doctors to
become doctors in the first place, or for them to treat patients with
potentially intractable problems every day (often inflicting pain and
suffering in the process), they must believe that what they do is likely
to create a better future for their patients than the patients would
otherwise have had. The patient and doctor thus search the medical
encounter for reasons to justify optimism. The beliefs and ideas underlying this need for optimism in turn influence how doctors formulate and communicate prognoses with patients and the decisions
they make.

Indeed, optimism—though it can be problematic, as we shall see—is as essential as other undercurrents of physicians' practice that have classically been identified, for example, the detachment physicians cultivate, the "gaze" with which they regard their patients, and the confidence they have in their power.[27] Moreover, I believe that optimism and an orientation toward the future more generally are previously overlooked elements of the "sick role" that *patients* adopt in response to disease.[28] Patients must not only try to get better, they must believe that they can get better.[29] Ambiguity is essential for these attitudes and behaviors in patients and physicians.

The belief that specific and direct communication is rude and harmful is widespread in non-American cultures and, as it turns out, prevalent in American medicine as well. Ambiguity permits a confusion, if not a conflation, between deception and tact. But more than a desire to be polite, American physicians may make use of ambiguity in prognosis "in order to express feelings and articulate realities which are too subtle for straightforward univocal representation."[30] Ambiguity is felt to capture philosophical truths about the world and, in the case of prognosis, may allegorically refer to the fundamental inability of human beings either to know the truth or to rework fate. In addition, just as the epistemology of clinical knowledge can drive prognostication to be ambiguous, so too, in a reciprocal fashion, can ambiguous speech be a way to express such knowledge. Ambiguity may not only be a passive way to conceal reality, but an active way to express it.

The *hope* that ambiguity cultivates in patients thus arises in two senses: hope in the sense of an optimistic expectation, and hope in the sense of a yearning desire. Patients are supposed to both wait for and want something that will occur in the future. Physicians tend to regard hope as something the doctor can give to the patient that the patient might lack. This perception reflects the asymmetry of the doctor-patient relationship more generally: the doctor is the giver and the patient the receiver of, for example, diagnostic information, drugs, therapeutic procedures, patience, and concern—and this asymmetric relationship persists in the domain of prognosis. Giving hope is seen as a way to show respect for and to dignify the position of the patient. Physicians' ways of speaking about hope reflect this perspective. Doctors repeatedly speak in terms of *giving* hope or, at a minimum, not taking hope away. For example, in a typical description, one physician observed, "It is very important to give as much hope as possible, even if you have to make it a little better than the reality of it." This hope, it turns out, is given by the cultivation, and not merely the preservation, of ambiguity.

Conversely, clarity is seen as the antithesis of hope and the precursor of fear. As one physician noted: "What happens in contemporary practice is that you really make patients fearful because you're obliged to tell them everything." Doctors believe that too much knowledge, especially of the future, is dangerous for patients and for the doctor-patient relationship. The consequences of clarity are typically characterized as follows:

> I had one very educated, sixty-five-year-old patient who had been all over the city, to every major medical center. He ended up with me because he liked my personality and because I came highly recommended. When he came to see me, his disease had relapsed and was no longer curable. And he came to me having been told by his physician that there was still treatment that he could receive and still be cured, and I very honestly told him right then and there that the only way that he could be cured was if we got his disease back under control and then if he had a bone marrow transplant—which at his age had a very high mortality. I said that the reality of the situation was that the chance of cure was very small, even though I was willing to treat him. And he essentially told me that I had taken all hope away from him, and that he couldn't be treated by a doctor who offered him no hope. He went elsewhere. And he died three months later.

This physician used this experience—of the patient losing his hope, his doctor, and his life in short order—to explain why she no longer is so blunt (so "honest" and "right then and there") with her patients. She is typical in her characterization of the adverse consequences of "taking away hope." It is out of such fears that physicians' commitment to ambiguity and indeterminacy, as well as their practical ways of prognosticating, arise.

Six

THE SELF-FULFILLING PROPHECY

I often had the distinct impression when I talked to patients that I was changing the future. I could never be sure whether presenting what I thought was going to happen would change what would in fact happen. And maybe the way I presented it was important too! So, if I said things one way, one thing would happen, and if I said them another, something else would happen. Because I am convinced that this is the case. The patient and I were changed by what I said: we thought differently and we acted differently. If I told the patient that I thought he would die, I felt strangely responsible, not just for what I said, but for what would happen. Maybe if I said the patient would die, then we would all act in a way that made this happen, in a sort of self-fulfilling prophecy. And I would be responsible.

— YOUNG GENERAL INTERNIST

Predictions, doctors believe, can affect outcomes through a kind of self-fulfilling prophecy. Indeed, the expression itself is occasionally part of physicians' self-conscious vocabulary. Physicians identify a broad range of ways that the self-fulfilling prophecy works, affecting both their own and their patients' attitudes and behaviors. Belief in the self-fulfilling prophecy and ideas about how it works are intriguing because they are found in a population of professionals who are ostensibly immune from such seemingly nonrational thinking. Nevertheless, the transcendent importance of the outcomes that preoccupy medical care, the malleability of these outcomes, and the interrelationship between technique and affect in medicine combine to provide fertile terrain for the emergence of such thinking.

Sociologist Robert K. Merton opens his seminal essay on the self-fulfilling prophecy by citing a sociological theorem attributed to W. I. Thomas: "If men define situations as real, they are real in their consequences."[1] Predictions about a given situation are not only an integral part of the situation but also, more important, they affect current behavior and subsequent outcomes. People can act on their predictions about the future in order to make the predictions come to pass. This *effectiveness* of predictions about the future is one of the main ways that social systems differ from physical ones—that is, they are purposeful rather than deterministic or stochastic.[2] Merton argues that the self-fulfilling prophecy is an initially *false* definition of a situation that evokes a new behavior that makes the originally false conception come true. However, in medicine at least, this need not be the case: self-fulfilling prophecies may be seen as reinforcing rather than just reversing prior expectations—for example, when actions accelerate death in a patient who would have died anyway.[3]

Prediction is effective on two levels. It may affect *present behavior* as a consequence of its articulation, and it may affect *future outcomes* through the change in behavior. These two effects are in turn enhanced by the conscious knowledge among actors that prediction has these consequences. People may in fact use predictions as a deliberate means to alter the future. In other words, it is the belief that predictions can alter the future (as well as beliefs about how predictions alter the future), more than the content of the predictions themselves, that is essential to the effectiveness of prediction. If people simply had impressions of what the future held (whether accurate or inaccurate), but did not believe that these impressions should or could influence the present or the future, then prediction would not have as much influence as it does.

Self-fulfilling prophecy may be divided into two types. *Positive self-fulfilling prophecy* refers to favorable predictions that cause corresponding favorable outcomes. *Negative self-fulfilling prophecy* refers to unfavorable predictions that cause corresponding unfavorable outcomes. Insofar as people believe that prediction is effective, their belief in these two sorts of prophecy should logically be coincident. Physicians' beliefs about the effectiveness of positive and negative self-fulfilling prophecy diverge, however, and this divergence provides a clue as to how predictions are thought to have their effect, at least in medical contexts.

The counterpart of the self-fulfilling prophecy is the self-negating prophecy, in which a prediction brings about its opposite. Self-negating prophecy may also be of two types. *Positive self-negating prophecy* refers to unfavorable predictions that cause favorable outcomes, as when a patient responds to an unfavorable prediction in a way that ultimately renders the prediction false.[4] And *negative self-negating prophecy* refers to favorable predictions that cause unfavorable outcomes. This categorization of types of self-fulfilling and self-negating prophecy, along with some simplified medical examples, is illustrated in figure 6.1.[5]

Here, I evaluate beliefs about self-fulfilling prophecy in medicine, the mechanisms of its action, its distribution and determinants, and its consequences for physicians and patients.

Prediction

	Favorable	Unfavorable
Favorable	**Positive self-fufilling prophecy** Example: prediction: patient will recover action: physician applies therapy vigilantly outcome: patient recovers	**Positive self-negating prophecy** Example: prediction: patient will die action: physician doubles efforts to save patient outcome: patient recovers
Unfavorable	**Negative self-negating prophecy** Example: prediction: patient will recover action: physician gets lax and is less attentive outcome: patient dies	**Negative self-fulfilling prophecy** Example: prediction: patient will die action: physician withdraws life support outcome: patient dies

Outcome (label on the left spanning Favorable and Unfavorable rows)

Figure 6.1. Typology of self-fulfilling and self-negating prophecy

How Self-Fulfilling Prophecy Works

Physicians explain how the self-fulfilling prophecy works in several ways. They believe that making a prediction can change the patient's attitudes or behaviors or physiology in a way that promotes the pre-dicted outcome. They believe that making a prediction can change the physician's attitudes or behavior in a way that promotes the predicted outcome. And they believe that making a prediction can directly pro-mote the predicted outcome in a way that seems almost magical.[6]

Effect on Patients' Attitudes, Behaviors, and Physiology

One explanation physicians commonly offer for the effectiveness of the self-fulfilling prophecy is that predictions may foster changes in patients' attitudes. In the case of negative self-fulfilling prophecy, the intermediary factor of depression is often invoked. For example, one physician observed:

> A physician gives someone a death sentence, saying, "You're going to be dead in six months," and that then brings on a depression, so that the patient doesn't eat, doesn't engage in anything vigorous,

and then becomes really debilitated. The patient may in fact die a lot sooner as a result of that erroneous information. I think it can do that, yes.

In this example, the depression brought on by the prediction has its negative effect in part by modifying the patient's behavior, subverting the patient's level of activity and effort to recover. The example also illustrates the confidence the patient is presumed to have in the physician's knowledge and power. It is because patients *trust* the physician that the unfavorable prognosis has its unfavorable impact.

A favorable prediction, conversely, may foster the patient's morale or decrease the patient's anxiety. One physician observed:

> Giving a favorable prognosis can probably lead to a favorable outcome, particularly if you consider patients, say, with far-advanced cancer, who often die of an infection superimposed on wasting. If you've got them in good morale, and they are eating and getting around, they will probably have better nutrition and be stronger and fight off that potentially fatal infection better than they might do otherwise. It is not going to cure the cancer. But if you're talking about duration of life, it may very well prolong that.

Similarly, another physician observed:

> I think that if the patient is relieved of his anxieties and has confidence that the doctor has done a thorough job assessing the situation, sure, I think this helps in making a good prognosis. It gives him a little better chance. The patient's mental attitude toward his disease is a big part of the disease, and if you're able to relieve him of anxieties and tell him that he can expect to have fewer or no symptoms in a few weeks or a few days or whatever, this, I think, will hasten his recovery. He is not going to be lying awake and tossing around and saying, "The doctor just doesn't know what's going to happen to me."

Here, relief of anxiety about the future of the disease is coupled with reassurance about the competence of the physician. Again, the confidence of the patient in the physician is central. Indeed, physicians believe that their ability to predict the future accurately is important to how they are perceived by their patients.

Physicians often believe that outcomes are sensitive to patients' general disposition and therefore to the predictions that engender particular thoughts and expectations in patients.

> I think there's so much we don't know about neuroimmunology and the healing power of good thoughts: "I'm going to get better," and therefore I get better. "This medicine is going to work," and therefore

it works. I think there are some cases where that might be true. There are a lot of cases where that's definitely not true—no matter what you think, the outcome's going to be the same—but I think there's probably truth to that. And I think that is one reason why oncologists that I've worked with are so hesitant to offer prognoses to people. They don't want to say "This won't work" or "This won't help" or anything like that because they fear the patient will lose hope. It's important to have a good positive outlook on everything.

Sometimes physicians describe this effect in more spiritual terms.

I think that there's something that can't be quantified called a "will to live," or a "living spirit," that can be affected by negative or positive comments or beliefs. Physicians have very great control— unfortunately—over whether that living will or living spirit thrives or dies. And I think that it is as important as antibiotics or chemotherapy. Physicians can influence how long patients live or die just by telling them a positive or negative prognosis.

This power that physicians have over patients is often viewed as regrettable or dangerous precisely because prediction is believed to be so effective. In the face of such effects, as we have seen, physicians not uncommonly raise religious or spiritual concerns when discussing the impact of prognostication on patients' lives.

Another way physicians think the self-fulfilling prophecy works, especially the positive type, is by changing patients' behavior—typically by increasing patients' compliance with therapeutic regimens. One experienced clinician gave the following illustration:

If you can inculcate positive feelings in a newly diagnosed, adolescent diabetic patient, the research data there is that one of the best predictors of good outcome—such as short-term blood sugar control—is if the person is upbeat and sanguine, interplays well, and is positive. The number of DKA [diabetic ketoacidosis] hospital admissions per two years and the hemoglobin A1c levels [a measure of sugar control] are better. But if the person is not upbeat, then it becomes the physician's job to try to change the negative feature of the appreciation of the illness.

Asked whether making an unfavorable prognosis can cause an unfavorable outcome, this physician continued:

Yes, I think that it can. If, because I say such an unfavorable thing, the patient then does not take proper care of himself in whatever area is ill or ailing, then I would submit to you that the chances of that organ having more problems is much greater.

The effectiveness of such behavioral change on the part of the patient can be expressed not just in chronic diseases like diabetes, but also in acute illnesses. This physician was asked whether similar reasoning would apply to an acutely and critically ill patient:

> If the patient gives up, and is neglectful and not attended to, then the answer is that I think it's possible. An example would be that if a patient on a respirator got the message that you thought he was all "washed up" or some other negative phrase, and then he got a mucus plug [in his trachea] and couldn't cough that up, and didn't bother to call anybody until he got obstructed, hypoxic, infected, whatever—then the answer is yes.

Similarly, some physicians note that predictions can become self-fulfilling by affecting the behavior of the patient's family—for example, by causing the family to increase their efforts as caregivers.

More generally, many physicians associate the effectiveness of the positive self-fulling prophecy with the patient's properly fulfilling the obligations of the "sick role," classically described by sociologist Talcott Parsons as including the duties of desiring to get well, cooperating with the doctor, and making an active effort to get better.[7] The effectiveness of the self-fulfilling prophecy thus in a sense depends on adherence to a specifically social role.[8] For example, one physician noted:

> With many patients, you can predict a good result and to a certain degree the individual will try to make that result really happen and might do more in the way of self-help than otherwise. They might force themselves to get out of bed, they might do more exercising, they might do more in the way of doing whatever you've told them to do in the way of being treated.

Another physician put it this way:

> Rendering a favorable prognosis helps the patient because most of the time patients are terrified about the likelihood that they will die, and I don't think that fear helps them go on about their lives and do what they have to do and be active and busy. Patients whose chemotherapy for breast cancer ends are particularly terrified: "Now the cancer is loose. Now nothing is being done." And I think that if you say, "Here is what the outlook is . . ." I think that is helpful in that setting. I think that telling someone with hypertension that if they continue to take their medicines, and if their blood pressure is under control, they are unlikely to experience major end-organ damage: I think this is helpful.

The self-fulfilling prophecy thus works by encouraging the patient to accept and comply with the doctor's therapeutic recommendations. And it works this way for both chronic and acute illnesses. In a sense, given the authoritative status of the physician with respect to the patient, the self-fulfilling prophecy works by reinforcing patient obedience and restraining deviance, as part of a broader professional function of controlling the patient's experience and behavior.[9] If patients are given a prognosis and are compliant as a result of it, they can avoid unfavorable outcomes. On the other hand, the power physicians believe they have over patients adds to their fear of making predictions. They dread the dangerous potential for unintended or misdirected and harmful effects, especially if their predictions are wrong.

These statements by physicians imply that being active and busy in confronting the adversity of illness is almost a duty of patients. Indeed, the sick role reflects a striving achievement orientation; patients can at least do something even if they cannot get better.[10] The sick role, in short, entails work, and it is through this work that the self-fulfilling prophecy is believed to be effective. Doctors in turn have the duty to support this work. Physicians' optimistic predictions reinforce patients' fulfillment of the sick role and reinforce their duty to be brave and to return to their normal state as quickly as possible. This emphasis on being active is so strongly a part of the American medical ethos that it appears even in circumstances in which it might seem superfluous—for example, when physicians encourage terminally ill patients to get out of bed or "do something." Physicians' responsibility thus extends not only to treating patients, but also to promoting optimism and, consequently, activity.

There is thus an aspect of the sick role that Parsons did not address. The sick patient also has the duty to remain hopeful and not brood. This is consonant with a larger theme in contemporary American society that stresses a positive, "can do" outlook. Physicians' belief in the self-fulfilling prophecy and also their related, systematic expressions of optimism support the performance of this social duty in patients.

Finally, physicians explain the effectiveness of the self-fulfilling prophecy as reflecting predictions' beneficial and detrimental effects on patients' immune function, nervous system, nutritional status, exercise tolerance, cardiovascular performance, and so forth. There is indeed empirical evidence that positive or negative beliefs can affect these parameters and subsequent biological outcomes, and physicians often refer to such data, though some do so in a skeptical and disparaging fashion.[11]

Effect on Physicians' Attitudes and Behaviors

According to many physicians, the self-fulfilling prophecy can also work by affecting physicians', and not just patients', attitudes and behaviors. For example, one critical care physician observed:

> I think that if you make a bad prediction, then you might curtail the care that you would give and limit things. . . . And on the opposite end of things, if you think that the patient is going to survive, then you might be more likely to spend your time and effort and resources on that patient to make them survive. So, yes, I think that the self-fulfilling prophecy is a clear possibility. In fact, I think that is one of the problems with using objective prognostic scoring systems: you get a probability estimate for survival, it looks horrible for the patient, and so you "lay the crepe" [prepare the patient for the worst] and talk to the family and limit your care, and sure enough that person gets worse the next day if you do that! And if you come across as pessimistic to the housestaff, nursing staff, and others who are working with you, then they too may limit what they do, and so have a real impact on the whole approach to the patient.[12]

Another physician suggested that the self-fulfilling prophecy might work by improving the physician's bedside manner (and might, consequently, optimize patient behavior):

> I think that, in terms of your attitude and information that you give the patient, and your concerns about the patient and the outcome of their disease, if these are communicated in a positive way, a way which has a certain amount of upbeat enthusiasm—I think that then allows patients to respond as well in the same way. This also allows the patient to be more open in terms of asking questions, and by asking questions to get better insight in terms of your care, in terms of the disease, in terms of knowing how to handle things. So in that sense I think the outcome can be better.
>
> I think there are certainly subtleties and interplay between the patient and the physician that the patient can perceive and pick up on. The physician sometimes doesn't recognize this. I had a patient once say, "Well, gee, if you're worried, I should be worried too." And it takes a fair amount of talking to make that clearer in terms of what they perceive and what you believe.

An unfavorable prediction could also come true if the physician were to become neglectful:

> If I have a negative feeling and I perceive some negative red flags in terms of the patient's clinical course, and if I fight it off and say, "It's

just too bad," then something bad can happen. The neglect would be
on my part, not the patient's part.

Thus, predictions may elicit acts of commission or omission on the part
of the physician that foster the predicted outcome, whether positive or
negative.

In several of these examples, the effectiveness of the self-fulfilling
prophecy depends on there being an *interaction* between the patient and
the doctor, in which each participant influences the other's behavior. The
fact that negative self-fulfilling prophecy can work through changes in
physicians' behavior is troubling to physicians, however. They may justify the role an unfavorable prediction plays in effecting an unfavorable
outcome—even death:

> We can say, "This patient is going to do very poorly," and as a result
> of that prediction take the patient off life support and he dies. But
> I don't know that that is really such a bad outcome. That might be
> the best outcome for that patient. So I don't know if making a bad
> prediction can cause a bad thing to happen after all. The patient may
> die, but that may not necessarily be the worst thing.

The deft rationalization that an unfavorable prediction that leads to an
unfavorable outcome (such as death) is really not so unfortunate is a
typical response of physicians faced with the potentially authoritative
influence of their predictions. Another physician described the following case:

> I had a patient who had a high cervical spine injury. This was a
> patient who was alert and awake. But he could barely communicate;
> his injury was high enough that it was hard for him to mouth his
> words. He was on the ventilator. We cared for him for a long enough
> time that, based on previous experience and our estimate of clinical
> outcome, we were confident that he was not going to recover his
> neurological function. We told him and his family that. And he said
> that he didn't want to continue to be ventilated. So we anesthetized
> him and took him off the ventilator and he died.
>
> So our estimate was that he wasn't going to recover neurological
> function. But my estimate would have been that he would have
> survived for—I don't know how long, but a pretty long time unless he
> got a complication from ventilation. There are a lot of quadriplegics
> who live on ventilators. And so, based on our probability estimate,
> after speaking to the patient, we were willing to discontinue care.

These two cases, which are typical, suggest that physicians are troubled
by the extent to which their prognostic assessments may contribute to

bringing about a dreaded outcome, namely, the death of a patient. The two physicians use different techniques, however, to disconnect their prognosis and the outcome. The first physician recasts the outcome as not being so unfavorable after all and transforms a negative self-fulfilling prophecy into a positive self-fulfilling prophecy. The second shifts attention to an unfavorable prediction about neurological recovery rather than a favorable one about survival, stressing an area where the link between his prediction and the observed outcome—the patient's death—is less direct and less threatening. A disconnection is cultivated between the thing predicted (neurological function) and the outcome observed (death).

Such strategies involve fundamental questions about what constitutes a favorable or unfavorable outcome and illustrate the point that the valence of an outcome is debated and defined socially.[13] But they are especially interesting because they reflect the dread among physicians of the effectiveness of predictions, especially unfavorable ones. An unfavorable prediction may lead to cessation of therapy, may thus cause death, and so may be fulfilled in a chain of action for which the physician feels responsibility.[14]

These comments also reveal a thinly disguised foreboding on the part of physicians about having to make decisions to withdraw life support at all; they would rather not acknowledge the connection between their actions and a patient's death. But even more remarkable, these comments suggest that physicians define prediction as an action in itself, so much so that to predict a patient's death is almost the same as to withdraw life support. The prediction itself has meaning, independent of its accuracy, independent of the thing predicted, independent of the actions it might foster, and independent of the outcomes it might engender. Prediction is not an idle, senseless, or trivial act, no matter how brief or offhand. When physicians make predictions—especially about death—they are grappling with their possible role in speeding death. Moreover, and quite beyond this importance, there is the very real belief that the act of articulating a prediction alone may be as effective at causing the outcome as the action it may (merely) trigger.

Direct Effect

Ideas about the workings of the self-fulfilling prophecy transcend the foregoing mechanisms involving patient and physician attitudes and behaviors. For many physicians, the mechanism of action is both more direct and more mysterious. One physician explained:

Death from illness, either acute or chronic, has a mystical nature. Not necessarily from a religious point of view, but from the point of view that it, on occasion, seems to be something that can be influenced.

Another physician observed:

I have to weigh how much giving people survival statistics changes their quality of life and changes what they would do with their life, because I also am convinced that if you tell somebody, "You have three months to live," they frequently die sooner. I've seen that happen where some oncologist told somebody, "You know you have a 30 percent chance of living out this year," and they up and die.

Still another physician explained:

I am reluctant to give specific prognoses to patients regarding time of survival. They will often live or die to meet that prediction. Rather, I encourage them to take each day one at a time, to tap into as many supportive resources as are available, and to live as fully as possible.

Although these observations reflect the notion that the self-fulfilling prophecy acts by modifying the physicians' or the patients' behavior, there is something more here: it is as if the action is *automatic*, as if the predictions truly are *self-fulfilling*. The presumption here is that the patient's response is very sensitive to the doctor's expectations—even unstated ones—about outcomes.

This sensitivity is very similar to the placebo effect. Placebos are generally defined as inert substances that are used as sham treatments in an effort to please the patient. The problem is, they often "work"—in the sense that, despite their inertness, they cause objective, biologically measurable changes in the patient. Indeed, some have proposed that mere contact with a doctor (or the doctor himself) is a sort of placebo.[15] Physicians are often troubled by the placebo effect, because it is hard to understand, because it suggests that some of the effect physicians have is neither deliberate nor rational, and because it suggests that what they do may be unnecessary. However, they also realize that the placebo effect is often beneficial and that part of their job is, in a sense, to maximize it.[16] A number of physicians I interviewed explicitly made the connection between the impact of predictions on outcomes, on the one hand, and placebos, on the other. Physicians realize that the placebo effect can also be used, advertently or inadvertently, in a harmful way. Indeed, some authors have defined a *nocebo* effect, or the causation of sickness or death by the expectation of same.[17] The classic example of this was provided by physician Walter B. Cannon in the 1940s in a paper aptly entitled "Voodoo Death," in which he discussed the "fatal power of the imagination."[18] Indeed, the placebo effect is to the nocebo effect what the positive self-fulfilling prophecy is to the negative self-fulfilling prophecy.

The connection between the self-fulfilling prophecy and the placebo/nocebo phenomenon is particularly apparent when it is realized that the way people detect and experience disease depends in part on their culture. Taxonomies of illness and of symptoms are first of all culturally specific *descriptions* of sickness events. But they are also a repertoire of permissible *expressions* of illness, and they may even become *prescriptions* in the right setting.[19] Physicians, as authorities on illness, have considerable power to call forth both placebo and nocebo processes. In a sense, they specify what to expect.[20]

Another physician described the effectiveness of prediction as follows:

> I think prediction was particularly powerful prior to the discovery of antibiotics and things like that, because it gave the patient a good deal of faith in the physician. Now there may be self-fulfilling prophecies. They are the *dangerous* side of prediction. For example: You see a patient; the patient's father has died; the patient is having some difficulty; and you point out, "You're going to be depressed, and this is how long you're going to be depressed. You are going to be depressed for three to six months, and then that depression will lift." The prediction has not only been a helpful thing, it may be that the prediction actually helps shape the illness. I don't know how it could do it. But it may do that. Maybe that's autosuggestion and control of behavior. But the patient can come in a few months later and say, "You know, you were right. I'm getting over this now, and I feel good about it; and I know that I'm going to feel better because *you laid out a course and the disease is following the course.*"[21]

The perception here is that the physician exercises power over the disease simply by articulating what the future holds. Moreover, there is the strong implication that the prediction has its effect by means of the self-fulfilling prophecy alone. But there is also an implicit danger, that the physician might as readily bring about unfavorable outcomes that would not otherwise occur, just by predicting them.

Typically, physicians divine a connection between their rendering of a prognosis and the patient's outcome, a connection to which they ascribe considerable meaning. One doctor recalled:

> After many weeks of working on this critically ill patient, I finally felt comfortable that the prognosis was poor and that the patient

wouldn't recover. I went to tell the nurse and to write the order to basically take the patient off the respirator. And the patient literally died that second! That was a really powerful experience.

Another physician told the following story, haltingly and with awe:

> I had a patient, an elderly man with prostate cancer, who was admitted complaining of a headache. On admission, he was engaged, animated, happy. His workup included a CT, which revealed metastases to his brain. I told this to the patient forthrightly, but with difficulty. The patient became very quiet, with sparse speech, and detached. And though there was no clinical change in him—in his tumor—he died in his sleep two nights later. I am convinced that the patient gave up and wanted to die and that the information I gave him caused his death. It was eerie and strange and mysterious, and I am sure that what I told him was connected to his death.

In a similar and remarkably powerful testimony, a young physician described a case involving a considerable amount of iatrogenesis. There is the feeling at the end of this case that when the physicians ultimately predicted that the patient would die—when they decided that the case was "hopeless"—they somehow caused the patient's death. There is the sense that the physicians' prognostic pronouncements iatrogenically hastened the patient's death, just as their therapeutic interventions had done previously.

> One of the hardest cases I ever took care of was when I was an intern in the CCU [cardiac care unit]. There was this guy who came in because he had some mid-epigastric burning. Turned out he had a gastric carcinoma. This was all as an outpatient. And they wanted to bring him in for a resection of his carcinoma. But he was an elderly guy, and there was a concern that he had angina, so they wanted to perform a cardiac catheterization to make sure that he could survive his gastric resection. So they catheterized him. On the table, he had a ventricular tachycardia. He infarcted. They brought him to the CCU. He eventually went to open heart surgery. He had an infarct after his surgery. He was on a ventilator. Had pneumonia, lung failure, and renal failure. And actually they had given him a medicine he was allergic to, so he had bone marrow failure as well! So here was a very healthy, functional man in his middle seventies who had the most minimal of symptoms which brought him to immediate attention as having a small, even curable, gastric carcinoma. And he goes through these amazing machinations of our medical facility and ends up with multisystem failure. It's unbelievable, isn't it? Now his gastric carcinoma is the *least* of his worries. He's on a ventilator and has a

heart that doesn't work, kidneys that don't work, and he's in bone marrow failure, and his lungs are shot. It's incredible!

So he's got four-system failure. He's going to die. There is no way he can live. And yet, I took care of him really from the first day I came to the CCU to the day I left about a month later. I think he died on the second-to-last day before I left the unit. So the entire time I took care of him, I began to—I began to hate him. This is the only patient I've ever had that I've ever truly hated. And it was because he wanted to live so badly.

Every day I had to take blood from him—new arterial lines, new central lines, feverish all the time, everything had to always be changed. He was blowing up like a balloon from poor nutrition. Edema everywhere. I would have to go in with a needle more than an inch just to hit a vein or an artery. You know, he would weep from his wound every time I would do it. I was clearly hurting him with everything I did. And it showed on his face. But he was *alive*. And, despite all these problems, which should have killed anyone else in just a few days, he lived an entire month. And I had to really hurt him day after day after day after day. And I wanted to quit weeks before he died.

But my superiors—who didn't have to go in with him every day and work with him—would not let me. Basically they told me that I "had to go culture him," or "he needs a new [intravascular] line." They're not the ones that have to do it. I'm the one that has to do it. And even despite my discussions with the family—and I think I was as capable of telling them his prognosis, even as a beginning physician, as anyone else—clearly he was not going to live. But the family was always optimistic because the attending physician always said every day that he was still alive. And the family hung on to that, like that was it. That was all they knew: that every day he was alive. And "When was he going to be able to come home?" Not "*could* he ever" but "*when*." And I couldn't understand: they couldn't see it. And so I had to hurt this guy every day.

Finally, they all saw that he wasn't getting any better. And they agreed to make him DNR [i.e., to enter a do-not-resuscitate order] and not to resuscitate him if he should have a final event. And the day they decided that, that very night he died. . . .

And the next day, the family came in to see him. He had died early in the morning. And they came in that morning to see him, and they saw me there, and I told them how very sorry I was. And they were furious—with me! His daughter told me that she hated physicians, that she hated me, and that she had a young boy who wanted to be a physician, and she would never let him. Never let him be a doctor—because of what we did to her father.

I think that was the hardest case I ever had. You know, I predicted—I knew he would die. It was remarkable that he—I never expected that he would die the day that they decided to make him DNR. And the patient didn't even know that we had made him DNR.

I can't believe that he carried on like this for a whole month. And yet he died the day his family and we made him a DNR. Even though he did not know that they had done that. Here he is, in this very controlled environment, and the attending is telling the family every day that the patient is alive another day. And all of a sudden we decide that it is hopeless, that he's not getting any better, let's just not push on any further—not *withdraw* life support, mind you, just not push any further—and that day he dies. The day that I don't have to put the defibrillator on him and resuscitate him if necessary, he dies.[22]

Physicians frequently mention strange coincidences in which unfavorable predictions seemed to accelerate, if not cause, a patient's death by unspecified and obscure means.

In addition to illustrating the physician's perceptions about the possible direct effect of prognostic assessments, even ones not communicated to patients, the foregoing case demonstrates the frightening and awesome power of medical care both to keep a nearly dead patient alive and to make a previously well patient nearly dead. In the face of such power, it is not surprising that the physician is troubled by the possibility that his prognostic assessments might have untoward and powerful effects similar to those of the diagnostic and therapeutic interventions. Moreover, the experience of caring for this patient—including the foreknowledge that he would die (acquired early in the patient's care) and the prognostic estimate that the case was "hopeless" (stated late in the patient's care)—was a very *personal* one for this physician. The physician was as troubled by his painful therapeutic interventions as by his ominous foreknowledge. What is more, he was ashamed.

This case, and several others considered here, also include another element of the self-fulfilling prophecy: in many instances, the patients are described as being relatively well, even "happy," *before* the rendering of the prognosis. The rendering of a prognosis, however, is associated with a reversal. The prediction hurts not only the patients' feelings but also their body and their prospects. It is an all-encompassing phenomenon, with the prediction being seen by physicians as something capable of taking hold of patients and causing them suffering, hopelessness, decrepitude, and even death.

These elements of prognosis—the shame, the fear, and the intimacy, as well as the sense of reversal and of powerfulness—are not uncommon, and are typically connected to cases where physicians believe their predictions can affect outcomes, perhaps by almost magical means.

Proof That Physicians Believe in the Self-Fulfilling Prophecy

The contention that physicians believe in the self-fulfilling prophecy is strongly supported by two randomized, controlled experiments that were incorporated into a survey of a random sample of practicing internists in the United States.[23] This experimental approach was employed in order to enhance confidence in the validity and generalizability of some of the qualitative findings from the in-depth interviews with individual physicians discussed above. The overall purpose of these experiments was to define and document certain beliefs physicians have about the self-fulfilling prophecy.

Self-Fulfilling Prophecy in Chronically Ill Patients

In the first experiment, physician respondents received one of six different versions of a hypothetical clinical vignette describing a seventy-two-year-old patient with metastatic prostate cancer. The patient was chronically ill and had a relatively long survival horizon. The versions differed only in terms of the predictions made by the hypothetical doctor and the outcomes observed (survival for two months or for two years). Respondents were randomly chosen to receive one version, and statistical comparison of responses to the various versions of the vignette confirmed the respondents' belief in the notion of self-fulfilling prophecy overall. Whereas the physicians studied definitely believed in *negative* self-fulfilling prophecy, however, they may or may not have believed in positive self-fulfilling prophecy. That is, in this setting of a chronic disease with a relatively long survival horizon, pessimism was more likely to be believed to have an impact than optimism. This probably results from the a priori expectation in this case that the patient would have a relatively favorable outcome (i.e., would live a relatively long time); while neither a two-month nor a two-year survival would be implausible, the two-year survival is actually more likely. Thus, a *pessimistic* prediction goes against the grain and may precipitate a decline in a patient otherwise likely to do relatively well.

There were at least two other important findings in this experiment. First, physicians were more likely to believe that making *no* prediction contributes to longer survival than to shorter survival. In other words, in this situation, physicians are more likely to believe that saying nothing will have a beneficent rather than a maleficent effect since the background expectation is of a relatively favorable outcome. Second, the experiment permitted an assessment of the extent to which physicians believe in the self-negating prophecy. It is hard to imagine that a patient in this setting would desire to live a *short* period simply to prove the physician's long survival prediction wrong; such a negative self-negating prophecy would be ridiculous here, and the experiment confirmed this. Physicians do not believe, in other words, that choosing to make a long prediction over making no prediction will itself hasten death. Similarly, physicians do not believe that making a short prediction over making no prediction will delay death. In short, there was no evidence that physicians believe in the self-negating prophecy, whereby predictions disprove themselves, either by the patient deliberately outliving the prediction or, less plausibly, living for a shorter duration than predicted. This belief regarding the self-negating prophecy is an additional reason, however, for physicians to make optimistic survival predictions, since optimistic predictions cannot harm patients.

Self-Fulfilling Prophecy in Acutely Ill Patients

In the second experiment, physician respondents received one of six different versions of a hypothetical clinical vignette describing a sixty-nine-year-old patient with a serious pneumonia in an intensive care unit. The patient was acutely ill and had a relatively short survival horizon. The vignettes again differed only in the doctor's prediction and the relevant outcome, in this case whether the patient recovered or died. Again, a statistical test confirmed that the physicians believed in the self-fulfilling prophecy. However, here physicians definitely believed in *positive* self-fulfilling prophecy whereas they may or may not have believed in negative self-fulfilling prophecy. That is, in this setting of acute life-threatening disease with a short survival horizon, optimism is more likely to be believed to have an impact than pessimism, probably because there is an a priori expectation in this case of a relatively unfavorable outcome. While neither recovery nor death would be unusual, death is actually considered to be more likely. Thus, an *optimistic* prediction goes against the grain and may foster improvement in a patient otherwise inclined to do relatively poorly.

In this experiment, physicians were more likely to believe that *not* making a prediction contributes to a shorter survival than a longer survival, though this observation did not quite reach statistical significance at the customary level. That is, physicians are more likely to believe that saying nothing will have a maleficent rather than a beneficent effect, perhaps because the background expectation is that the patient will die.

Again, the experiment found no evidence of belief in the self-negating prophecy: physicians did not believe that predicting survival would hasten death or that predicting death would foster recovery. Choosing to predict recovery over choosing to say nothing was thus a no-lose proposition—at least with respect to the patient's prospects for recovery—since it would not adversely affect survival. This belief, then, is an additional reason for physicians to make optimistic survival predictions in such circumstances.

The Meaning of Saying Nothing About the Prognosis

Beyond documenting physicians' belief in the self-fulfilling prophecy, these two experiments reveal that the meaning of saying nothing—that is, making no prediction about the outcome of a clinical case—may depend on what physicians' background expectation about the outcome is. In the case of the patient with prostate cancer and a long survival horizon, more physicians believed that saying nothing was associated with a favorable outcome. In the case of a patient with serious pneumonia and a short survival horizon, more physicians believed that saying nothing was associated with an unfavorable outcome.

This asymmetry is consonant with aphorisms such as "no news is good news" for patients with a long-standing, chronic illness.[24] Conversely, for a critically ill patient, physicians (and probably patients as well) appear to interpret failure to make an explicit prognosis as bad news. Failure to volunteer reassurance when there is a material threat of death is ominous—intensive care physicians, for example, have the aphorism "no step forward is a step back." Thus, the background expectations in a particular situation inform the meaning of failure to offer predictions. Physicians' silence tends to be taken to mean that they expect the most likely outcome to come to pass; if physicians say nothing about the future, it suggests that they think things are on course, whether for a favorable or unfavorable outcome.

Differences between Long and Short Survival Horizons

In general, physicians believe in the effectiveness of the self-fulfilling prophecy not only in situations of chronic disease with relatively long expectations for survival but also, more remarkably, in situations involving acute illness and threat of imminent death. There is, however, an important difference in their beliefs about the self-fulfilling prophecy in these two types of situations. In a situation with a relatively long survival horizon (and chronic illness), physicians were more likely to believe in the effectiveness of unfavorable predictions; in a situation with a relatively short survival horizon (and acute illness), they were more likely to believe in the effectiveness of favorable predictions.

This difference between belief in negative and positive self-fulfilling prophecy suggests that physicians find the self-fulfilling prophecy especially effective when the prediction runs *counter to expectations*. Thus, a patient with prostate cancer who is likely to live a reasonably long time is more harmed by an unfavorable prediction than he is helped by a favorable one. Conversely, an intubated patient with a serious pneumonia who has a high chance of dying within a very short period is more helped by a favorable prediction than she is harmed by an unfavorable one. Physicians appear to believe that predictions that are consistent with expectations are less powerful and less effective than those that are inconsistent with expectations.[25]

Physicians explain this somewhat paradoxical result by noting that when predictions are consistent with a patient's illness trajectory, they are less likely to be "influential" with respect to a patient's clinical care, management, and, ultimately, outcome. But predictions that are not consistent with the patient's trajectory are more likely to have an impact. For example, in the case of a chronic disease, the expectation is generally favorable (that is, death is generally not imminent), so unfavorable predictions can be more damaging than favorable ones. One experienced physician described the differential effectiveness of favorable and unfavorable predictions in such a setting as follows:

> If I'm cruising at a given level of care and get neglectful, then the care and quality can fall. And I'm saying that if I'm cruising at the high level I like to think I am, then no matter how much more enthusiastic or optimistic I get, I can't do better than that. So the elbow room on the plus side is much less than the elbow room on the minus side, at least—hopefully—in my practice.

In other words, there is more room for physicians to do worse than there is for them to do better, and the harmful effect may be couched in terms of the impact of predictions on the physician's behavior—a fairly commonly articulated explanation for how the negative self-fulfilling prophecy works. Physicians generally believe that they are providing the best care possible, and fear that an unduly unfavorable outlook could adversely affect their attitudes and behavior and, consequently, the quality of care they deliver. This explanation also highlights another point: whereas physicians are expected to show confidence when it comes to therapy or diagnosis, they are expected to avoid a presumptive, potentially dangerous confidence in prognosis.[26]

Physicians' Attributes Associated with Belief in the Self-Fulfilling Prophecy

In addition to responding to the experimental vignettes, all physicians participating in the survey were asked direct questions about their belief in the effectiveness of predictions. A majority expressed belief in both positive and negative self-fulfilling prophecy: 73 percent believed that "All else being equal, predicting a favorable outcome to a patient can help a favorable outcome come to pass," and 61 percent believed that "All else being equal, predicting an unfavorable outcome to a patient can help an unfavorable outcome come to pass." It is noteworthy that more physicians believed in positive than negative self-fulfilling prophecy. In general, however, those who believed in positive self-fulfilling prophecy were highly likely also to believe in negative self-fulfilling prophecy.

Although the belief in self-fulfilling prophecy is widespread among physicians, it is not uniformly distributed, at least with respect to positive self-fulfilling prophecy. A number of professional and demographic factors are associated with belief in positive—but not negative—self-fulfilling prophecy.[27] Older physicians, with more years in clinical practice, were more likely to believe in the positive self-fulfilling prophecy.[28] Compared to specialists such as oncologists, generalist physicians were much more likely to believe in a positive self-fulfilling prophecy, but did not differ from specialists with respect to negative self-fulfilling prophecy. Gender, board certification (a credential suggesting advanced study and skill), and physicians' belief that their training regarding prognostication was adequate were not associated with belief in either the positive or negative self-fulfilling prophecy. Neither was physicians' feeling that their patients "accept the prognoses" that the physicians offer; this suggests that physicians believe that the self-fulfilling prophecy might work regardless of the patient. Physicians who considered themselves optimists were much more likely to believe that favorable predictions can help to bring about favorable outcomes in their patients.[29]

Finally, physicians who are asked for prognostic information more frequently were less likely to believe in the positive self-fulfilling prophecy. That is, greater exposure to situations calling for prognostication (at least as self-reported) decreases physicians' belief in the effectiveness of positive self-fulfilling prophecy. There are several possible explanations for this impact of greater exposure. Physicians who are asked for prognostic information more frequently may be somehow more "realistic" and thus less likely to believe in the self-fulfilling prophecy. And such physicians may practice in subspecialties, such as oncology or intensive care, where the outcome may be less modifiable by the articulation of a prediction. However, there may be something more here. Physicians practicing in circumstances where they are asked to offer serious prognoses—about how long patients have to live—are under great pressure; they cannot avoid prognosticating since the patient has asked for the information. Under such circumstances, physicians may avoid the unsettling belief that they can alter the outcome of the patient's disease (whether favorably or unfavorably) and are in some way responsible for the outcome. As we shall see, it is professionally threatening when a belief in the self-fulfilling prophecy is coupled with an unavoidable obligation to render a prognosis.

The Danger of Prophecy

Most physicians agree that "it is dangerous to make prognoses in caring for patients." But what specifically do they consider dangerous? And why should prognosis be any more dangerous than diagnosis or therapy? Certainly, one important reason is that prognostication involves dealing with the unknown and with uncertainty. However, the belief that prognostication is dangerous also results partly from a belief in the self-fulfilling prophecy and partly from a belief in the quasi-magical properties of prediction. Physicians tend not to consider diagnosis as dangerous or dreadful except insofar as it implies a prognosis. Indeed, physicians may take intellectual pleasure in cleverly deducing a diagnosis, but they take no such pleasure in prognosis, as noted in chapter 2. Quite the contrary, they are fearful of the casting forth of ideas and possibilities that prognostication represents. Prognosis gives diagnosis its affective component, striking fear in physicians and patients alike.

Insofar as physicians believe that their predictions are effective, it is not surprising that they feel somewhat responsible for patient outcomes. The negative self-fulfilling prophecy raises the frightening prospect that physicians might—through the formulation and articulation of a prognosis, however accurate clinically or probabilistically—harm, or even kill, their patients. The belief in the negative self-fulfilling prophecy

consequently places a powerful constraint on making unfavorable predictions. Belief in the positive self-fulfilling prophecy is only slightly
less of a problem, however, in that it raises the unsettling prospect
that physicians might be expected to cause whatever favorable outcome
they might predict: once again, patients might hold physicians responsible for the outcome. Favorable predictions—whether volunteered by
physicians or elicited by patients—considerably increase the pressure
on physicians. Belief in positive self-fulfilling prophecy raises the possibility that physicians are omnipotent and omniscient—notions that
are both hubristic and frightening. The rendering of prognoses is thus
not benign, for the patient or for the physician, and this is part of what
physicians mean when they say prognostication is dangerous.[30]

The danger is compounded, however, by the possibility of a quasi-
magical direct action of the self-fulfilling prophecy. By "quasi-magical"
I mean that the effectiveness of prediction depends simultaneously
on rational, explainable mechanisms and on nonrational, inscrutable
mechanisms.[31] In this light, the aversion to articulating an unfavorable
prognosis within earshot of the patient can be construed as a form of
"sympathetic taboo" or "negative magic."[32] Certainly, physicians often
offer explicit motives for such behavior, including the desire to preserve
hope in the patient, to avoid injuring the feelings of the patient, and to
protect the physician's reputation for effectiveness. But the prohibition
against articulating unfavorable prognoses may also result from the fear
that the unfavorable utterance might have a quasi-magical effect.

The existence of a latent belief in a magical process in prognostication is not unexpected, because prognosis typically involves both high
stakes in the outcome (for both the patient and physician) and high
uncertainty. As Talcott Parsons has argued:

> The health situation is a classic one of the combination of uncertainty
> and strong emotional interests which produce a situation of strain
> and is very frequently a prominent focus of magic. But the fact that
> the basic cultural tradition of modern medicine is science precludes
> outright magic, which is explicitly non-scientific.[33]

The prohibition against an explicit belief in magic drives beliefs about
a possible direct effectiveness of the self-fulfilling prophecy under the
surface and makes physicians extremely reluctant to admit them. But
they are no less present, transmuted into biases or rituals rather than
magic per se.

This type of magical thinking about prediction is consistent with
certain other behaviors seen in medicine. Renée Fox suggests that "sci-

entific magic" consists of "essentially magical ways of behaving that simulate medical scientific attitudes and behaviors, or that are hidden behind them, and that help physicians and nurses to face problems of uncertainty, therapeutic limitations, and meaning."[34] Fox offers several examples, including ritualized wagering on the outcome of medical interventions and the naming of laboratory animals. Speaking of the latter, Fox argues that this is "an emblematic way of trying to achieve greater control over their experimental situation and, in so doing, to symbolically curtail untoward happenings, reduce 'failure' (especially the death of the animals), and increase the probability of research and clinical success."[35] These forms of scientific magic are ironic, protesting, self-mocking, yet hopeful rituals.

Elaborating on this phenomenon, Fox includes the "ritualization of optimism" as a form of scientific magic, noting

> the tendency of medical practitioners to favor demonstrably vigorous ways to treat patients, and their accentuate-the-positive inclination to be staunchly hopeful and tenaciously confident about the success of their active intervention—even when, and often especially when, a positive outcome is unlikely. Trying hard to "do something" effective about a serious medical problem can have a "self-fulfilling prophecy"-like impact on health professionals, patients, and patients' families alike. Particularly in an energetically melioristic culture like our own, with its "we shall overcome" outlook, it can encourage all concerned to endure, persist, and continue to believe, in ways that can contribute to the stabilization of a patient's condition, to its improvement, and beyond that, to his or her recovery.[36]

The belief in the self-fulfilling prophecy—and perhaps the belief in its quasi-magical effectiveness—is a major determinant of the ritualization of optimism in medicine and, in certain well-defined circumstances, of pessimism as well.

What then is the relation between the quasi-magical means by which prediction might be effective and the danger that prediction poses? The prospect that predictions might fulfill themselves in a quasi-magical way makes them all the more dangerous in that, if they are effective in a nonlogical way, then they are that much harder to understand and to control. Predictions might "take on a life of their own," to quote one physician. Physicians are much less threatened by the prospect that a prediction might lead to changes in a patient's behavior, which then might lead to a fulfillment of the prediction—a mechanism which makes logical sense—than they are by the possibility that the prediction itself, directly and obscurely, might lead to its own fulfillment. Indeed, the three mechanisms of effectiveness of the self-fulfilling prophecy may be ordered from least to most dangerous as follows: the effect on patients, the effect on physicians, and finally the quasi-magical effect. This order reflects a gradient in which the physician's *responsibility* for the patient's outcome steadily increases. It is one thing for physicians' predictions to affect patients (and thus outcomes), another for them to affect the physicians themselves (and thus outcomes), but something else entirely for predictions to affect (and effect) the outcomes directly.

In their thinking about how the self-fulfilling prophecy works, physicians are partaking of a common understanding of causation in which those predicates of an outcome that an actor is able to control are privileged as the *causes*. That is, if several events precede and are related to an outcome (such as the death of a patient), the ones that are at least potentially modifiable by the physician are seen as the ones that cause it. Thus, even if physicians realize that the patient's physiology or behavior are essential to the progression of a disease and a patient's death, they may still consider their own actions as absolutely instrumental.[37] More-over, like all people trying to understand cause and effect, physicians tend to notice the predicates that are seen as "abnormal." Implicitly, therefore, such notions of causation seek to "attribute responsibility and to assign fault in a world of events presumed to be caused by 'free and deliberate' acts by 'conscious and responsible' agents."[38] In such a world, if the physicians' predictions change patients' behavior, the physicians are responsible for the outcome; if their predictions change their own behavior, they are responsible; and if their predictions cause the outcome directly, they are still responsible. These beliefs, in turn, are powerful sources of the professional norms regarding the avoidance of prognosis.

There are two final ways in which prediction is dangerous. One involves the connection of prognosis to death. The effectiveness of pre-diction raises troubling questions for physicians about whether they can cause or prevent, hasten or delay death. Physicians are concerned with what causes death, who causes it, and who might be held responsible for it. They describe making a prediction as being "like handling a bomb," "like navigating the shoals," or as merely "treacherous." Physicians are unsettled by the notion that they have either too much or too little control over death. It is quite understandable that, under such circumstances, professional norms have developed that discourage making predictions and suggest saying nothing about the future.

Finally, the perceived dangers of prediction include not only the danger that physicians feel prediction poses to the patient (e.g., in fostering unfavorable outcomes), but also the danger it poses to physicians' own professional status and feelings of rational control. As we have seen, this threat takes a number of forms, including the feeling that both patients and colleagues will hold prognostic errors against physicians who make predictions.

The Self-Negating Prophecy

Although the survey results suggest that physicians do not in general believe in the self-negating prophecy, some physicians described their belief in this phenomenon. For example, one physician recounted the following example we saw in chapter 3:

> There was a fifty-year-old guy who came in from another hospital with Wegener's disease. . . . By all rights, his mortality approached 100 percent. And after three weeks on the ventilator, . . . it seemed rather hopeless. And we told the family that, and we were entirely ready to start withdrawing support. Then, for whatever reason, in one day, we noticed that all of his chest tubes stopped having air leaks. The very next day, his oxygen requirements turned around and he was requiring much less mechanical ventilation. And within an amazing ten days, he was off the ventilator. And he left the hospital!

It is hard to disentangle such a positive self-negating prophecy from sheer coincidence, especially when the mechanism of action is not specified.[39] Sometimes, however, physicians provide a rationale for the self-negating prophecy. One physician observed that "some patients derive satisfaction from proving their doctors wrong," and he noted that "this can be a very useful means of motivating certain patients." Similarly, sometimes physicians themselves deliberately try to show that a prediction—often one they themselves have made—was wrong, in a sort of test of mettle. For example, one physician described a colleague of his as follows:

> There was one guy in particular in that ICU who thought his mission in life was to save the patient who he thought was going to die. And he did fool me a few times, and salvaged patients that I thought had a very unfavorable prognosis.

The self-negating prophecy also underlies the folkloric tales (discussed in chapter 4) that physicians tell about favorable and unfavorable predictions that turn out to be wrong, as if the prediction brings about its own undoing.

Consequences of the Belief in the Self-Fulfilling Prophecy

The fact that physicians believe in the self-fulfilling prophecy, that this belief is widespread, and that it works in so many different ways, is deeply consequential. Physicians both hope and fear that their predictions will shape patient outcomes. How does this set of beliefs affect how physicians interact with patients and how they view their work?

First, as we have seen, physicians believe that articulating a prognosis is a way to control patients' conduct. This is indeed one of the main ways that the self-fulfilling prophecy is believed to work, and physicians often consciously choose to articulate prognoses—or modify how they articulate prognoses—in order to improve patient compliance. It should be noted that this effect on patient compliance is seen as desirable not only for its presumed salutary impact upon the patient's health, but also in that it supports the doctor's authority.

Beliefs about the self-fulfilling prophecy and its modes of action also have important implications for what physicians communicate to patients, families, and colleagues, and for how they communicate it. The classical reason physicians offer for not communicating bad news to patients is a desire to "protect" the patient. Over the last few decades, this rationale has come under withering criticism as paternalistic and self-serving. But there is another reason that physicians do not communicate unfavorable news: the belief in the self-fulfilling prophecy. This belief helps explain both the withholding of information from patients and the widespread practice of giving different information to the patient and the patient's family.[40] Although these communicative behaviors are a product in part of the difficulty and unpleasantness of sharing bad news with patients, they also reflect a desire to avoid contributing to a patient's decline through the mechanism of the self-fulfilling prophecy. Physicians do not wish to be responsible for patients' deaths, whether through iatrogenesis involving therapy or iatrogenesis involving prognostic pronouncements.

A belief in the self-fulfilling prophecy also strongly contributes to what may be called the "ritualization of optimism."[41] Insofar as physicians believe that favorable predictions can cause favorable outcomes, they naturally shade their prognoses toward the optimistic end of the continuum, favor positive ways of thinking about and interacting with their patients regarding their prognosis and treatment, and choose to say nothing, if possible, rather than offer an unfavorable prediction. Moreover, they have fewer reservations about articulating a favorable prognosis when appropriate, not only because this enhances their feelings of professional effectiveness and relieves the patient's anxiety, but also because they believe that such an articulation directly serves therapeutic objectives and helps the patient. More generally, however, the belief in the self-fulfilling prophecy supports the norm that physicians should avoid prognosticating altogether. Because the self-fulfilling prophecy makes prognostication "dangerous," physicians often have much to lose by making predictions. If physicians did not believe in the self-fulfilling prophecy, they would be much more willing to make and state their predictions.

The asymmetry between belief in the positive and negative self-fulfilling prophecy and also the belief in the special effectiveness of prediction when it is counter to expectations are consonant with physicians' belief in their ability to influence the course of disease. In other words, physicians feel able to alter a future that might otherwise occur, whether favorably or unfavorably. Paradoxically, however, this asymmetry also betrays a professional understanding that there is indeed an intrinsic biology of disease that physicians cannot influence. Disease, such beliefs suggest, does, after all, have an innate course, which is the object of the alteration by the articulated prognosis.

Making predictions—especially given the conviction that they influence the outcome through self-fulfilling prophecy—is a source of role strain and anxiety for physicians. The tension is this: to have optimistic, positive expectations may be hubristic but to have pessimistic and negative ones may indicate helplessness and ill will. On the one hand, physicians are afraid of being omnipotent; on the other, they are afraid of not being powerful enough. The necessity of prognosticating in medical practice can, given physicians' belief in predictions' effectiveness, be seen to conflict with the professional obligation to "do no harm."

Prophecy poses a more general problem for the secularized role of the healer in modern society, however. The reason is that prognosis is usually applied, either manifestly or latently, to a concern that has retained its transcendence, namely death. While the role of the physician has become progressively more secularized in American society, death has retained its mystical and religious properties. To the extent that prognosis is concerned with death, and to the extent that the practice of physicians in general remains concerned with death, the act of prognostication cannot avoid highlighting the ineradicably nonsecular nature of healing. The problematic nature of prediction in modern medicine is only augmented by the dangerous, effective, or even quasi-magical properties that physicians attribute to it. The self-fulfilling prophecy is a troubling aspect of being a physician, and serves as a reminder of the ever-present prophetic dimension of even a modern physician's role, a dimension physicians have not escaped, much as they might wish to.

THE RITUALIZATION OF
OPTIMISM AND PESSIMISM

*The classic time when I shade my prognosis to make it more optimistic
is when I make a diagnosis of Alzheimer's disease. The disease has
such connotations of loss of self, devastation, complete dependence,
death in a special care unit of a nursing home. It's got so much
baggage around it, it's like the cancer of the 90s. So, while I would
never say, "Oh, this is a wonderful disease. I'm so happy about it," I
do try to frame a notion of what we're doing now and what's to come.
And just talking about Alzheimer's disease in a rational way can cool
people off. I try to talk optimistically about Alzheimer's disease, and
demystify it.*

— GERIATRICIAN

Physicians are supposed to positively influence human experiences that
are as common as they are immutable and transcendent: birth, illness,
suffering, death. Physicians and patients alike attach great existential
and moral significance to these experiences; the stakes in their outcomes
are high. As Renée Fox has argued:

> However familiar and routine [medical work] may be, or seemingly
> unthreatening and non-tragic, no medical action that involves a pa-
> tient is trivial or completely ordinary. Below their scientific surface,
> medical acts and events intersect with the human condition of pa-
> tients and their relatives, and of medical professionals themselves—
> with some of their most profound aspirations, hopes, and fulfill-
> ments; their deepest worries, anxieties, and fears.[1]

Further complicating the position of the physician is the high degree
of uncertainty about these serious concerns. Physicians confront situations that have transcendent meaning, involve important outcomes,
and manifest considerable uncertainty—and in all this, the physician is
supposed to make a difference.

What is more, physicians are supposed to be able to make prognoses
about these concerns. The necessity of prediction in uncertain circumstances is a distinctive stress associated with physicians' work. How
do physicians cope with this uncertainty? One way, as we have seen,
is simply to avoid prediction altogether. But when avoidance is neither
possible nor desirable, they use strategies such as being optimistic and

speaking in statistical generalities. However, physicians need ways not only to develop and communicate prognoses, but also to cope with their stressfulness and uncertainty. That is, physicians respond to the need to prognosticate on two levels: the practical level of actually making and communicating the prediction and a more symbolic level that addresses the importance and meaning of prediction. They cope with the stress of prognosticating, especially with the uncertainty it entails, by adopting one of two strategies: the *ritualization of optimism* or, under certain specific circumstances, the *ritualization of pessimism*.

By "ritualization," I mean that the prognostic behavior manifested by physicians, along with its attendant communication and consequent actions, is systematic, widespread, socially patterned, and symbolically meaningful. In general, behavior is ritualized partly to fulfill a specific purpose, whether implicit or explicit; this is indeed the case in the ritualization of optimism or pessimism in medical prognostication. But behavior is also ritualized partly to fulfill a symbolic function. With respect to prognosis, ritualization serves to reaffirm both physicians' decisions and professional role and certain underlying social values. The ritualization of optimism *stands for* the favorable outcome of the patient's problem and for the effectiveness and knowledge of the physician. The ritualization of pessimism *stands for* an unfavorable outcome and for the powerlessness (and thus exculpation) of the physician. And both serve, in a symbolic though illusory fashion, to provide certainty where there is none—for the patient and the doctor.

The process of ritualization serves a redressive function even when the object of the ritual is not attained. That is, while people may engage in ritual acts with some specific purpose in mind (such as when physicians make a prediction in order to choose a therapy), the true purpose of the ritual may be subserved by the mere performance of the acts. Ritualization, in short, is the transformation of ideological and idealized social norms into emotionally felt individual desires. To borrow anthropologist Clifford Geertz's phrase, it fuses "the world as lived and the world as imagined."[2]

The emergence of such patterned mechanisms to cope with unpredictability—notwithstanding the strongly scientific and logico-rational orientation of modern medicine—is not surprising. The situation faced by physicians when caring for patients is analogous to other situations that involve high stakes for the participants as well as a considerable amount of uncertainty. The prototypic examples of this were provided by anthropologist Bronislaw Malinowski in his study of how the Trobriand Islanders engaged in activities such as gardening and fishing.

The outcome of these activities can clearly be strongly influenced by the application of practical knowledge and hard work. But it is nevertheless possible—indeed, it is common—that the play of chance might eclipse such efforts. Malinowski observed that:

> [The islander's] experience has taught him . . . that in spite of all his forethought and beyond all his efforts there are agencies and forces which one year bestow unwonted and unearned benefits or fertility, making everything run smooth and well, rain and sun appear at the right moment, noxious insects remain in abeyance, the harvest yields a superabundant crop; and another year again the same agencies bring ill-luck and bad chance, pursue him from beginning till end and thwart all his most strenuous efforts and his best-founded knowledge.[3]

How did the islanders cope with the influence of these "agencies" and the resultant uncertainty? They used magical rituals. Indeed, Malinowski argues that the function of magic is to address the impact of uncertainty on human actions directed at practical goals. Malinowski showed that the Trobriand Islanders used magic for deep-sea fishing (which involved voyages out to the open sea, considerable danger, and uncertain success) but *not* for lagoon fishing (where their technical knowledge and expertise were adequate and success was more certain). Only when their science was inadequate to the magnitude and uncertainty of the task did they turn to magic.

In thinking about the role of magic in contending with the uncertainty inherent in human action, Malinowski was primarily concerned with the way magic serves to "ritualize man's optimism, to enhance his faith in the victory of hope over fear [and to express] the greater value . . . of confidence over doubt, of steadfastness over vacillation, and of optimism over pessimism."[4] It is hard to imagine, in circumstances similar to those Malinowski considered, that a situation of high stakes and high uncertainty could exist in which the normative social response would be anything other than the ritualization of optimism—because people are ordinarily invested in the salutary outcome of their efforts. However, in modern medicine, circumstances involving a ritualization of *pessimism* also arise.

The Ritualization of Optimism

When they must formulate or communicate a prognosis, physicians certainly tend to favor optimism, which they justify on the basis of practical utility: optimism is useful both to patients and to physicians. For patients, it can promote health.[5] Physicians appreciate this fact, but may also encourage optimism to avoid unpleasantness and to keep patients happy and compliant. For example, one study of fifty-one oncologists revealed that more than 75 percent believed that a "positive attitude" affects outcomes in both early and late stages of cancer, affects whether patients experience complications, and affects how patients view their doctors.[6] Given such beliefs about the benefits of positive thinking, 88 percent of these physicians "usually made an effort to change their patients' attitudes to a more optimistic view" with respect to their disease. These physicians gave several specific reasons for encouraging optimism, including enhancing patients' ability to tolerate adversity (63 percent), making them easier to manage (24 percent), and improving the doctor-patient relationship (31 percent). Physicians frequently use optimism quite consciously; in another study, 75 percent of physicians reported that they find it "helpful to shade their prognoses to the positive.[7] Optimism preserves hope, provides encouragement, fosters treatment, and engenders confidence.

But the optimism we are considering here transcends the foregoing, in terms of degree, scope, and function. Ritualized optimism is the favorable outlook held by physicians in spite of, and as a result of, the uncertainty inherent in the patient's predicament—and often in spite of, or even as a result of, evidence suggesting an unfavorable prognosis. This outlook, ritualized on both cognitive and behavioral levels, states: "When in doubt, suspect recovery, and act accordingly." This is an optimism about the future that is out of proportion to the objective reality of the case. It is an optimism that has origins apart from the patient's physiology and that serves different purposes than simply recounting the clinical truth. Physicians not only communicate prognosis optimistically but *internalize* this perspective. This optimism, in other words, penetrates to a deeper level of physicians' attitudes and behavior than just the superficial aspects of how they communicate prognoses. And it has deeper symbolism.

As with the Trobriand Islanders, physicians are especially likely to ritualize optimism when the stakes and the uncertainty are high, and when they are not sure whether their technical or scientific know-how is adequate to the challenge. Uncertain prognoses may both permit and demand optimism.

In addition to physicians' need to cope with uncertainty, one of the most fundamental causes of the ritualization of optimism is their belief in the self-fulfilling prophecy. Insofar as physicians believe that favorable predictions can cause favorable outcomes, they will—especially when the situation is sufficiently uncertain as to leave open a range of possible outcomes—tend to shade their prognoses toward the favorable end of that spectrum. Physicians offer a favorable prognosis not only if they believe that such an outcome seems certain but also if it seems uncertain, because they believe that offering such a prognosis actually serves therapeutic purposes. Physicians who believe in the positive or negative self-fulfilling prophecy are approximately twice as likely as those who do not to shade their prognoses to the positive.[8] Moreover, in keeping with Malinowski's conception, physicians who find it troubling to make prognoses when either the stakes or the uncertainty in a situation are high are also approximately twice as likely to shade their prognoses to the positive. When the future is at risk, physicians are generally more likely to be optimistic than pessimistic.

The thoroughgoing impact of optimism is illustrated in the way one physician handled the prognosis of a breast cancer patient:

> I was able to communicate the prognosis in honest terms when I first saw her a few years ago. "There is no denying the fact that you have breast cancer. There is no denying the fact that your breast cancer, despite very good early treatment, has unfortunately done what a lot of breast cancer does: it has spread and become metastatic. That means that there is no longer any standard treatment that can cure your breast cancer. So what we're left with, then, is a disease which by any modern medical standards is incurable. All that is true. But that doesn't mean that there's nothing we can do about the breast cancer. We can find drugs or combinations of drugs and see if we're successful in stopping the progression of the disease. You know it's in your bones, but it has not yet moved, so far as we know, to any solid organs." And I talked to her about my view of metastatic cancer— even her own metastatic cancer—as being a kind of chronic disease. A chronic disease which has a better prognosis than some chronic diseases, and a worse prognosis than other chronic diseases.
>
> Then, about a year ago when her cancer first appeared in her liver, I said that this was the first solid organ involvement that we knew about. The fact that it now had a metastatic deposit in the liver indicated that the disease was progressing despite our efforts at chemotherapy, and that meant that we had to rethink the therapy program. But again, knowing what I knew about my patient, I told her all of this, since it was true, but I used the information to plan the next step in the treatment and the management, *not* to say something like: "This is further evidence that your disease is terminal and that you'll be dead in twelve or eighteen months." It's been a little over a year since we found the liver metastases, and we came up with

an interesting new combination of drugs. And she's done extremely well. Liver function remains normal; the two liver metastases that we spotted a year ago have not disappeared, but they have regressed in size somewhat. And we're continuing.

So I don't think I've ever lied to this lady, or deceived her even in terms of the prognosis that she has a disease which is progressive and which is incurable. I've repeated these facts to her, but I've not used numbers or days to hammer the point home. I've avoided doing this in part because others had done so before and had generated such a negative, hostile response from her. It was not what she wanted to hear. It's not that she wants to be deceived, or that I deceived her, but that the way you offer prognosis, what you mean by prognostication, seems to me to include a broad spectrum of prediction.

This physician's optimistic reframing of what, in more objective terms, is an extraordinarily bad prognosis (breast cancer metastatic to bone and liver, unresponsive to chemotherapy)—a fact the physician recognized on one level by using terms like "incurable," "terminal," and "progressive"—affects his interaction with this patient and his choice of treatment. The physician is clearly choosing words carefully and optimistically, a technique we have identified in other such conversations. But the physician goes beyond this and volunteers that he has internalized his own "view" of metastatic cancer as being a chronic disease.[9] The physician's optimism here not only colors how he communicates the prognosis but permeates his management of the case and his very conception of the disease. The ominous metastases in the liver are "deposits," the patient's impending death is on a "spectrum" of possible outcomes, the toxic drug therapy is "interesting," and the patient has done "extremely well."

The extent to which physicians internalize, and act on, such optimistic perceptions is also evident in studies comparing physicians' predictions about the survival of terminally ill patients to actual outcomes. As we saw in chapter 3, the predictions showed a systematic and substantial optimistic bias, and doctors who knew their patients better, saw them more often, or knew them longer, more commonly overestimated patient survival. It would seem that when physicians are invested in the outcome of their activities, when the "stakes" are especially high, they tend to favor especially optimistic beliefs in a setting of uncertainty. A similar pattern is seen in physicians' estimates of the success of cardiopulmonary resuscitation; whereas survival to hospital discharge after this intervention is in fact 10 to 20 percent overall, American physicians estimate it to be about 40 percent.[10]

The ritualization of optimism in prognosis is thus overdetermined. It results not only from the belief in the self-fulfilling prophecy, the desire to influence patients and their disease, and the expectations patients have regarding what is told to them. It also results from a professional desire to maintain control over the patient's clinical course, both by encouraging patients to follow the doctor's recommendations and by bolstering physicians' perceptions of their own effectiveness. Making favorable predictions reinforces physicians' perceptions that they can and will cure the patient, as they are trained and socialized to do. Among other things, the ritualization of optimism in physicians' attitudes and practices symbolically stands for their ability to positively shape the future when it is uncertain and when the stakes are high.

The Ritualization of Pessimism

Sometimes, however, physicians are willing to communicate pessimism in their prognoses. For example, 35 percent of internists report that they sometimes find it useful to "shade their prognoses to the negative."[11] And most physicians admit to finding pessimism helpful in some circumstances. On the other hand, there are practical problems with being deliberately pessimistic, namely, it is unpleasant to give bad news to patients, patients might become distressed, or patients might leave their physician.

Nevertheless, physicians recognize the practical and symbolic utility of pessimism, again, in circumstances of prognostic uncertainty, especially when the stakes are the life or death of the patient. Under such circumstances, optimism or neutrality may exact an unacceptably high price, because physicians believe that an unduly favorable prediction is more professionally threatening than an unduly unfavorable one. Unexpectedly bad outcomes after favorable predictions make physicians feel that they have made a mistake.[12] One physician described the situation as follows:

> When something unexpectedly good happens, I think that it is to the patient's good and I think, really, that even though I've said that maybe this is going to be a severe illness or something, and then it doesn't turn out to be that, I guess I'm glad that it doesn't turn out to be that. But, if I think something good is going to happen and it turns into something bad, I feel that somehow I've made a *very bad mistake* which has not been to my benefit and not to the patient's benefit. Moreover, when something unexpectedly bad happens, I question my clinical abilities. When that happens, it's always very humbling.

The belief that unexpectedly bad outcomes call physicians' clinical abilities into question, whereas unexpectedly good ones do not, strongly discourages giving favorable prognoses, and thus discourages optimism in prognosis. Consequently, physicians may use pessimism to prepare themselves, their patients, and their patients' families for what is to come.

When both the stakes and uncertainty are high, being pessimistic is perceived by physicians as in some ways a no-lose strategy. As one physician noted, "It is of use to be optimistic, but *professionally* it may often be better to be pessimistic because if the outcome proves poor, the outcome is not unexpected; and if the outcome proves good, you are a hero." Another explained: "It's much easier to explain a situation in which a patient recovers unexpectedly than vice-versa. If one is pessimistic, the patients are more grateful if a good outcome occurs and more accepting if it doesn't." Physicians refer to this technique as "hanging crepe," a reference to the black crepe that used to be hung at funerals, and deliberate pessimism is thereby presented as a means of preparing the patient for death.[13] Hanging crepe thus converts an uncertain situation fraught with risk into one that is regarded as less problematic: if the patient does poorly, the physician may conveniently avoid not only self-doubt about professional effectiveness but also recriminations by the patient and the patient's family. Many physicians cite the possibility of a lawsuit in cases of unexpected, unfavorable outcomes, and they note that it is therefore prudent to be pessimistic. Conversely, if a gravely ill patient does well after a pessimistic prediction, the physician gets credit for his rescue. Thus, when the prognosis is uncertain and the stakes are high, physicians may find it convenient to err on the side of pessimism.

Pessimistic predictions are driven by more than the protection of professional self-interest, however. Physicians note that pessimism is especially useful if they have practical objectives that might, in fact, be clinically beneficial to patients. A prototypic and common example is if they wish to withdraw or withhold life support or to persuade a patient to forego resuscitation should it be needed (that is, to establish "do not resuscitate," or DNR, status).[14] Prior to reaching such a point, physicians may have displayed considerable optimism in the care of the patient; but a change in objectives calls for a change in outlook. A pessimistic prediction in such circumstances serves at least two purpose. First, it helps to enlist patient and family support for the proposed action. And second, it protects the physician's self-perception by assuaging the physician's guilt about withdrawing life support, by configuring the unfavorable outcome in the particular patient as aberrant or inevitable, and by distancing the physician from the notion that his actions are causing a patient's death.

A young physician with considerable ICU experience gave a typical description of the ritualized use of pessimism:

> In a person who is doing so terribly that I think the situation is hopeless, if the family doesn't understand and they still have all these hopeful, hopeful questions and haven't heard what I have said, then I go a step further and I make it even worse. Not that I lie about the situation at all. But I actually tell them in more graphic detail exactly what's wrong. And I make some predictions for them. If they say, "Yes, I want my family member resuscitated," and if I clearly know that person is going to die, whether they are resuscitated or not, and if I am as near 100 percent certain as I can be that I can predict this, then I will tell the family member exactly what resuscitative efforts include. And if it hasn't sunk in, I can tell them even further. I go through a scenario with them in detail. Not in true morbid fashion, but I make them understand exactly what it is to be resuscitated. How almost futile it is to do that, to pursue that route. I even at times go on to both sympathize and empathize with them, saying that if it was my grandfather, I would not do that.

This account is typical in its inclusion of the following elements: the deliberate exaggeration of the unfavorableness of the prognosis, the use of graphic detail that would generally be withheld, the use of bluntness that is ordinarily condemned by physicians, the review of what resuscitation is really like (as compared with its generally favorable presentation in the popular media), and the reference to the decision the physician would make if this were a member of his own family.[15] Most patients succumb to such an onslaught. This physician, however, like the one cited earlier discussing his patient with breast cancer, is at pains to characterize his approach as not being deceitful or mendacious. For them, this type of attitude and behavior is not about veracity; rather, it transcends the facts of the case and becomes about their function as a physician and about their patients' experience.

In short, the ritualization of pessimism seeks to normalize expected failure. Whereas the ritualization of optimism expresses the belief in the primacy of hope over destiny, the ritualization of pessimism expresses the belief in the primacy of destiny over action.

Balancing Optimism and Pessimism

Though optimism predominates in prognosis, physicians employ both optimism and pessimism as means of handling unpredictability. Physicians' belief that they can, after all, do something for their patients, their belief in the self-fulfilling prophecy, and their desire to encourage patients all militate toward optimism when physicians must render a prognosis, especially in uncertain circumstances. Conversely, the threatening nature of unexpectedly unfavorable outcomes and professional disapproval of favorable predictions that are seen as hubristic militate toward pessimism. One physician reflected on the complexity of these decisions as follows:

> In making a prognosis, there is always the fear of giving false hope. You don't want to give false hope and say, "Everything is going to be OK." You want the patient's family to know—you want to be honest with them—that things look very, very bad. But I guess you don't want to be wrong, so you're not going to say that the patient is going to die either—even if you know the patient will. It's a fine line. You want to give just enough hope, but not too much. You want to be honest and you don't want to be wrong.

Physicians may thus be pulled in opposite directions, and they need to carefully decide whether optimism or pessimism is in order in rendering prognoses when the patient's condition is uncertain and when both would seem reasonable.

The ritualization of optimism in medicine calls for an aggressive interventionist stance consistent with physicians' socialization, with professional norms dictating active effort to confront disease, with institutional and bureaucratic exigencies, and with cultural expectations. Conversely, the ritualization of pessimism generally (but by no means always) occurs in situations wherein the intention is to stop treating the patient. Such circumstances call for a minimalist stance on the part of physicians, in keeping with physicians' recognition that they are indeed not omnipotent and should not be expected to be so.[16]

Factors other than the valence or relative certainty of the prognosis may also elicit these behavioral and cognitive strategies. It is not simply a matter of optimism being applied when the most likely outcome is favorable (despite the uncertainty) and pessimism when the most likely outcome is unfavorable (again, despite the uncertainty), in a sort of reinforcing, augmentative fashion. When deciding whether to communicate optimism or pessimism, physicians are also influenced by their own clinical objectives, by the type of person to whom they are speaking, by the patient's explicit predictions, and by characteristics of the patient. Because all of these factors may be independent of the patient's true prognosis, the actual communication of prognostic information and its shading to one or the other extreme may symbolically reflect certain further needs and values.

The clinical objectives at hand are a strong determinant of whether physicians are optimistic or pessimistic in their formulation and communication of prognoses. As we have seen, a desire to stop life support for a patient with an unfavorable prognosis may elicit systematically pessimistic prognostication. Conversely, a patient who is ambivalent about the risks and benefits of chemotherapy may be encouraged to take the drugs if the physician makes optimistic predictions. In addition, optimism may be used to keep the patient sufficiently happy that he continues in the care of the physician, which might benefit the physician professionally, financially, or emotionally. Thus, the choice between pessimism and optimism is influenced by objectives that may have only a slight relationship to the patient's true prognosis. In short, physicians make decisions not only about whether to offer a prognosis at all but also about its valence, and they may shade their prognoses to serve therapeutic objectives or, more generally, to get the patient to conform with their views.

The person to whom the physician is communicating the prognosis also strongly influences whether the physician expresses optimism or pessimism. The same expected outcome can be cast in altogether different lights depending on whether they are interacting with patients, families, or colleagues. Moreover, as we saw in chapter 5, patients' own predictions about their disease also influence whether physicians are optimistic or pessimistic, though in variable and complex ways. For example, many physicians adopt the strategy of counterbalancing patients' expectations; others reinforce patient perceptions. In either case, the patients' expectations are an important, and at times determinative, factor with respect to the optimism or pessimism that physicians have and communicate.

Finally, patient social attributes, such as age or parental status, constitute an important heuristic for choosing between optimism and pessimism in a situation of prognostic uncertainty. Youth or responsibility for a family may raise the stakes, increasing both the patient's and the physician's investment in the outcome, and so encourage optimism. For example, one physician described her behavior as follows:

I had a forty-year-old female patient with sarcoid [an unusual immunological condition] that affected her brain, and she had skin and bone infections as a result of it as well. She was just a disaster and was in the hospital for four months. And everybody thought for sure that this woman would never, ever leave the hospital. That she'd never unspike [return to normal body temperature], that she'd develop antibiotic-resistant germs, that she couldn't have physical therapy, couldn't have her wound handled, couldn't have this stuff done. I thought in my heart that she probably wouldn't get out of the hospital.

However, this is one of those examples where I thought it was worth it, in a young woman who had two children whom she primarily supports at home, to get her a specialist consultant from Johns Hopkins. And to make a long story short, she's better. She's at home with her kids. And she's been out of the hospital for over a year.

Despite initially making a prediction for her own use that this patient "probably wouldn't get out of the hospital," this physician decided that she should be optimistic and act as if she had rendered a favorable prediction because the patient was young and responsible for two children. In acting this way, the physician believes that she had a salutary impact and was vindicated in her actions. Another physician makes a similar point:

Whether I am optimistic or pessimistic totally depends on the scenario. Right now we have a situation in the intensive care unit with a twenty-four-year-old. She has Wegener's [an immunological condition that affects the lungs and kidneys], and she's doing terribly. Every day that she is alive is a small miracle. By all rights she should be dying. I fully expect that she will die. There is nothing that we can do to bring her back. But I hope I'm wrong. She is *twenty-four.* She's not a ninety-five-year-old woman who's been through multiple hospitalizations or admissions, or even had a full life. She is a twenty-four-year-old woman with a family and a little daughter.

There are two things going on with the family. Every day I see them I tell them that every day she's in this situation is not a day of stability but a day that a step backwards has been taken. A day she's not getting better is a day she's getting worse. Because that is truly what it is in the unit. And, you know, they still ask me, "Is there a chance?" and I still say, "Yes."

Asked if he would still say yes if the patient were older, the doctor continues:

No I wouldn't. I would say, "No." I would say, "Probably not," "Almost certainly no." I would not say, "Definitively no," because,

again, I can't say that. "Almost certainly no." But she's twenty-four,
so I say yes. I say she's getting worse everyday, but I say, "Yes, there
is a chance that she will get better."

The patient's age and serious condition distress this physician so much
that he cultivates optimism about the patient's chances for recovery. One
has the sense that the physician wishes to delude even himself.[17]

Both the ritualization of optimism and the ritualization of pessimism
are means of handling uncertainty, though the two strategies often serve
countervailing purposes. Uncertainty that cannot be resolved by scientific and technical means is resolved by symbolic means: the ritualization
of optimism fosters a symbolic *connection* between physicians' actions
and favorable outcomes, and the ritualization of pessimism fosters a
symbolic *disconnection* between physicians' actions and unfavorable
outcomes. When the patient is young, for example, ritualized optimism
symbolizes the physicians' commitment to caring for the patient and
hope that the patient will recover. When the goal is, say, the withdrawal
of life support, ritualized pessimism symbolizes physicians' recognition
of their limitations and their fear that the patient will not recover. The
heuristics for choosing between optimism and pessimism all connect the
expression of optimism to other socially meaningful objectives, whether
they be the sanctity of young life or the effectiveness of physicians,
further confirming the symbolic importance of these practices.

The choice between optimism and pessimism is thus an implicit
reflection of social values. Physicians sometimes realize this and observe
that "it comes down to one's personal values as to how to best prognosticate." One way to cope with the problematic nature of such value
judgments is to let the patient make the decision; this, after all, is what
physicians do when they base their choice of optimism or pessimism
on what patients say about the prognosis. Another way is to avoid
prediction altogether.

More generally, the coexistence of optimism and pessimism illustrates Robert Merton's discussion of the ambivalence within social roles.
As Merton argues, paired norms and counternorms may evolve as
social devices for helping people in certain social positions cope with
the contingencies they face in trying to fulfill (potentially conflicting)
functions: "This is not merely a matter of social psychology but of role-
structure. Potentially conflicting norms are built into the social definition
of roles that provide for normatively acceptable alternations of behavior
as the state of a social relation changes. This is a major basis for that oscillation between differing role-requirements that makes for sociological

ambivalence."[18] The ritualization of optimism and the ritualization of pessimism thus may exist simultaneously in the medical profession, in individual physicians, and even in individual cases, and can serve as a particularly powerful inducer of ambivalence and hence strain.

Moreover, the processes of optimism and pessimism are not as oppositional as they might at first appear. Both are rooted in uncertainty: the future course of a patient's illness cannot be known but a prediction must be made. So cognitive mechanisms that support and influence the physicians' perspective and hopes are called into play. These mechanisms bring meaning and order to this otherwise uncertain domain.

Complementary Approaches to Diagnosis and Prognosis

In coping with uncertainty in *diagnosis*, physicians have an institutionalized norm of preferring to judge a well patient to be sick over judging a sick patient to be well.[19] In short, "When in doubt, suspect illness." This pessimistic bias serves several useful purposes—not the least of which is an enforced vigilance. Describing this suspicious attitude about diagnostic possibilities, one experienced physician observed:

> I've always been interested in obscure fevers and have written some things about them. I've got a tendency to think of malignant disease as a cause of such fevers without very good grounds for it, and I often say to the housestaff that we've got to be sure this isn't a cancer in the pancreas or somewhere that we haven't found. I have overdiagnosed malignant disease a good many times. I don't know why it is. It's a quirk of mine to look at things from a bad standpoint sometimes.

Pessimistic bias in diagnosis is widespread.[20] Yet, with the important exceptions discussed above, physicians appear overall to have a complementary, optimistic bias in prognosis: in short, as we have seen, "When in doubt, suspect recovery." Among other purposes, this complementary attitude may indeed correct for the pessimistic bias in diagnosis. Patients are judged to be sicker than they are but are reassured that they will get better than they might.

Both of these perspectives are consistent with the professional role of the physician in society: the approach to diagnosis suggests that there is something for physicians to do (sickness abounds), the approach to prognosis, that there is something they can do (recoveries are possible). These beliefs both support the need for, and the effectiveness of, physicians. Diagnostic pessimism is a consequence of vigilance and prognostic optimism a consequence of hope.

Physicians learn in their training that they are more culpable if they dismiss a sick patient than they are if they retain a well one; with respect to diagnosis, they should err on the side of unduly *unfavorable* assessments. In prognosis the case is largely the reverse. Physicians judge other physicians to be poorer clinicians if they predict an unduly unfavorable outcome than if they predict an unduly favorable outcome. With respect to prognosis, physicians should err on the side of unduly *favorable* assessments.

Optimism and the Therapeutic Imperative

Despite the benefits of the ritualization of optimism, it may have adverse consequences. Physicians facing prognostic uncertainty may systematically assume that patients are likely to live longer than they are and, acting on this assumption, may overuse or misuse certain treatments. Prognostic optimism may reinforce the already strong imperative in the medical profession to treat patients at all costs. This imperative leads physicians to overrate the success of their interventions, to overlook side effects of treatments, to prefer certain responses to therapy over others, and to favor demonstrably vigorous treatments.

The problem of timing the referral of terminally ill patients for hospice care illustrates one way ingrained optimism may lead to detrimental consequences. Hospice referral is one of the few clinical decisions in modern medical practice in which a concrete intervention explicitly hinges on a prognostic assessment. Hospice is a type of terminal care whose primary goal is to mitigate patients' physical and mental pain and suffering; referral usually entails a switch in the management of a patient from a primarily curative to a primarily palliative approach. Hospice care, which is generally provided by trained nurses who visit a patient's home, has several advantages over traditional, hospital-based terminal care: it facilitates at-home death,[21] optimizes pain relief,[22] is cost-effective,[23] and is associated with greater patient and family satisfaction.[24]

Partly in anticipation of such advantages, Medicare started covering hospice care in 1982; by 1997 over a quarter of a million beneficiaries were receiving hospice care annually, and persons covered by Medicare constitute approximately 75 to 80 percent of all hospice patients in the United States.[25] According to Medicare regulations, a person is eligible for the hospice benefit only if the patient's doctor and the hospice medical director certify that the patient is "terminally ill," that is, that "the individual has a medical prognosis that the individual's life expectancy is six months or less."[26] By electing the hospice benefit, beneficiaries waive all rights to Medicare payment for curative treatment of their terminal condition; in exchange, they receive noncurative medical and support services, many of which would not otherwise be covered.

To reap the maximum benefit from hospice care, then, the decision to refer a patient should be properly timed. Unfortunately, research has shown that the decision to refer is not always made optimally—many patients die quite soon after referral, and, conversely, some live for quite a long time after referral.[27] Such "inappropriate" stays may have adverse experiential, clinical, and financial implications for patients. On the one hand, if patients are referred to hospice too early, they may forgo potentially beneficial therapy aimed at curing their disease.[28] On the other hand, if they are referred too late, they may experience a death that is needlessly painful or problematic. Overall, late referrals are more common: most patients die within about a month after the initiation of hospice care, and many receive hospice care for only a few days before their deaths.[29]

Some editorialists, concerned especially with the problem of late referral, have remarked that "in the absence of objective criteria, the only patients referred to the hospice may be those who are so obviously close to death that the hospice's palliative care will be offered too late."[30] These concerns are justified, as we have seen. Excessive prognostic optimism may thus deprive patients of optimal access to advantageous hospice services. Similarly, excessive optimism about the prospects of critically ill patients may lead to an overuse of life support technology, possibly to their detriment.

Thus, the ritualization of optimism, although useful in many respects, can also have negative effects. It may lead physicians and patients to make choices that are ultimately harmful to patients and their families. At its starkest, too much optimism near the end of life may mean patients never see the end coming, never prepare for it, and fight vainly against it. Although optimism may symbolize the role of hope over destiny, it should not lead to the supplanting of destiny by desire.

Eight

A DUTY TO PROGNOSTICATE

The words coming out of my mouth feel like a proclamation. They can make things happen. Prognoses are powerful. They can be helpful or harmful, and good physicians know this. They should feel responsible and should act responsibly.

— EXPERIENCED GENERAL INTERNIST

A view of life that casts events as either random or predetermined makes the world uncontrollable, experience meaningless, and events amoral. But in an indeterministic world—one in which at least some elements of the future can be *purposefully* realized—the future and statements about it are controllable, meaningful, and moral.

Prognostication in seriously ill patients has moral overtones, which, coupled with the various functions of prognosis in medical practice, cast the physician in the role of a prophet. The similarity between prognosis and prophecy is illuminating because it further highlights the nontechnical and interpersonal aspects of prognostication. As a form of prophecy, prognosis is morally, and not merely biologically or even socially, encoded. As a consequence, physicians may be seen to have an obligation to prognosticate and to do so as accurately and empathetically as possible. There is a moral duty *in* prognostication and a moral duty *to* prognosticate. This duty can be supported by—but should not be delegated to—either patients themselves or statistical protocols. Thus, the avoidance of prognosis represents the shirking not only of a clinical but also of a moral responsibility, a responsibility that pertains both to individual physicians and to the profession as a whole.

Prophecy and Morality

Prognosis resembles prophecy in its functional, structural, and symbolic uses, through which prognostication transcends being merely a technical part of medical care and becomes a creative and meaningful act for patients and physicians alike. Prognoses often carry the implication that their articulation can change the future and bring about the desired end. This theoretical and metaphorical argument about the resemblance of prognosis to prophecy in turn has practical implications for how we regard physicians' role obligations.

Prognosis, as we have seen, serves numerous *functional* purposes. It influences physicians' decisions about whether and how to conduct diagnostic evaluations, administer therapy, or communicate information. Deliberate prognostication is also a means of coping with unpredictability, working to decrease uncertainty and to make collective action possible.[1] That is, prognosis forms a basis for planning: like a shared value system, the collective foretelling of the future stabilizes and integrates the behavior of individuals.[2] Finally, insofar as it offers a sense of control and foreknowledge, the act of prognostication may be a source of reassurance, satisfying the fundamental need to convert an insubstantial and uncertain future into a concrete and certain, even if undesirable, one. In short, like prophecy, prognosis influences—or is believed to influence—present behavior, future outcomes, or both.[3]

Prognosis can also serve a *structural* purpose supporting a hierarchical relationship between patients and physicians. Predictions that prove true (or that are believed to have proven true) may reinforce a belief in the predictor's understanding of the world and bolster claims to authority by individual physicians and the medical profession as a whole. This effect highlights the differing positions and perspectives of the patient and the doctor. In articulating a vision of the future, a zone of authority is mapped out and a set of ideas is endorsed. The physician doing the predicting is either suggesting or demanding that the patient conform with a particular perspective and act in a particular way.

The hierarchical nature of the relationship becomes obvious when the patient actively solicits a prognosis from the doctor. In so doing, the patient acknowledges the expertise and the authority of the physician. Patients intend, after hearing the prediction, to act accordingly, that is, with deference to the prediction.[4] The relationship between physician and patient is no less hierarchical, however, when the patient does not actively solicit a prediction and when the physician asserts his authority unilaterally, an authority that in large measure rests on superior training and knowledge. Insofar as physicians are better able to predict the outcome of a patient's disease than the patient or any other professional or occupational group, physicians' authority is maintained.[5] Professing knowledge of the future may even become a basis for claims to expertise and authority in other areas of medical practice. Such a use of foretelling in medicine has been appreciated since ancient times; Hippocrates, for example, remarks:

> It seems to be highly desirable that a physician should pay much attention to prognosis. If he is able to tell his patients when he visits

them not only about their past and present symptoms, but also to tell them what is going to happen, as well as to fill in the details they have omitted, he will increase his reputation as a medical practitioner and people will have no qualms in putting themselves under his care.[6]

Prognosis thus becomes a "weapon in the struggle for public recognition."[7]

Predictions need not be falsifiable for a claim to authority to be made by a physician or respected by a patient. Authority and status may arise from the act of prediction itself. Indeed, there is a reciprocal relation between prediction and authority: authority is accorded to those who make predictions (especially predictions that prove accurate); conversely, prediction is the prerogative of those with authority. In some sense, the authority of the foreteller is separate from the factual rightness or wrongness of the prediction. Thus, the relationship between doctor and patient that prognostication creates is analogous to that between prophet and supplicant. It can be seen as an example of an archetypal relationship in social systems, one involving complementary roles in which each participant's actions define the other's.[8]

Beyond its functional and structural roles, prognosis may also provide a *symbolic* medium for the expression of profound wishes, hopes, and expectations, as well as the confrontation of uncontrollability, meaninglessness, and randomness. The expression of a specific vision of the future helps fulfill—even if only in an illusory fashion—the human desire to avoid failure and to achieve success.[9] In both its content and form, prognosis lends meaning to patients' experience of illness. With respect to content, prognostication can symbolize the recovery of the patient, the scrutability of the illness, or the competence of the doctor. With respect to form, predictive speech has two key axes that have symbolic meaning: ambiguity versus clarity and optimism versus pessimism. Ambiguity may symbolize the uncertainty inherent in the world; it reflects the gap between expectation and outcome and the limits of human knowledge. Optimism in the expression of a prognosis may be symbolic of hope, and pessimism symbolic of destiny.

In its symbolic function, prognosis again resembles prophecy. To say that patients' experience of illness is random is to deny fundamentally that it has meaning and to deny that events can be predicted, much less accommodated or controlled. According to sociologist Max Weber:

Prophetic revelation involves for both the prophet himself and for his followers . . . a unified view of the world derived from a consciously integrated and meaningful attitude toward life. To the prophet, both the life of man and the world, both social and cosmic events, have a certain systematic and coherent meaning. To this meaning the conduct of mankind must be oriented if it is to bring salvation, for only in relation to this meaning does life obtain a unified and significant pattern.[10]

The orientation of prophecy toward meaning and order—toward prospectively bridging the gap between expectation and outcome—is further supported by the observation that prophecy is generally not directed toward causing disorder.[11] If the prophetic vision anticipates disorder, it does so to engender changes in the present that might avert—or at least vitiate—the calamity. Prophecy involves descriptions and prescriptions of behaviors that, if enacted, would purportedly bring about (or at least increase the chances of) a favorable outcome. Taking action in accordance with prophecy, then, is a bid to right the disorder, disequilibrium, and meaninglessness experienced in the present and feared about the future. It can thus restore a semblance of order even if the prophetic vision is not ultimately realized.

Unpredictability and the Meaning of Patients' Experience

Physicians have evolved mechanisms to contend with unpredictability; they expend effort to cope with it; and they modify their behavior to account for it. But unpredictability is important for reasons that transcend such practical, operational responses. The potentiality of an uncertain world contributes profoundly to the human condition; indeed, unpredictability can be construed as a predicate for experience. While unpredictability can be a source of suffering and senselessness in medicine, it can, paradoxically, also be a source of relief and meaning, as patients and physicians capitalize on uncertainty to hope for the best, and to act as if the best outcome were indeed likely.

Anthropologist and psychiatrist Arthur Kleinman has argued that

> the meanings of chronic illness are created by the sick person and his or her circle to make over a wild, disordered, *natural* occurrence into a more or less domesticated, mythologized, ritually controlled, therefore *cultural* experience.[12]

Making meaning out of illness is partly about understanding and controlling disease, metaphorically if not biologically. Elsewhere, Kleinman has argued:

> Biomedicine . . . employs a thoroughly disenchanted rationality for which the question of ultimate (or really any human) meaning lacks

legitimacy. For biomedicine, disease processes have no purpose; illness experiences no teleology; and death, no mystery. Biomedicine's
technological triumphs are its defining image.[13]

Kleinman argues that when "meaning" is understood as simply a "cognitive response to the challenge of coherence," and when it neglects
the teleology (and, I would add, eschatology) of illness, it is missing a
critical aspect to its definition. It places too much value on "knowing
the world" and too little on inhabiting it, acting in it, or wrestling with
it. Accepting uncertainty and unpredictability—and even manipulating them—is a key aspect of the latter process of finding meaning. In
other words, unpredictability provides a counterpoise to the energetic
triumphalism and cognitive certitude of modern medicine, and makes it
possible both to endure its failings and to understand its limitations. This
does not mean that patients and physicians do not crave accurate and
precise prognoses; rather, it means that such prognoses have sometimes
multifarious, often paradoxical, and usually moral implications.

Thus, prediction can shape both the biological and cultural course
of disease. It shapes it biologically in that it results in the physician
and patient making certain choices (e.g., to administer chemotherapy)
that then influence the patient's biology (e.g., by shrinking the tumor)
and hence outcome. Moreover, prognostication can itself have biological
effects on patients (e.g., by affecting their mood). Prediction shapes
disease culturally because there is an interdependence between the act
of predicting the course of an illness and a patient's experience of the
illness.[14] If prognostication consists of revealing to the patient the usual
course of a disease, then it is a way of validating, both initially and
continuously, the patient's subsequent experience of this course. In other
words, prognostication is a way of modifying the course of disease both
objectively and subjectively.

As we have seen, when physicians prognosticate, they also modify
their own and their patients' behavior. This itself is another reason
prediction has meaning. Predictions affect not only experience but also
actions. The articulation of a particular vision of the future typically has
as its consequence the duty to take certain actions, whether to avoid or
to achieve the stated outcome. When a prediction is articulated, a choice
must be made about what the future holds in two senses: what to say
about the future, and what consequent actions to take in the future. This
effectiveness of prognosis makes it meaningful.

The privileging of the future as a source of meaning and as a choate
domain of human experience is in keeping with a trait that philosopher

Hans Jonas has argued more generally characterizes modern thought, namely, that the present is regarded as a derivative and deficient mode of existence compared to the past or the future.[15] Both past and future are seen as *defining* the present. Certainly, this is the case insofar as anticipation about the future dictates present courses of action. But it is also the case that the future is a source of meaning for experiences in the present: it is where hope of relief and of understanding lies. If the future were certain and predictable, it would be much less meaningful.

"True" and "False" Prophets

The way prophecy manipulates the unpredictability of the future to make the future scrutable and meaningful raises interesting questions about the integrity of the prophecy and of the prophet. In a religious setting, the problem of accuracy and morality (which are linked) focuses on the threat of "false" prophecy. This suggests a more general insight about prediction in social life and about prognosis in medicine. The essential feature of "true" prophets is that, as faithful and transparent conduits of divine knowledge, they are accurate: their predictions come true. Conversely, "false" prophets offer predictions that do not come true. There is a problem, however, with using outcome as a criterion for evaluating the "truth" of prophecy, since whether a prediction will be realized is not apparent at the moment it is offered and, indeed, may remain unrealized precisely because the prediction is effective in modifying present actions.[16] This problem of knowing whether a prophecy is true and the prophet virtuous has led to certain observable attributes of the prophecy and the prophet being used as proxies for accuracy and morality. Unlike the accuracy of the prediction, these attributes are evaluable at the time the prediction is made. These characteristics fall into three categories: the content of the prediction, the form of the prediction, and the nature of the predictor. Most of these traits have their analogues in medical prognostication.

With respect to the content of predictions, true prophets are expected to confine themselves to specific areas. They are also expected to render predictions that are what people ought to hear rather than what they want to hear. With respect to the form of prediction, true prophecy "makes sense"—it conforms to cultural tradition. Moreover, true prophecy makes use of an established rhetoric and style and is developed using "proper" techniques or processes. Finally, true prophets themselves must display specific attributes. They should have undergone some formal training or initiation and should have high moral character. They should act in a disinterested fashion; people expect that predictors will report what they believe the future holds rather than manufacturing or manipulating an image of the future for the purpose of profiting themselves.[17]

In sum, prognosis resembles prophecy in that it is effective (in terms of changing behavior and perhaps outcome), involves a hierarchical and socially structured relationship, and conveys symbolic meaning. These aspects of prognosis each contain moral elements and suggest important duties on the part of physicians. The role of a prognosticator is a deeply moral one, governed by obligations of truthfulness, disinterestedness, completeness, accuracy, and empathy. Patients soliciting or receiving prognoses put their faith and trust in physicians, who have a great technical and moral responsibility as a result.

Avoidance and Dread of Prognosis: A Synopsis

When such a fundamental and important aspect of medical care is absent, it raises the question of why this is so, whether this is inevitable, and whether this is justifiable. The relative absence of prognosis in modern medical thought and practice certainly cannot be explained by an absence of patient need or interest. When patients are sick, their interest in diagnosis and therapy is often secondary to their interest in prognosis; indeed, diagnosis and therapy derive their importance primarily from the implications they have for the prognosis.

The absence of prognosis is neither accidental nor incidental, for, as we have seen, there are powerful norms militating against both the development and communication of prognoses. Physicians are reluctant prophets. They are socialized to avoid prognostication. The invisibility of prognosis, however, is best characterized as a submersion. Prognostication is in fact not so much absent as it is latent and implicit in medical care. This is one of the key paradoxes about prognosis: it may inform physicians' clinical work even if they do not articulate it explicitly.

We have examined numerous reasons for the avoidance of both inward and outward prognostication in medical practice, including the fact that prognostication is objectively difficult; the uncertainty and error inherent in prognostication; the consequential nature of such error for the patient's care and the physician's reputation; and the troublesome feelings prognosis can evoke for patients and physicians alike. This avoidance is further promoted by the fact that a patient's prognosis may depend on social factors that physicians consider to be imponderable; diagnosis and therapy, in comparison, are felt to be more directly linked to biological factors, which are considered to be more appropriately the province of physicians. Finally, prognostication is generally avoided because of the complementary relationship between therapy and prognosis in both the theoretical and practical consideration given to disease; when therapy is available, as it usually is, prognosis is avoided.

But physicians do not merely avoid or neglect prognosis; they dread it. This dread primarily arises from two sources. First, physicians believe in the phenomenon of the self-fulfilling prophecy. The fact that predictions may cause outcomes—especially, on occasion, by quasi-magical, automatic means—makes them appear dangerous. Unfavorable prognoses are feared for their potential to harm patients, and favorable ones are feared for the expectations of omniscience and omnipotence they might raise. The second source of dread of prognosis is its identification with death. When physicians are asked about the role of prognosis in clinical practice, they almost invariably reply that it is to predict mortality. When physicians predict mortality, they are struggling with their role in forestalling or hastening death, and they unavoidably confront their relationship both to the individual patient's death and to death in general. To the extent that prognosis is linked with death, prognostication is necessarily mysterious, dangerous, and, therefore, dreadful.

The dread of prognosis, in turn, fosters magical and religious sentiments in physicians, both of which are fundamental ways of coping with the strain posed by the limits of human ability and of science, especially in the face of death. The combination of high uncertainty, high stakes, and high emotional interest in medicine in general—and in prognostication in particular—produces a situation strongly conducive to magical ways of thinking. Physicians adopt optimistic rituals that reflect a desire to cure the patient and that symbolically enact their hopeful expectations. Physicians also allude to the role of religion. Dramatic turnabouts evoke a recognition of the "miraculous" or "tragic"— in either case uncontrollable—nature of medical practice; the knowledge that such events can occur lightens the enormous burden physicians feel they must shoulder in caring for patients and in predicting the course of disease.

The Difficulty of Changing Prognostic Behavior

Given the extent to which physicians avoid prognosis, especially in the care of patients at the end of life, it is clear that it will be difficult to change their behavior. This difficulty was demonstrated by a recent landmark

study, the Study to Understand Prognoses and Preferences for Outcomes and Risks of Treatment (SUPPORT), which showed not only that
physicians' practice with respect to prognosis and end-of-life care was
poor but also that giving physicians prognostic statistics did not change
whether they communicated a prognosis to patients or what decisions
they made. The study involved a total of 9,105 adults hospitalized in five
American hospitals with various life-threatening illnesses, each of which
was associated with a 50 percent chance of death within six months.[18]
The initial part of the study, involving the first group of 4,301 patients,
documented substantial defects in the care of seriously ill patients in the
United States, including possibly excessive use of high-technology care,
substantial levels of untreated pain, and significant disregard for patient
preferences. It confirmed the fact that Americans often die bad deaths.[19]

In a subsequent part of the study involving the second group of
4,804 patients, the investigators randomly specified half of this group to
receive an intervention "aimed to improve communication and decision
making by providing timely and reliable prognostic information, by
eliciting and documenting patient and family preferences and understanding of disease prognosis and treatment, and by providing a skilled
nurse to help carry out the needed discussions, convene the meetings,
and bring to bear the relevant information."[20] That is, the physicians
caring for the "intervention" group received reliable, individualized,
computer-generated prognostic information and were informed about
the patients' preferences for end-of-life care as elicited by a specially
trained nurse. They were not, however, required to accept or use this
information. The physicians for the control group did not receive this
prognostic or preference information, though they were free, of course,
to talk to their patients or estimate prognoses on their own. The statistical
prognoses provided for the intervention group were not, of course,
perfect; nevertheless, their accuracy probably approximates the best that
can currently be achieved.[21]

On the basis of a comparison between the intervention group of
patients and doctors on the one hand and the control group on the
other, the investigators concluded that the intervention did not have
an impact on *any* of the several prognostically relevant outcomes it
sought to influence, including physician-patient communication, timing
of do-not-resuscitate orders, physicians' knowledge of their patients'
preferences regarding resuscitation, number of days spent receiving
high-technology interventions in intensive care, frequency and level of
reported pain, or use of hospital resources. This lack of effect was as
disheartening as it was unexpected.

The investigators noted that while physicians treating patients in the intervention group received prognostic information provided by the research nurse 94 percent of the time and were informed about patient preferences 78 percent of the time, they acknowledged or remembered receiving the prognostic information only 59 percent of the time and reported receiving the preference information only 34 percent of the time. More remarkably, only 15 percent of the physicians reported having discussed this specific prognostic and preference information with patients or their families. The patients likewise reported a relatively low rate of discussion by their doctors of either their prognosis or their preferences. In *both* the intervention and control groups, about 20 percent of patients reported that their doctor had discussed their preferences for end-of-life care and about 40 percent reported discussing their prognosis. The authors do not clarify how it could be that 40 percent of *patients* reported a discussion of prognosis while only 15 percent of *doctors* did. It is possible that patients may have been confused about the source of prognostic information they were given; perhaps some patients thought they or a family member had discussed the prognosis with their doctor whereas, in fact, they had discussed it with the research nurse or some other party. Or perhaps patients did not realize what a real discussion of prognosis would entail and so overreported such discussions. In any case, there is no data in the published reports about what patients considered to constitute a "discussion of prognosis."

Regardless of how it is defined, it is clear that discussion of prognosis occurred insufficiently frequently, since a majority of these seriously ill patients said they would have desired a discussion of the prognosis. Moreover, all had an objectively high risk of death within a few months, so the prognosis was material to their care, and there was ample opportunity for them to be provided with prognostic information, given that they were in a hospital being seen daily by physicians. The patients in this study went on to have deaths that, as the investigators documented in rich detail, were deeply unsatisfactory in numerous respects. But it is not very surprising that giving physicians prognostic information failed to avert this outcome, since it had failed in its more basic goal of changing physician behavior in communicating with patients regarding their prognosis.

Such communication might indeed have been helpful. Another study drawn from the SUPPORT project showed that patients generally had substantially unduly optimistic expectations about their prospects for recovery. These false prognostic impressions apparently influenced the choices patients made, tilting patients in favor of active treatment of their illnesses rather than palliative care.[22] This study of 917 patients with advanced lung and colon cancer found that only 58 percent of those patients who estimated they had a 90 percent or greater chance of surviving to six months actually lived that long; of those estimating a 50 percent chance, only 21 percent did. These unduly optimistic estimates were in turn associated with a greater preference on the part of the patients for ostensibly life-extending therapy. As it turned out, however, this therapy did not extend the patients' lives and their deaths may have been made worse as a result of it (more, for example, died in an intensive care unit on a ventilator rather than peacefully at home).[23] Despite the patients' misestimates, and the apparently consequential nature of these misestimates in the SUPPORT study, the problem did not appear to result from a gross inability on the part of the physicians to predict mortality; that is, the study found that the physicians were better able to estimate prognosis than the patients. Instead, the problem appeared to have resulted from the physicians failing to communicate prognoses. The study concluded that

> to achieve the goals of making care at the end of life consistent with patient values and [to minimize] futile therapy, we may need to change what physicians tell patients about their prognoses and be sure that patients hear and understand what their physicians have said.[24]

While I agree that we need to change what physicians tell patients, I also believe that this will not be easy.

Part of the problem is that, when interviewed, physicians sometimes claim that they do indeed communicate prognostic (and other) information but that patients simply do not remember it: patients are "bald-faced deniers," as one physician put it.[25] Given the stressful nature of such discussions for patients, this propensity certainly seems plausible, and no doubt sometimes this is the case. However, it is unclear whether it is the physicians or the patients who are remembering encounters correctly. Did the physician really communicate the prognosis and the patient not hear it or misunderstand it? Or did the physician fail to communicate the prognosis? Studies comparing physician and patient recollections about conversations regarding cancer diagnosis, treatment, and prognosis generally reveal significant disagreement.[26] For example, one study of one hundred lung cancer patients found that only 36 percent of the patients agreed with their doctor regarding their prognosis for cure, with patients holding systematically more optimistic views than their doctors.[27] The one study that I am aware of that has sought to objectively clarify this discrepancy (e.g., by recording the conversations and subsequently evaluating them independently) found that physicians are *not* communicating as much information as they think.[28] It is well to ask who can justifiably be held responsible for this discrepancy in prognostic knowledge in any case. Even if it were the case that patients were not retaining the information being communicated, physicians would clearly need to assume substantial responsibility for trying to improve this state of affairs.

In short, the especially poor quality of the information patients have in such circumstances may be adversely affecting their care, perhaps leading them to make choices contrary to their interests. Certainly, to the extent that patients desire prognostic information, they deserve at least to be privy to what information physicians have available (which, while often in error, is at least more accurate than what they appear to have been told).

Overall, in the core SUPPORT study involving all 9,105 patients, the investigators concluded that

> we are left with a troubling situation. The picture we describe of the care of seriously ill or dying persons is not attractive. One would certainly prefer to envision that, when confronted with life-threatening illness, the patient and family would be included in discussions, realistic estimates of outcome would be valued, pain would be treated, and dying would not be prolonged. This is still a worthy vision. However, it is not likely to be achieved through an intervention such as that implemented by SUPPORT.[29]

It is easy after the fact to be critical of the design of the intervention employed in this remarkable study. We have seen that physicians' reluctance to make use of prognostic information has multiple, compelling sources; it is therefore not surprising that SUPPORT reached the conclusions that it did. Given the variety and origins of the reasons physicians avoid prognosis, how could the provision of statistical information to physicians by nurses change patient outcomes, especially if it did not enhance physician-patient communication or address physicians' underlying reservations about prognosis? The failure of the SUPPORT intervention highlights how ingrained are physicians' patterns of practice. Physicians avoid discussing prognosis, and they offer treatment to patients as if the prognosis is better than it is, even—perhaps especially—when the patient is seriously ill. Unfortunately, patients' lack of reasonably accurate prognostic information may significantly affect the decisions they make at the end of their lives and the quality of care they receive.

The Way Forward

One of the most important sources of the duty to prognosticate is thus the fact that patients' lack of prognostic information may be consequential. Achieving a good death, that is, one consistent with the patient's wishes, often depends on some advance warning. Patients' desire for prognostic information is often greater than their interest in treatment options or diagnostic details, and they certainly expect physicians to be willing and able to provide it when asked.[30] Of course, not *all* patients want *all* the information *all* the time. Though most patients want to be informed, this predilection varies, and physicians should respect patient wishes.[31] However, variation in *physician* preferences for communicating prognostic information seems less defensible.

Moreover, the patient's request for a prognosis is a query not only about what the doctor thinks will happen, but also about what actions the doctor can take to avoid, assure, or modify the predicted outcome. The request for a prognosis is an invitation for the physician to take responsibility for implementing appropriate actions, as well as, to some extent, for the ensuing outcomes. Because prognostication can materially affect the actions that patients and physicians take on behalf of the patient, and because these actions are consequential, physicians have an obligation to clarify the prognostic predicates of these actions, inwardly if not also outwardly.

Another important source of the professional duty to prognosticate is the involvement of prognosis with transcendent concerns. Death is a focus of ethical, religious, existential, and moral attention whenever and however it occurs. Similarly, the existence and remission of suffering are also foci of moral examination. Did the patient do anything to bring about the suffering? What sort of life has the dying person led? What are the implications of an awareness of death? What meaning does the individual see in their death?[32] The salience of these questions is heightened by the fact that, in modern times, it is possible to influence the course of illness and the manner of death as never before. This raises still further moral questions. What is the meaning of this influence and how might it best be exercised? What sorts of actions should the patient or doctor engage in to modify the course of the illness? Insofar as prognostication is linked with suffering and death, it is inextricably connected to moral action and to the most consequential and meaningful of concerns. To predict death is to engage the foregoing questions, and to engage these questions entails the realization that death is near.

The necessity of prognostication is heightened by the asymmetry in knowledge that exists between the patient and the physician. As a result of this asymmetry and of the trust patients put in them, physicians hold power over patients and—literally and metaphorically—over their futures. The patient is sick, perhaps with a terminal illness; the doctor has technical knowledge and therapy that the patient is seeking. The physical and emotional vulnerability of patients who are seriously ill, coupled with the professional authority of the physician, suffuses the entire clinical encounter with the strongest possible obligations, prognostic obligations no less than diagnostic and therapeutic ones. The burden of prediction justly falls to the one who is best able—by virtue of expert training, lack of vulnerability, and claims to authority—to bear it.[33]

Finally, as we have seen, physicians believe that, when they must articulate a prognosis, they should shape patient expectations about their disease, for example, through the careful use of language or the cultivation of optimism. This obligation originates in part from the very unpredictability of the future; in a deterministic world, "shaping" would be both less necessary and less possible. However, this obligation also originates in one of the key functions of the professions, including medicine, which is to bring to bear expert knowledge to decrease uncertainty. Physicians' predictions, in a sense, represent a social mechanism to manage a biological reality. Physicians are obligated to develop and apply expertise to prognosis as much as to diagnosis or therapy.

If physicians are to fulfill this duty, and thus enhance the use of prognosis in clinical practice, certain obstacles clearly must be overcome. Patients do not always want or benefit from prognostic information, and physicians will have to be sensitive to this. Physicians are currently not very accurate in the prognoses they offer. Information regarding prognosis in educational venues and materials is currently minimal. And physicians resist generating prognostic information. These practical obstacles to prognostication, however, do not subvert the moral obligation to prognosticate. Individual physicians and the profession as a whole can do much better than current practice would suggest.

At the level of the individual physician, there are several opportunities for improvement. Physicians should make efforts to improve both their inward and outward prognostication. Inwardly, they should strive to more formally and routinely incorporate prognostic thinking into their management, much as they currently incorporate a patient's symptoms or test results. They might keep mental track of the accuracy of their prognoses, much as they track the accuracy of their diagnostic and therapeutic decisions.[34] If physicians were to begin a process of self-calibration in this respect, their accuracy and confidence in prognosis might both increase. Physicians might also make greater efforts to avail themselves of prognostic resources that do exist; information is increasingly available on how to formulate and evaluate prognostic information in many clinical situations.[35] However, most physicians whom I interviewed were unaware of such information. Certainly, no matter how difficult it may be for physicians to *foretell* the future, they can make more of an effort to *foresee* it.

The obstacle posed by the existence of error in prognostication deserves special attention. The error rates currently seen in prognosis (characterized in chapter 3) should be reducible. The most general problem is that physicians are often miscalibrated. That is, they are making systematic errors in one direction. If, as is the case, physicians caring for terminally ill patients routinely overestimate duration of survival by a factor of three or more, it seems reasonable to expect them to be able to recalibrate themselves for the group as a whole, even if errors in individual cases unavoidably persist. In other words, if physicians were simply to divide their prognostic estimates by three, they would be estimating the survival of terminally ill patients as a group more accurately. Beyond this, there are other techniques available to physicians to enhance prognostic accuracy. For example, disinterested parties might be sought to render prognoses, as there is evidence that the less well a physician knows a patient, the less likely the physician is to misestimate survival.[36] In addition, physicians might formulate predictions in ways that offer methodological advantages; there is evidence, for example, that physicians perform better at estimating the duration of survival if the prediction is formulated in units of probability rather than units of time.[37] Furthermore, prognostic estimates might be averaged across practitioners, thereby decreasing the error, as is often done in meteorological and business forecasting.[38] Finally, prognoses might be supplemented by actuarial models, since there is evidence that the combination of physicians' and computer estimates of survival are often superior to either alone.[39] Certainly, both individual physicians and the profession as a whole could invest in finding ways to increase prognostic accuracy.

Greater attention to the communication of prognoses, or outward prognostication, is also clearly in order. Physicians have a very hard time communicating prognoses and they do so poorly. Yet good resources to enhance their communication exist.[40] Such poor performance, in other words, need not be tolerated. With respect to the articulation of prognosis, physicians should give greater attention to how to acknowledge the uncertainty in prediction. If, despite their best efforts, significant uncertainty remains, they need to develop ways to sensitively communicate this to patients as well as ways to help patients cope with the uncertainty. Finally, individual physicians would benefit from seeking feedback from their patients on how they are doing with respect to communicating prognoses.

However sympathetic we might be to individual physicians who avoid prognosis or respond inadequately to the need for prognosis, we should not excuse the profession as a whole. The avoidance of prognosis at the level of the profession is particularly deplorable since there is no *interpersonal* justification for the absence here. Research and education regarding prognosis cannot by any means harm patients, nor can coverage of prognosis in textbooks and journals. From a policy perspective, whatever allowance we might accord to individual physicians for their avoidance of prognostication, there should be none at the professional level.

Several steps might be taken to enhance the amount and quality of prognostication in the profession. More basic research on the prognosis of specific diseases is needed: For any given disease, what are the key prognostic variables? How should these be weighted and combined? How much variance do they explain? Which outcomes are most relevant to patients? Moreover, more applied research is needed on how such prognostic information might best be integrated into clinical care. Some physicians recognize this need. For example, Alvan Feinstein, a physician who is an authority on ways to enhance the science of clinical care, noted in 1983:

> The omission of prediction from the major goals of basic medical science has impoverished the intellectual content of clinical work since a modern clinician's main challenge in the care of patients is to make predictions.[41]

My impression, however, is that this impoverishment has still not been adequately addressed, nor is it likely to be unless concerted efforts are made to address the barriers to prognostication we have been considering.

Prognosis should assume a more explicit role in medical pedagogy. Students and trainees need to become more familiar with the development and use of prognostic information. One way for the medical profession to highlight the importance of prognosis is to incorporate it into formal assessments of knowledge and performance. Nonwritten clinical evaluations of students and trainees should stress both the factual knowledge and the interpersonal skills needed to develop and communicate prognoses. So should written examinations. Why is it often deemed more legitimate, for example, to ask a student which type of cell is affected by colon cancer, which drugs might be used to treat it, how the drugs work, or what the anatomy of the surgery is, than to ask what the median survival is, what the spread in survival times is, what tests might be done to decrease prognostic uncertainty, or what the features of the disease that modify the prognosis are? Such questions could be incorporated into tests at the level of both medical schools and postgraduate certification and licensing exams—from where they are often neglected.[42] The topic of prognosis should also be stressed in postgraduate clinical training. An illustrative example of the way prognosis is neglected at this level is provided by the following item- ization of knowledge "required to function as a medical oncologist," as stipulated by the American Board of Internal Medicine Subspecialty Board in Medical Oncology in 1988:

> knowledge of tumor biology; an understanding of the natural history of the various malignancies; the staging and post-treatment evalua- tion of patients; criteria for response; the pharmacology of anti-cancer drugs, including pharmacokinetics, drug interactions, and therapeu- tic drug level monitoring; indications for and uses of radiotherapy, surgery, hematologic supportive care, and biological compounds in the management of patients; management of the complications of malignancy, including pain and neurologic, infectious, metabolic, and endocrine problems associated with malignancy or its treatment; and interpretation of diagnostic imaging tests, laboratory tests, and pathologic studies.[43]

Knowing, collecting, synthesizing, or communicating prognostic infor- mation is lacking from this admittedly demanding list.

Equally important, physicians need to rethink the professional norms regarding the avoidance of prognostication. Whose needs are being served by these norms? Are they truly helpful to patients? Are they really consistent with physicians' professional duties? Furthermore, physicians should legitimate discussions regarding prognosis not only with their patients but also with each other. Discussions of cases should explicitly address not only the differential diagnosis and therapeutic options, but the likely prognosis as well. This would throw prognosis open to discussion and afford the opportunity to decrease error.

Finally, physicians need to modify their prognostic expectations. To predict death is not to be defined by it. If physicians are to enhance the care of the dying in modern American settings, settings in which chronically ill older patients are increasingly the norm, they need to stop viewing the death of their patients as a personal or professional failure. They need to stop viewing death as something to be avoided not only clinically, but also rhetorically. Physicians are profoundly motivated to heal. Yet the reality is that the majority of deaths occur in elderly patients known to be seriously ill; in such circumstances, death is a normal and unavoidable life passage. A recognition of this fact by physicians would certainly make it more acceptable to predict death. But it would also allow physicians to broaden their horizons concerning outcomes that might be relevant to optimal patient care at the end of life. Quality of life, not only death, might then become a more important object for prediction and action. In changing their thinking, physicians might realize that there is much that patients can hope for even when death is inevitable.

Better prognostication is called for on the basis not only of moral considerations but also of practical ones. As we noted in chapter 1, ongoing changes in how medicine is practiced are likely to drive an increased demand for prognostication. For example, the imminent explosion in information about the human genome, and the consequent development of tests for genes that put people at risk for disease, will provide a whole new class of medical information that will be specifically prognostic in nature. Whatever the merits or demerits of this change, it is easy to imagine that genetics will become a critical model doctors use both to understand disease and to explain it to patients. In some ways, the use of genetic information for prognostic purposes will be more palatable for physicians than the current clinical bases for prognosis. They may feel more comfortable telling patients with a gene associated with lung cancer, for example, that they are at increased risk for lung cancer—or even that they *will* develop cancer—than they do telling a patient who smokes that they will develop lung cancer, even if the risks are mathematically identical, because the genetic information will appear to be biologically preordained, scientifically fixed, unsusceptible to individual or social influences, and unmodifiable by physicians.[44] The perception that genetics is a fundamental cause of events will help physicians to feel less responsible for either the prediction or the outcome. Moreover, physicians may feel that genetic prognostication will be less prone to error. Finally, as genetic tests initially come to market, they will have few, if any, therapeutic implications; in keeping with the reciprocal relation between therapy and prognosis, they will therefore primarily find prognostic use. Thus, many of the reasons we have considered that act to restrain physician prognostication will likely be less prominent when genes underlie the prognosis.

Nevertheless, some of the reasons physicians avoid prognosis will persist even in the application of genetic tests. There will still be the problem of uncertainty.[45] There will still be questions regarding the actions patients and physicians should take in response to the prediction. There will still be the link to death, and the fear and emotion it engenders. And, if anything, the use of genetic information will only increase the link of prognosis to concerns about the role of individual destiny, concerns that may readily assume existential or religious overtones.

Better Ways to Prognosticate

Physicians are taught in medical school to elicit the "history of the present illness," that is, the patient's story about when and how the illness began and how it has progressed. This information is deemed essential to determining diagnosis and therapy.[46] Following this subjective narrative, physicians customarily examine the patient and conduct lab tests, after which they formulate a diagnosis, institute therapy, and inform the patient about these items. However, the discourse about the patient's illness need not end there. I see prognosis as a sort of "future of the present illness," the articulation of which is no less relevant to the management of the patient's condition than is the review of the past.

I see optimal prognostication at the individual level as involving a number of steps. When caring for patients who are seriously ill, physicians, if they lack the requisite knowledge, should identify objective measures of prognosis in the literature, where available, and assess their validity, utility, and relevance. They should evaluate how the patients' unique clinical or social attributes affect the prognosis, then consider how the prognostic assessment and the patients' values and preferences regarding outcomes (which must themselves be explored) inform the decisions to be made. Physicians should also consider how their own attributes or values may influence the prognosis that is formulated and the way it is communicated (since, as we have seen, physicians may vary in these respects). Finally, physicians should give thought to how best to discuss the prognosis with the patients and their families; they should pay attention to the words that they use and the way they communicate quantitative information.[47] As with good medical care more generally, all this should be done with the utmost probity and compassion.

In the course of my discussions with physicians about prognosis, I encountered examples of prognoses that were sensitively, accurately, and usefully communicated to patients. Some of these can serve as a template for what I have in mind regarding the fulfillment of a duty to prognosticate. For example, one oncologist provided the following description:

> If someone is newly diagnosed, I'll sit down and first ask them what their understanding of their disease is. I hear what they have to say, and usually it's right. But if it's not, I tell them what *my* understanding is. And I tell them the prognosis if this is relevant.
>
> Recently, a man was referred to me by the surgeons. He had a gastric cancer that was metastatic to lymph nodes and tissue in the peritoneum. That has a terrible prognosis, and it's terrible even with chemotherapy. It's one of these things where you can't really justify giving them chemotherapy and radiation because it's going to make them so sick and not really help them. This was a middle-class man whose mother also had just died of gastric cancer. When he came, he wanted this experimental therapy, but he had no health insurance, so he wanted to pay out of pocket. It was going to cost $20,000 a cycle, and it was not likely to work: at best, 8 percent of people will have some kind of shrinkage (though not elimination) of their tumor. And it was going to make him sick. It probably wouldn't have extended his life. He probably only had eight months to live.
>
> So that was a case in which we really talked long and hard about the treatment options. We talked about experimental therapy, and we talked about hospice, and we talked about standard of care, and I basically explained that the outcomes were all going to be the same, but that with this therapy he was going to feel worse. He wanted to know how much it was going to cost. We worked all that out. We had a very frank discussion. But I think he needed to know all this prognostic information to make a decision—to help him decide if he was going to bankrupt his family to do this therapy that really had little chance of helping. And he decided not to.

This physician employed prognosis on numerous levels, and she did not shy away from her responsibility. Indeed, the entire clinical encounter was basically about prognosis, in the broadest and most commendable sense. The doctor chose the correct outcomes to predict, predicted them with precision ("8 percent," "eight months"), predicted the outcome of the disease with and without treatment, foretold the expense and suffering associated with treatment, helped the patient to understand his plight, and showed respect and sympathy for the patient. The doctor and patient "had a very frank discussion," and worked through all the questions that arose. To me, this is a sterling example of how prognosis can be used optimally in clinical practice, and not just because it involves the avoidance of potentially painful therapy.

Another example was provided by a physician experienced in the care of the terminally ill who was asked how he thought prognoses should ideally be communicated. He responded that he would tell the patient something like this:

> Most patients with disease like yours live about three months, even with treatment, though I have seen exceptions. However, I can promise you that I will not abandon you. There is much that I can do for you, even if we are powerless to stop your disease. I am confident that we can respect your wishes as to how you want to live the rest of your life and that we can make sure that you do not have pain or other worrisome symptoms. Is there something more that I can tell you about your condition?

He would typically follow up such a statement by urging the patient to tell him about "your hopes and dreams" or "what your days are like now." In his experience, such requests almost always led to a meaningful and relevant discussion about the patient's future.

Both of the above physicians, by their actions and words, communicate an essential element when they are rendering the prognosis: one of the most important gestures that a doctor can make, especially when giving a prognosis during a serious illness, is to promise that the patient will not be abandoned, symbolically or literally. Such a gesture uncouples the prognosis itself from the care and concern the patient will receive. This would be easier for physicians to do if they indeed could change their own perceptions about the meaning of death.

A Duty to Prognosticate

The role of prognostication in medicine is thus multifarious. Like prophecy, prognostication affects what people feel, think, and do, and what happens as a result. Like prophecy, it addresses issues of meaning and explanation: it seeks order in apparent randomness, good in seeming evil, and hope in inevitable death. The uncertainty and gravity of the future in patients who are suffering from life-threatening illness heighten the need for prognosis, but have on balance militated toward its avoidance. The balance might beneficially be shifted. For although physicians avoid prognostication, they are nevertheless called to it.

ORIGINAL SOURCES OF DATA

The data collected and analyzed to support the arguments in this book were drawn from surveys and interviews of hundreds of physicians, as well as other sources. Some of these sources and the methods used have been described in greater detail in other publications.

Survey of a National Sample of Internists

Details about the methodology of this survey have been previously published.[1] Using the 1994 American Medical Association Masterfile, a directory of virtually all American physicians,[2] I drew a simple random sample of 1,500 internists from the 94,381 internists who had completed their training and were in active practice. The sample included both general internists and subspecialty internists in population-representative proportions. Of the 1,500 names, 189 were excluded prior to the survey for various reasons. The final sample thus consisted of 1,311 internists.

A total of 697 physicians responded to the survey, yielding an unadjusted response rate of 53 percent. This response rate compares favorably to response rates achieved in comparable lengthy surveys of physicians.[3] Assuming that subjects who did not respond were eligible to participate in the same proportion as those whose eligibility status could be ascertained, the estimated denominator for the survey may be adjusted downward to 1,179; consequently, the adjusted response rate is 59 percent.[4] Because of occasional missing data, and because a few subjects returned unusable surveys, totals in the analyses do not equal 697.

Two techniques were used to evaluate nonresponse: (1) respondents and nonrespondents were compared along several demographic variables that were available for all 1,500 subjects, and (2) the pattern of responses across time was assessed. In keeping with previous research examining response rates based on Masterfile samples,[5] the respondents did not differ from nonrespondents in terms of age, specialty, or geographic location. Moreover, time to response was not associated in a statistically significant fashion with any of the variables reported here (for example, age, sex, specialty, percent of time in patient care, experience with life support withdrawal, finding prognostication difficult, finding prognostication stressful, or feeling that one's training in prognostication had been inadequate). Thus, the incremental addition of respondents to the survey sample had no observed effect on sample representativeness.[6]

Survey subjects received a twelve-page, confidential survey instrument requiring about twenty minutes to complete, a cover letter, a small financial incentive, and a prepaid return envelope. The survey instrument solicited demographic data, attitudes and self-reported practice with respect to prognostication and attendant clinical decisions, responses to hypothetical vignettes, and open-ended comments. The precise wording of the vignettes was varied across random subsets of the subjects, as described in appendix 2; these results are summarized in chapters 3, 5, and 6.

Respondents had a mean (± s.d.) age of 45.8 ± 10.7 years and had spent a mean of 18.9 ± 11.0 years in practice; 77.6 percent spent 90 percent or more of their time in clinical practice; 80.7 percent were male; and 79.8 percent were board-certified. Their specialties were as follows: 47.8 percent general internists, 12.5 percent cardiologists, 9.5 percent gastroenterologists, 6.9 percent pulmonologists, and 6.6 percent oncologists, with the remaining 16.7 percent in other internal medicine subspecialties. This distribution of subspecialties and of demographic and professional features parallels that for internal medicine physicians in the United States.

Open-Ended Interviews and Written Comments

I collected qualitative data regarding physicians' attitudes and practice with respect to prognostication from two sources. First, I conducted in-depth interviews with a convenience sample of thirty physicians, whose characteristics are summarized in table A1.1; twenty-two of these interviews were conducted by me, the remainder by two trained interviewers. Twenty of the subjects (67 percent) were internists, of whom nine were subspecialists (mostly oncologists) and eleven were generalists. The remaining ten (33 percent) were physicians outside of internal medicine, including surgeons, pediatricians, and psychiatrists. Twenty-one subjects (70 percent) had an academic affiliation. The subjects came from the states of California, Pennsylvania, Washington, Massachusetts, New Mexico, and Illinois. Their average age was 43.2 years and 60 percent were male. The interviews lasted an average of eighty minutes and were conducted in accordance with a semistructured interview instrument.[7] Most of the interviews were recorded and complete written transcripts

Table A1.1. Characteristics of interview subjects

	Specialty	Age	Sex
1	cardiology	70	M
2	endocrinology	64	M
3	general internal medicine	28	F
4	general internal medicine	29	F
5	general internal medicine	30	F
6	general internal medicine	30	F
7	general internal medicine	36	F
8	general internal medicine	36	M
9	general internal medicine	46	F
10	general internal medicine	57	M
11	general internal medicine	64	M
12	general internal medicine	76	M
13	general surgery	40	M
14	geriatrics	30	M
15	infectious disease	80	M
16	neurosurgery	33	M
17	obstetrics/gynecology	56	M
18	oncology	31	F
19	oncology	47	F
20	oncology	52	M
21	oncology	57	F
22	orthopedic surgery	50	M
23	pediatric nephrology	30	F
24	pediatrics	31	F
25	pediatrics	32	M
26	psychiatry	28	M
27	psychiatry	32	F
28	pulmonology/intensive care	32	M
29	pulmonology/intensive care	34	M
30	radiology	35	M

were prepared. In choosing how many physicians to interview, I was guided by Renée Fox's admonition that the proper number of interview subjects would be determined if I "continued interviewing until I no longer heard anything new." While I cannot say that by the end of this series of interviews I was no longer hearing *anything* new or interesting, I can report that the amount of new information being gathered with relevance to the problems I had put before myself was approaching zero. Minor details in the passages quoted in this book have been changed to preserve confidentiality or to clarify the exposition (e.g., by changing identifying details, deleting or paraphrasing medical jargon, clarifying pronouns and antecedents, and reordering sentences).

Second, I obtained physicians' written comments on the survey described in the previous section. These comments were elicited via an open-ended question on the survey form ("Is there anything else you would like to tell us about how you feel about the role of prognosis in clinical practice?"); 162 respondents out of 697 (23 percent) offered comments, which ranged in length from a couple of sentences to several paragraphs. In approximately fifty of these cases, the comments were quite substantial and insightful. All of these respondents were internists, of diverse specialties.

Prospective Study of Prognostic Accuracy in Terminally Ill Outpatients

In this project, I asked physicians to make specific mortality predictions for 504 patients when they were referred to one of five Chicago hospices during a three-month period in 1996. The patients were then prospectively followed for more than two years to observe the duration of their survival, and the physicians' predictions and the observed outcomes were compared (as summarized in chapter 3). Prognostic accuracy could thus be quantified, and patient and physician attributes associated with prognoses that proved unduly favorable or unfavorable could be assessed.

The 504 patients in the study had the following attributes: their mean age was 68.6 ± 17.4 years; 44.6 percent were male; 67.8 percent were white; 77.0 percent had diagnoses of cancer or AIDS; and they had been diagnosed with their condition an average of 1.6 ± 2.6 years previously. The patients were referred to hospice care by a total of 365 physicians, who had the following attributes: they had been in practice an average of 16 years; 80 percent were male; 80 percent were board-certified; and 31.8 percent were general internists, 17.0 percent oncologists, 19.9 percent other internal medicine subspecialties, 15.4 percent family practitioners, 7.5 percent geriatricians, 5.0 percent surgeons, and the remainder various other specialties.

Among other questions, referring physicians were asked to predict survival in two ways: (1) as a point estimate of survival in units of time ("How long does this patient have to live?") and (2) in units of probability ("What are the patient's chances of survival at 7, 30, 90, 180, and 360 days?"). Physicians were also asked what prognosis, if any, they would offer to the patient (to examine the phenomenon of "discrepant communication," discussed in chapter 5). Physicians provided these mortality predictions, along with other information about themselves and their relationship with the patients, during a four-minute telephone survey typically administered within forty-eight hours of the patient's admission to the hospice. In the course of these interviews, approximately fifty of the respondents offered unsolicited opinions about the role of prognosis in their practice, and these remarks were noted. In most cases, these remarks deplored the difficulty and stressfulness of prognostication.

Analysis of Textbook Entries

Two content analyses were performed. Details regarding the first have been previously published.[8] Briefly, in order to study the bases of medical thinking about prognosis, I performed a content analysis of a series of textbook entries regarding lobar pneumonia spanning the century from 1892 to 1988, with special attention to the period between 1892 and 1947. There were two rationales for this strategy. First, this early period largely precedes the advent of effective therapy for pneumonia, and outcomes were often quite bad. When little could be done to treat this life-threatening disease, we might expect that patients and physicians alike would be concerned with identifying which patients would do well and which would not. Second, since this period includes the introduction of effective antibiotic therapy for pneumonia, in the late 1930s, I was able to test whether prognosis becomes effaced when therapy becomes dominant and to assess how soon after antibiotics were discovered textbooks came to adopt the "modern" form of entry (that omits information about prognosis).

I selected lobar pneumonia since its recognition and diagnosis have not changed much over the period under consideration, whereas its treatment and prognosis have. Since this condition is readily recognizable across time, it was possible to follow the evolution in clinical thinking about prognosis while holding constant the particular disease (along with its clinical manifestations, recognition, and diagnosis). An additional reason for the selection of pneumonia was that it was a leading cause of death throughout the period from 1892 to 1947, and remains so today.

The texts I examined were all the editions of a highly regarded and standard textbook initially authored by William Osler, *The Principles and Practice of Medicine.* Twenty-two editions of this textbook appeared between 1892 and 1988; I comprehensively reviewed the entries for lobar pneumonia in all of them, and quantified the proportion of chapter length devoted to different aspects of the clinical management of pneumonia in certain editions. These aspects were grouped into seven categories: (1) etiology, (2) presentation (including signs and symptoms), (3) pathology, (4) diagnosis, (5) therapy, (6) prognosis, and (7) complications.

The second content analysis involved looking at a single leading textbook: J. D. Wilson, et al., *Harrison's Principles of Internal Medicine,* 12th edition (New York: McGraw-Hill, 1991). Details are available elsewhere.[9] The purpose of this analysis was to identify the extent to which prognosis, as compared with other cognitive clinical tasks, receives explicit, demarcated attention in the discussion of various diseases. The textbook has 380 chapters; a systematic selection scheme was employed, and 45 chapters that address diseases or clinical syndromes were analyzed.

Boldface headings and subheadings were examined in particular. These headings were felt to reflect the major cognitive organization of the chapter and the categorization by the authors of the relevant aspects of the disease under consideration. While the vast majority of chapters reviewed had explicitly demarcated sections in which information relevant to the etiology (80 percent), pathogenesis (80 percent), clinical manifestations (82 percent), diagnosis (80 percent), and treatment (98 percent) of the conditions was considered, only 27 percent had explicitly demarcated sections relevant to prognosis, and these sections were usually quite brief. Moreover, as expected, such sections tended to occur in chapters on conditions for which treatment options were relatively limited.[10]

Audiotapes of Advance-Directive Discussions

Details regarding this data collection effort have been previously published.[11] As part of a study of how physicians discuss advance directives,

Dr. James Tulsky and his colleagues collected audiotapes of conversations between fifty-six attending internists and fifty-six of their established patients in five practice sites in North Carolina and Pennsylvania. Conversations lasted an average of about 5.5 minutes. In contrast to the sample described below, these patients were generally chronically ill; the mean estimated five-year survival of these patients, as estimated by their physicians, was 64 percent (range 9–97 percent). The authors graciously made transcripts of these conversations available for my analysis of prognostic content.

Audiotapes of Routine Clinical Encounters

Details regarding this data collection effort are available elsewhere.[12] We conducted a study which sought to identify the nature, extent, and purpose of prognostically relevant interactions within *routine* medical and surgical visits using a database of taped encounters between 125 physicians (66 surgeons and 59 primary care physicians) and patients in their own offices in Oregon and Colorado.[13] Patients and physicians were well known to each other in this sample, having seen each other a median of six previous times. In the case of surgeons, the encounters centered around topics such as knee surgery, breast biopsy, trigger finger release procedures, varicose vein removal, and shoulder muscle repair. In the case of primary care physicians, the encounters centered around topics such as asthma, hypertension, and minor respiratory or urinary infections. The encounters lasted an average of about fifteen minutes.

We used quantitative and qualitative methods to examine the nature of these encounters and to characterize the patient and physician factors associated with prognostically relevant information being discussed. In our examination of these encounters, we noted whether *any* future-oriented statement was made. We considered a statement, made by either the doctor or patient, to be "prognostic" if it involved a more than abstract reference to the future course of the patient's illness and its treatment. We drew a distinction between discussions of the risks of a disease or therapy or of hypothetical possibilities, on the one hand, and predictions about outcomes, on the other. There are two major ways we drew this distinction: (1) an endorsement by the physician of one or a few *particular* outcomes out of several that might have been discussed (e.g., when the physician states, "This is the most likely thing to happen"), or (2) the *personalization* of the outcome by the physician (e.g., when the physician states, "This is what will happen to *you*"). The following, for example, is a verbatim statement by a physician about the risks of a procedure *without* prognostic content: "The procedure works best if you keep the leg wrapped for a couple of weeks, because if you don't, there's a tendency for it to get lumpy, hard spots." If the physician, on the other hand, had said something like "After the procedure, you will have to wrap your leg; if you do that, you most likely will not get any lumpy or hard spots," the statement would be considered prognostic since it would be both more definitive and more personal. Indeed, discussing risks and possibilities in an abstract or neutral way ("these are the risks of this procedure") can be seen as a means of *evading* prognostication.

Participant Observation

Finally, I made observations and kept notes about aspects of clinical care that were relevant to prognosis during my own clinical training. This training, beginning with my graduation from medical school in June 1989, consisted of two years as a houseofficer in internal medicine at the Hospital of the University of Pennsylvania, from July 1989 to June 1991, and three years of fellowship, from July 1991 to June 1994 (during which time I was primarily responsible for the supervision of other physicians). Over the course of this training, and since then, I have had countless discussions with physicians about the role of prognosis in their practice and their attitudes toward it. While less formal than the interviews described above, these conversations have also informed this work.

During my training, out of both a professional commitment and a personal interest, I was especially careful to make efforts to participate in the care of terminally ill (and hence vulnerable) patients who died in the hospital; I made note of the role, if any, of prognostication in their care. I was personally present and certified death in more than twenty such cases. In two cases, I personally withdrew life support, after a prognosis about the likelihood of recovery had been made and at the patient's request, and death ensued within an hour. These clinical experiences with terminal care were supplemented by informal work at several hospices. During my clinical work, I also had the privileged opportunity to discuss with several patients and their families what they regarded the role of prognosis to be, particularly in the care offered at the end of life. These data, while meaningful, have not formed a significant part of the arguments in this book since I have chosen to focus exclusively on the attitudes and behaviors of physicians.

DETAILED SURVEY EXPERIMENT RESULTS

The findings about physicians' feelings of accountability for prognostic errors, about their beliefs in the self-fulfilling prophecy, and about their responses to patients' own prognostic expectations were strongly supported by four experiments that were incorporated into a survey of a random sample of practicing internists in the United States. This experimental approach was deliberately employed in order to enhance confidence in the validity and generalizability of insights gleaned from in-depth interviews with individual physicians. The conduct of the survey is summarized in appendix 1. The general methodological approach of such survey experiments is described elsewhere.[1] Here I provide more detailed results for the survey experiments summarized in chapters 3, 5, and 6.

Findings for Chapter 3: The Consequences of Prognostic Error

Experimental Design

In the first experiment, subjects were randomized into six groups and received one of six versions of the hypothetical clinical vignette reproduced, with the accompanying questions, in figure A2.1. The clinical details of the case were carefully chosen so that two different survival outcomes were plausible: the patient might have had a relatively favorable outcome and lived a long time (twenty-four months) or an unfavorable outcome and lived a short time (two months). Versions of the vignette varied only on two points: the prediction offered by "Dr. Brown" (no prediction, prediction of short survival, or prediction of long survival) and the outcome (short or long survival).[2]

In the second experiment, subjects received one of six versions of the clinical vignette reproduced in figure A2.2. The clinical details of the case were again carefully chosen so that two different outcomes (recovery or death) were plausible. Vignettes again varied only in terms of the prediction offered, this time by "Dr. Jones" (no prediction, prediction of death, or prediction of recovery), and the observed outcome (death or recovery).[3]

Dr. Brown is an internist. One of Dr. Brown's patients is a 72-year-old man with a two-year history of prostate cancer. The patient had been well until two years before, when Dr. Brown had noted a nodule on the patient's prostate on routine exam. The patient was found to have metastatic disease to his pelvis and ribs, and he was treated with antiandrogen therapy consisting of leuprolide and flutamide. Except for intermittent bony pain managed with oral narcotics, the patient's course was satisfactory until five days ago, when he was admitted for considerable pain at his right femur. X-rays showed metastatic disease without fracture in this area, and treatment with local radiation was initiated. The patient and Dr. Brown decided that subsequent management should consist solely of narcotics and palliative radiation, regardless of the prognosis.

At this point, Dr. Brown predicted to the patient and to colleagues that the patient would probably live *about two months*. The patient lived for *twenty-four months* before dying.

[Please circle a response for each of the following questions.]

	strongly disagree	somewhat disagree	undecided	somewhat agree	strongly agree
1. The observed survival outcome is unusual.	1	2	3	4	5
2. What Dr. Brown told the patient about the patient's prospects for recovery contributed to the observed survival outcome.	1	2	3	4	5
3. Dr. Brown appears to be a good clinician.	1	2	3	4	5
4. In view of Dr. Brown's statement about the patient's prognosis, other patients would have confidence in Dr. Brown.	1	2	3	4	5
5. Dr. Brown appears to be adept at making prognoses.	1	2	3	4	5
6. Dr. Brown would have to explain the observed survival outcome to the patient's family.	1	2	3	4	5

Figure A2.1. Survey case involving a chronically ill patient. Versions of this vignette varied only at the points emphasized: "Dr. Brown" would offer one of three predictions ("about two months," "about twenty-four months," or "no prediction") and one of two survival outcomes would be observed ("two months" or "twenty-four months").

Dr. Jones is an an internist. One of Dr. Jones' patients, a 69-year-old woman with no past medical history, presented to the emergency room complaining of progressive non-productive cough, malaise, and fever for 10 days, along with dyspnea for one day, and was admitted by Dr. Jones. An admission chest x-ray revealed right-sided infiltrates. Treatment with intravenous cefuroxime and high-dose erythromycin was initiated, and a number of blood, urine, and sputum specimens were taken. An HIV test was negative.

On the third hospital day, the patient's urine test came back positive for *Legionella* urinary antigen. Despite being an appropriate antibiotics, the patient's clinical picture had progressed until, by the third hospital day, it was consistent with the adult respiratory distress syndrome, and the patient required intubation and mechanical ventilation. By the eighth hospital day, the patient required significant ventilatory support, including 80% oxygen and positive end expiratory pressure. On the eighth day, the patient also required initiation of low-dose intravenous vasopressors. She was sedated but responsive. As of the twelfth hospital day, there was no change in the patient's condition or treatment.

At this point, Dr. Jones predicted to the patient and to colleagues that the patient would *probably not recover*. A few days later, the patient did *recover* and was ultimately discharged in her premorbid state.

[Please circle a response for each of the following questions.]

	strongly disagree	somewhat disagree	undecided	somewhat agree	strongly agree
1. The observed survival outcome is unusual.	1	2	3	4	5
2. What Dr. Jones told the patient about the patient's prospects for recovery contributed to the observed survival outcome.	1	2	3	4	5
3. Dr. Jones appears to be a good clinician.	1	2	3	4	5
4. In view of Dr. Jones' statement about the patient's prognosis, other patients would have confidence in Dr. Jones.	1	2	3	4	5
5. Dr. Jones appears to be adept at making prognoses.	1	2	3	4	5
6. Dr. Jones would have to explain the observed survival outcome to the patient's family.	1	2	3	4	5

Figure A2.2. Survey case involving an acutely ill patient. Versions of this vignette varied only at the points emphasized: "Dr. Jones" would offer one of three predictions ("probably not recover," "recover," or "no prediction") and one of two survival outcomes would be observed ("not recover" or "recover").

For both experiments, the six subject groups are identified here with two-letter codes corresponding to the version of the vignette they received, in which the first letter (*N*, *U*, or *F*) indicates whether *no* prediction, an *unfavorable* prediction, or a *favorable* prediction was made and the second letter (*U* or *F*) indicates which outcome was observed, *unfavorable* or *favorable*.

All subjects in both experiments were then asked a series of identically worded questions in response to the vignettes, followed by five-point Likert-type scales of agreement. Differences in response patterns to the questions can logically only be attributed to differences in the group assignment of the subjects, an assignment under experimental control. For simplicity, the results presented here show the percentage of physicians "agreeing" with various statements.[4] The results presented in chapter 3 relate, in particular, to physicians' responses to four statements: (1) "In view of [the doctor's] statement about the patient's prognosis, other patients would have confidence in [the doctor]"; (2) "[The doctor] appears to be a good clinician"; (3) "[The doctor] appears to be adept at making prognoses"; and (4) "[The doctor] would have to explain the observed survival outcome to the patient's family." These statements correspond to questions 4, 3, 5, and 6 respectively in figures A2.1 and A2.2.

Physicians' Perceptions of Patients' Judgments

Physicians believe that an erroneous prediction by a physician would lead to a decrease in patients' confidence in the physician. Figure A2.3 summarizes the results for the first experiment, involving "Dr. Brown" and a chronically ill patient with cancer. As shown, 40.6 percent of physicians thought that patients would have confidence in Dr. Brown in version NU, in which no prediction is made and an unfavorable outcome was observed. Fewer respondents, 25.5 percent, thought that patients would have confidence in Dr. Brown when a favorable prediction was made and the same unfavorable outcome was observed, as in version FU. This difference demonstrates that physicians, not surprisingly, believe that patients will lose confidence if a physician chooses to make a prediction that proves to be unduly favorable.[5] More remarkably, however, they also thought that patients would judge a physician adversely for an unduly unfavorable prediction, where the outcome was *better* than predicted; in version UF only 9.7 percent of subjects believed patients would retain confidence in their physicians, compared to 40.6 percent in version NF, where the doctor made no prediction. A direct comparison of versions FU and UF reveals that, if the physician is to make an error in prediction, an optimistic error is to be favored over a pessimistic one, at least in terms of patient confidence.

Physicians believe that patients are more likely to forgive them for an overly optimistic prognosis than for a symmetrically overly pessimistic prognosis. The reason may be that respondents believe that, in addition to having made a mistake, a physician making an unduly unfavorable prediction must bear the cost of the unfavorable prediction itself: nobody likes to hear or offer bad news, especially, as we have seen, if it proves false. An optimistic error, on the other hand, may be interpreted as an appropriate and legitimate expression of hope by the physician.

A comparison of versions NU with UU and NF with FF in figure A2.3 illuminates an additional finding. Physicians believe that patients are even more likely to have confidence in them if a prediction is both articulated and accurate. In the opinion of physicians, they get credit from patients for *both* calling the future and calling it accurately, though this is especially the case if the outcome is favorable.[6]

Similar results regarding loss of patient confidence in physicians who make prognostic errors are obtained in the vignette involving "Dr. Jones" and an acutely ill patient receiving intensive care, as shown in figure A2.4. However, here, if the physician is to make an error, there is a slight, although not statistically significant, preference for pessimistic rather than optimistic error, as illustrated by the comparison of version FU with UF.

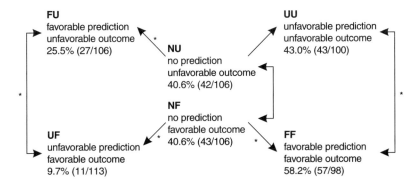

Figure A2.3. Percentage of physicians receiving each of six versions of a vignette depicting a *chronically* ill patient who agreed that *patients would have confidence in the physician* (fig. A2.1, question 4). Absolute numbers are shown in parentheses. Significance of pairwise comparisons: *$p < 0.05$ by Fischer's exact test.

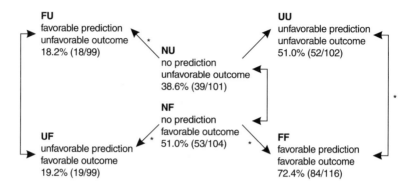

Figure A2.4. Percentage of physicians receiving each of six versions of a vignette depicting an *acutely* ill patient who agreed that *patients would have confidence in the physician* (fig. A2.2, question 4). Absolute numbers are shown in parentheses. Significance of pairwise comparisons: *$p < 0.05$ by Fischer's exact test.

Taken together, the experiments show that physicians believe patients would lose confidence in them if they were to make prognostic errors of either the unduly favorable or unduly unfavorable type, but especially the latter.[7] Inaccurate predictions compromise patient confidence. In addition, the experiments suggest that physicians believe patients affirmatively desire to be given (accurate) prognostic information. Finally, comparing the results across the two vignette experiments suggests that physicians believe patients are likely to be especially confident if the physicians makes an accurate prediction for an acutely ill patient (e.g., comparing version FF in figure A2.3 and A2.4).

Physicians' Perceptions of Colleagues' Judgments

The two experiments also show that physicians feel that prognostic errors would be held against them by their colleagues. The key observations here are once again made by comparing version NU to FU and NF to UF. Substantially fewer respondents agreed that the doctor in the vignette was a "good clinician" when the doctor made a prognostic error of either the unduly favorable or unduly unfavorable type. As shown in figure A2.5, 62.3 percent of physicians thought that "Dr. Brown" was a good clinician in version NU, in which no prediction is made and an unfavorable outcome was observed, compared with 39.0 percent who thought the doctor was a good clinician in version FU, when an unduly favorable prediction was made. An unduly unfavorable prediction caused an even sharper drop in approval, from 62.6 percent in version NF to 20.2 percent in version UF. It is remarkable that respondents held

unduly unfavorable (that is, pessimistic) predictions against the doctor
to a greater extent than unduly favorable ones (that is, optimistic ones).
That is, the difference between NF and UF is greater than the difference
between NU and FU.

With respect to prognostic behavior, however, accuracy is *not* the
only determinant of physicians' assessments of the hypothetical doctor's clinical ability. The mere fact of whether a prediction was offered
is also important. This is illustrated most convincingly in figure A2.5.
Physicians were more likely to feel that Dr. Brown was a good clinician
if the doctor made *no* prediction than if the doctor made an *accurate*
prediction, regardless of the outcome ultimately observed. For example,
while 62.3 percent of physicians thought Dr. Brown was a good clinician
if no prediction was made and an unfavorable outcome was observed
(version NU), substantially fewer physicians, 43.0 percent, approved of
the doctor's correctly predicting this outcome to the patient (version
UU). The situation is similar even if the outcome is favorable, though
this decrease does not reach statistical significance at the customary
level; while 62.6 percent of physicians thought that Dr. Brown was a
good clinician if no prediction was made and a favorable outcome was
observed (version NF), only 53.6 percent felt the doctor was a good
clinician when a favorable outcome was correctly predicted (version
FF). In short, physicians judge a hypothetical colleague adversely merely
for offering a prediction to a patient, even if the prognosis proves to be
accurate, but especially if the prognosis is accurate and the outcome is
unfavorable.[8] This is in stark contrast to physicians' understanding of

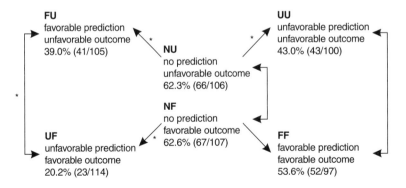

Figure A2.5. Percentage of physicians receiving each of six versions of a vignette
depicting a *chronically* ill patient who agreed that *the physician is a good clinician*
(fig. A2.1, question 3). Absolute numbers are shown in parentheses. Significance of
pairwise comparisons: *$p < 0.05$ by Fischer's exact test.

patient preferences, which, as discussed above, is that patients would prefer to be given an (accurate) prognosis than not.

As shown in figure A2.6, very similar results regarding perceptions of other physicians' clinical ability are obtained in the vignette involving "Dr. Jones" and an acutely ill patient. In this situation, however, articulating an *accurate* prediction was *not* judged to be worse than avoiding prediction. Neither was it deemed better, however, as shown by comparing version NU with UU and NF with FF. That is, there is still no advantage to prediction.

This propensity to hold the making of a prediction against a colleague—even if it is accurate, but especially if it is inaccurate—occurs despite a recognition that a colleague is *technically* proficient at making predictions. Figures A2.7 and A2.8 show the extent to which physicians believe the two hypothetical doctors were "adept" at making prognoses. Comparing version FU to UU and UF to FF in each figure reveals that physicians find other physicians to be most adept at prognostication if they make correct predictions and least adept if they make incorrect predictions. Physicians are thus able to recognize clinical acumen in this area, even if they believe that it may be applied only at risk to the clinician's standing. In both experiments, making a correct prediction was recognized as a positive attribute, despite the fact that choosing to offer a prediction at all was seen as compromising (or at least adding nothing to) the physician's reputation as a clinician among other physicians (though it might indeed enhance his standing with patients). The data in these figures also document that physicians in both

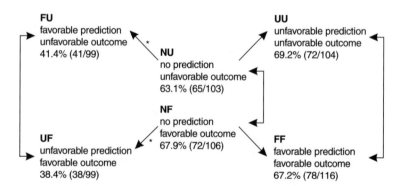

Figure A2.6. Percentage of physicians receiving each of six versions of a vignette depicting an *acutely* ill patient who agreed that *the physician is a good clinician* (fig. A2.2, question 3). Absolute numbers are shown in parentheses. Significance of pairwise comparisons: *$p < 0.05$ by Fischer's exact test.

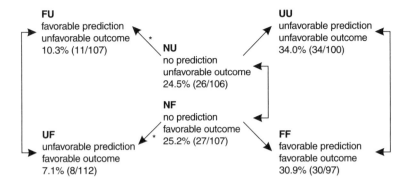

Figure A2.7. Percentage of physicians receiving each of six versions of a vignette depicting a *chronically* ill patient who agreed that *the physician is adept at making prognoses* (fig. A2.1, question 5). Absolute numbers are shown in parentheses. Significance of pairwise comparisons: *$p < 0.05$ by Fischer's exact test.

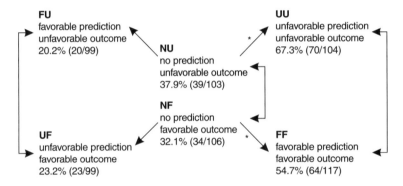

Figure A2.8. Percentage of physicians receiving each of six versions of a vignette depicting an *acutely* ill patient who agreed that *the physician is adept at making prognoses* (fig. A2.2, question 5). Absolute numbers are shown in parentheses. Significance of pairwise comparisons: *$p < 0.05$ by Fischer's exact test.

cases viewed an unduly favorable and unduly unfavorable prognosis as approximately equivalently bad *technical* errors, although the unduly unfavorable error was judged to be more detrimental to a physician's standing as a clinician.

Contrasts between Acutely and Chronically Ill Patients

The contrasts in respondents' various opinions of "Dr. Jones" and "Dr. Brown" suggest some further interesting observations. In general, Dr. Jones received more credit for an accurate prediction, whether favorable or unfavorable, than Dr. Brown—in that greater percentages of respondents expressed favorable opinions. Dr. Jones is felt to warrant more confidence, to be a better clinician, and to be more adept at making predictions (comparing versions UU and FF across the two cases for each of the three questions). These differences are attributable to the different types of cases confronted by the two physicians: Dr. Jones's patient is in an ICU and has a high risk of death in a short time frame. Dr. Brown's patient is chronically ill, with a relatively long survival horizon. Thus, Dr. Jones' patient is more "challenging."

Physicians' Need to Explain

Physicians believe that it is necessary to explain unexpected outcomes and erroneous predictions, regardless of whether they were favorable or unfavorable. Figure A2.9 summarizes the results for the experiment involving a chronically ill patient with cancer. As shown, 43.8 percent of physicians thought the doctor would have to "explain the observed outcome" in version NU, in which no prediction was made and an unfavorable outcome was observed. Thus, nearly half of physicians feel that an outcome should be explained even if no prognosis is made. By comparison, however, many more respondents, 84.1 percent, thought the doctor would have to explain an unfavorable outcome when a favorable prediction was made, as in version FU. Respondents also felt the doctor would have to explain an unexpectedly favorable outcome; 59.3 percent felt an explanation was in order in version UF, where the doctor made an unfavorable prediction and a favorable outcome was observed, whereas only 34.0 percent felt this way in version NF, where no prediction had been made.

While error in prediction calls for explanation, expected outcomes following a (correct) prediction require no more explanation than situations where no prognosis was made. Comparing version NU with UU and NF with FF reveals that a correct prediction does not meaningfully increase or decrease the necessity for explanation. Indeed, comparing FU with UU and UF with FF reveals that it is the *inaccuracy* of the prediction, rather than the valence of the outcome, that causes the need for explanation. Finally, an unduly favorable prediction is much more likely to require explanation than an unduly unfavorable one (comparing version FU with UF), supporting a predilection for pessimism on the part of physicians if error is unavoidable (so as to avoid, relatively speaking, the necessity of an explanation).[9]

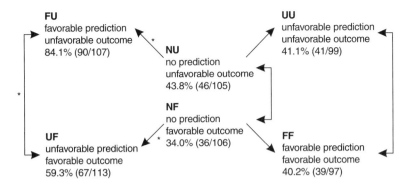

Figure A2.9. Percentage of physicians receiving each of six versions of a vignette depicting a *chronically* ill patient who agreed that *the physician would have to explain the observed outcome* (fig. A2.1, question 6). Absolute numbers are shown in parentheses. Significance of pairwise comparisons: *$p < 0.05$ by Fischer's exact test.

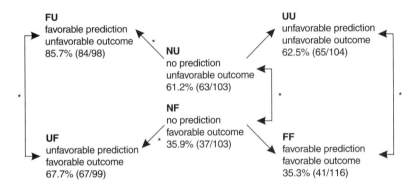

Figure A2.10. Percentage of physicians receiving each of six versions of a vignette depicting an *acutely* ill patient who agreed that *the physician would have to explain the observed outcome* (fig. A2.2, question 6). Absolute numbers are shown in parentheses. Significance of pairwise comparisons: *$p < 0.05$ by Fischer's exact test.

Similar results regarding the need for explanation are obtained in the vignette involving an acutely ill patient, as shown in figure A2.10, though in this case there is a somewhat smaller *marginal* need for explanation of errors (comparing versions FU and NU, for example) than in the case involving a chronically ill patient. Nevertheless, the absolute percentages for five of the six versions of the vignette are higher in figure A2.10 than in figure A2.9, suggesting a greater need for explanation (regardless of prediction behavior) in acute than in chronic situations. Acute illness poses more of a threat to the patient and is more problematic for the doctor.

Findings for Chapter 6: The Self-Fulfilling Prophecy

Belief in Self-Fulfilling Prophecy in Chronically Ill Patients

In the first experiment, as outlined above, all subjects received a version of a clinical vignette describing a seventy-two-year-old patient with metastic prostate cancer being cared for by a "Dr. Brown." Figure A2.11 summarizes another result of this experiment. The percentage of physicians who agreed with the statement "What Dr. Brown told the patient about the patient's prospects for recovery contributed to the observed survival outcome" is shown for each of the six groups. Groups NU and NF are the control versions of the vignette, versions in which the Dr. Brown made no prediction and in which unfavorable or favorable outcomes were observed, respectively. Respondents' belief in the ability of predictions to influence outcomes may be seen by comparing other prediction/outcome situations with the controls.

In version NU, the doctor makes no prediction about how long the patient will live, and the patient is noted to have lived for a relatively short period (two months); in this version, only 17.9 percent of the respondents agreed that this prognostic behavior "contributed to the observed survival outcome." By comparison, 40.0 percent of respondents who received version UU, in which the doctor predicted a short survival (and a short survival was in fact observed), agreed that this prognostic behavior contributed to the outcome. Thus, in this situation, respondents believed in the effectiveness of the self-fulfilling prophecy with respect to a relatively unfavorable outcome.

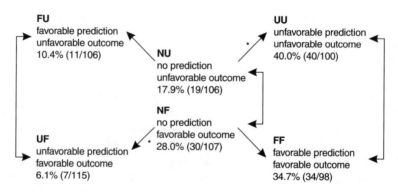

Figure A2.11. Percentage of physicians receiving each of six versions of a vignette depicting a *chronically* ill patient who agreed that *the prediction contributed to the outcome* (fig. A2.1, question 2). Absolute numbers are shown in parentheses. Significance of pairwise comparisons: *$p < 0.05$ by Fischer's exact test.

In version NF, the doctor makes no prediction but the patient is noted to have lived for a relatively long period (twenty-four months); in this version, 28.0 percent of the respondents agreed that the prognostic behavior contributed to the observed survival outcome. By comparison, 34.7 percent of respondents who received version FF, in which the doctor predicted a long survival (which was then observed), agreed that this prognostic behavior promoted the observed outcome. Thus, in this situation, respondents believed in the effectiveness of the self-fulfilling prophecy with respect to a relatively favorable outcome.

A statistical test of the hypothesis that physicians believe that un-favorable predictions help to cause unfavorable outcomes (comparing versions NU and UU) *and* that favorable predictions help to cause favorable outcomes (comparing NF and FF) suggests that physicians believe in the self-fulfilling prophecy.[10] However, in this case, involving a chronic condition with a long survival horizon, physicians definitely believe in the *negative* self-fulfilling prophecy, whereas they may or may not believe in the positive self-fulfilling prophecy. That is, the pairwise difference between NU and UU is statistically significant, whereas the pairwise difference between NF and FF is not.[11]

Not only is the difference between NF and FF smaller than the difference between NU and UU, but a higher percentage of physicians believe in the effectiveness of the doctor's behavior in version UU than do so in version FF (40.0 percent versus 34.7 percent), though this difference does not reach statistical significance. More physicians, that is, agreed that a short prediction contributes to a short survival than that a long prediction contributes to a long survival, again suggesting that the strength of the belief in the positive self-fulfilling prophecy is lower than the belief in the negative self-fulfilling prophecy.

Thus, in this setting of a chronic disease with a relatively long survival horizon, pessimism is more likely to be believed by physicians to have an impact than is optimism, probably because there is an a priori expectation that the patient will have a relatively favorable outcome in this case; while neither a two-month nor a two-year survival is implausible or "unusual," the two-year survival is actually more likely. Thus, a *pessimistic* prediction goes against the grain and may precipitate a decline in a patient otherwise likely to do relatively well.

At least two other important comparisons illustrated in figure A2.11 illuminate physicians' beliefs in this area. Comparing the two control versions (NU versus NF) reveals that physicians are more likely to believe that making no prediction contributes to longer survival than that it promotes shorter survival, though this difference did not quite reach statistical significance at the customary level.[12] In the case of a chronically ill patient with an expected survival on the order of two months to two years, making no prediction is associated with a relatively favorable outcome. In other words, in this situation, physicians are more likely to believe that saying nothing will have a beneficent rather than a maleficent effect since the background expectation is that the patient will have a relatively favorable outcome.

Comparing version NU with FU and version NF with UF permits an assessment of the extent to which physicians believe in the self-negating prophecy, whether positive or negative. In this setting, it is hard to imagine that a patient would desire to live a shorter period (assuming such a choice could be made) simply to prove the physician's long survival prediction wrong. Such a negative self-negating prophecy would be ridiculous here, and the comparison between versions NU and FU confirms this: while 17.9 percent of the controls agreed that not articulating a prognosis led to a short survival, only 10.4 percent of those receiving version FU believed the doctor's long prediction fostered a short survival. Similarly, comparing versions UF and NF reveals that physicians do not believe that making a short prediction rather than no prediction will delay death—indeed, quite the opposite. There is no evidence that physicians believe in the self-negating prophecy, either positive or negative. These beliefs regarding the self-negating prophecy are an additional reason for physicians to make optimistic survival predictions, since optimistic predictions cannot hurt patients.

In summary, the pattern of responses to different versions of this vignette revealed (1) that physicians believe in the ability of predictions to contribute to survival outcomes and (2) that unfavorable predictions are deemed more likely to influence events than are favorable predictions, at least in this situation, wherein the baseline survival expectation is indeed relatively favorable.

Belief in Self-Fulfilling Prophecy in Acutely Ill Patients

In the second experiment, all subjects received a version of a clinical vignette describing a sixty-nine-year-old patient with a serious pneumonia in an intensive care unit being cared for by a "Dr. Jones." Figure A2.12 summarizes the relevant portion of this experiment. The percentage of physicians who agreed with the statement "What Dr. Jones told the patient about the patient's prospects for recovery contributed to the observed survival outcome" is shown for each of the six groups. Groups NU and NF are again the control versions of the vignette, versions in which Dr. Jones made no prediction. Respondents' belief in the ability of predictions to influence outcomes in the setting of an acutely life-threatening illness may be seen by comparing other prediction/outcome situations with the controls.

In version NU, the doctor makes no prediction about whether the patient will live, and the patient is noted to have died; in this version, 14.6 percent of the respondents agreed that this prognostic behavior contributed to the observed survival outcome. By comparison, 21.2 percent of respondents who received version UU, in which the doctor predicted death and death occurred, agreed that this prognostic behavior contributed to the outcome. Thus, in this situation, respondents believed in the effectiveness of the self-fulfilling prophecy with respect to a relatively unfavorable outcome.

In version NF, the doctor again makes no prediction but the patient is noted to have recovered; in this version, only 7.6 percent of the respondents agreed that the prognostic behavior contributed to the patient's survival outcome. By comparison, 41.9 percent of respondents who received version FF, in which the doctor predicted recovery (and the patient recovered), agreed that this prognostic behavior fostered the observed outcome. Thus, in this situation, respondents tended to believe in the effectiveness of the self-fulfilling prophecy with respect to a relatively favorable outcome.

As in the previous experiment, a statistical test of the hypothesis that physicians believe that unfavorable predictions help to cause unfavorable outcomes (comparing versions NU and UU) *and* that fa-

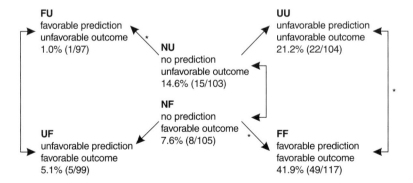

Figure A2.12. Percentage of physicians receiving each of six versions of a vignette depicting an *acutely* ill patient who agreed that *the prediction contributed to the outcome* (fig. A2.2, question 2). Absolute numbers are shown in parentheses. Significance of pairwise comparisons: *$p < 0.05$ by Fischer's exact test.

vorable predictions help to cause favorable outcomes (comparing NF and FF) suggests that physicians believe in the self-fulfilling prophecy. However, in this case, involving an acute condition with a short survival horizon, physicians definitely believe in the *positive* self-fulfilling prophecy, whereas they may or may not believe in the negative self-fulfilling prophecy. That is, the pairwise difference between NF and FF is statistically significant, whereas that between NU and UU is not.[13]

Not only is the difference between NF and FF greater than the difference between NU and UU, but a higher percentage of physicians believe in the effectiveness of the doctor's prognosis in version FF than do so with respect to version UU (41.9 percent versus 21.2 percent). That is, significantly more physicians agreed that a favorable prediction contributed to recovery than thought an unfavorable prediction contributed to death, suggesting that the strength of the belief in positive self-fulfilling prophecy is higher than the belief in the negative self-fulling prophecy.

In this setting of acutely life-threatening disease, then, optimism is considered more likely to have an impact than is pessimism, probably because there is an a priori expectation that the patient will have a relatively unfavorable outcome. That is, while neither recovery nor death would be thought "unusual," death is considered to be more likely. Thus, an *optimistic* prediction goes against the grain and may foster improvement in a patient otherwise expected to do relatively poorly.

In this vignette, comparing the two control versions (NU and NF) reveals that physicians are more likely to believe that not making a prediction contributes to a shorter survival than that it fosters a longer survival, though this difference did not quite reach statistical significance at the customary level.[14] In the case of an acutely ill patient with a significant chance of death within a few days, making no prediction is associated with the background expectation of a relatively unfavorable outcome. Physicians are more likely to believe that saying nothing will have a maleficent rather than a beneficent effect, perhaps because the background expectation is that the patient will likely die.

Comparing version NU with FU and version NF with UF permits an assessment of the extent to which physicians believe in the self-negating prophecy. While 14.6 percent of the respondents to version NU agreed that the absence of a prediction contributed to the patient's death, only 1.0 percent of those who received version FU believed that Dr. Jones's favorable prediction contributed to the patient's death. Physicians do not believe, in other words, that predicting survival will hasten death. Comparing versions NF and UF reveals that physicians are as likely to believe that predicting death fosters recovery as to believe that making no prediction fosters recovery. Again, there is no evidence that physicians believe in the self-negating prophecy. Thus, choosing to predict recovery over choosing to say nothing is a no-lose proposition—at least with respect to the patient's prospects for recovery—since it cannot adversely affect survival.

In summary, the pattern of responses to different versions of this vignette revealed (1) that physicians believe in the ability of predictions to contribute to survival outcomes and (2) that favorable predictions are considered more likely to influence events than are unfavorable predictions, at least in this situation, wherein the baseline survival expectation is relatively unfavorable.

Physicians' Attributes Associated with the Belief in Self-Fulfilling Prophecy

In addition to responding to the experimental vignettes, physicians participating in the survey were asked direct questions about their belief in the effectiveness of predictions; these questions were not coupled to any clinical vignettes. A majority indicated belief in both positive and negative self-fulfilling prophecy: 73 percent believed that "All else being equal, predicting a favorable outcome to a patient can help a favorable outcome come to pass," and 61 percent believed that "All else being equal, predicting an unfavorable outcome to a patient can help an unfavorable outcome come to pass." Physicians believing in positive self-fulfilling prophecy were highly likely also to believe in negative self-fulfilling prophecy ($p < 0.001$).

The fact that the percentages of physicians acknowledging these beliefs in response to direct questions are even higher than those reported in the two vignettes probably reflects the willingness of physicians to endorse the notion of the self-fulfilling prophecy in general, even if they had some reservations about its relevance to those two particular cases.

Bivariate and multivariate logistic regression models were estimated to assess the relation of various attributes of physicians to their belief in positive and negative self-fulfilling prophecy. The bivariate results are summarized in table A2.1.

Findings for Chapter 5: Responding to Patient Expectations

To evaluate the generalizability of the qualitative findings regarding the manner in which physicians respond to patients' perceptions about their own prognoses, two additional experiments were incorporated

Table A2.1. Bivariate relations between selected variables and the belief in positive and negative self-fulfilling prophecy (SFP)

Variable	Belief in positive SFP Odds Ratio (95% CI)	Belief in negative SFP Odds Ratio (95% CI)
Age (five-year increment)	1.14 (1.03–1.25)*	1.08 (0.99–1.17)
Male gender	0.93 (0.57–1.51)	0.98 (0.63–1.51)
Board-certified	0.81 (0.50–1.32)	0.91 (0.59–1.40)
Generalist	1.61 (1.10–2.36)*	1.11 (0.79–1.56)
Optimist	1.78 (1.10–2.88)*	1.52 (0.96–2.41)
Adequate training in prognostication	1.10 (0.75–1.61)	1.14 (0.80–1.61)
Patients accept prognoses when offered	0.71 (0.35–1.45)	1.29 (0.72–2.30)
Experience with requests for prognostic information (number of patients per year, ten-patient increment)	0.95 (0.91–0.99)*	0.97 (0.93–1.01)

*$p < 0.05$

into the survey. These experiments involved altogether different clinical vignettes and questions from those discussed above; more detail is available elsewhere.[15] Partial results for one experiment are summarized here.

In this experiment, all subjects received a clinical vignette describing a hypothetical sixty-six-year-old man with chronic obstructive pulmonary disease and pneumonia necessitating ICU admission. At the end of the vignette, this seriously ill patient, who has a substantial chance of dying, expresses an opinion about his "prognosis for being discharged from the hospital and returning to his previous baseline." Physician respondents were randomized to receive one of five different versions of the vignette, which varied only in the degree of optimism, pessimism, or neither expressed by the hypothetical patient. Respondents were then asked a series of identically worded questions about how much optimism or pessimism about the patient's prognosis they would communicate to the patient himself and to their professional colleagues. Differences in responses to these questions can logically only be attributed to differences in the group assignment of the subjects, an assignment under experimental control.[16]

Table A2.2 summarizes the results of one question. If the patient expresses neither optimism nor pessimism about his prognosis, 40.9 percent of the physicians would express optimism to the patient. However, if the patient expresses optimism, a larger percentage, 51.5 percent, express optimism. Similarly, if the patient expresses pessimism, a slightly larger percentage, 44.2 percent, express optimism. Overall, what the patient says to the physician about his prognosis is statistically significantly associated with what the physician would say to the patient. The pattern, however, is a U-shaped one, with physicians expressing increased levels of optimism in response to *either* patient pessimism or optimism.

Moreover, physicians appear to believe in the ability of optimism in the patient to materially improve the chances for a favorable outcome: not only do they increase the optimism they express to the *patient* in such a situation, but in other questions connected to this vignette and not detailed here, they also increase the amount of optimism about the (truly unfavorable) prognosis that they would communicate to *colleagues*. Patient optimism affects both personal and impersonal prognosis.[17]

Physicians are always substantially more optimistic with patients regarding the patient's condition than they are with professional colleagues, consistent with the data regarding discrepant communication reviewed in chapter 5. These results are given in table A2.3 for the special case of situations where the patient in the vignette expressed neither optimism nor pessimism.[18] For any given level of optimism a respondent may have expressed about the patient's prognosis to a colleague (an indication of the respondent's "objective" assessment of the gravity of the patient's illness), respondents were substantially and significantly more likely to be more optimistic when talking to patients.

These patterns document the presence of optimism in physicians' discussions of prognosis out of proportion to their objective assess-

Table A2.2. Relation between expressions of optimism or pessimism by a hypothetical patient to the physician and by the physician to the patient.

	Patient's statement to physician (experimentally controlled)		
	pessimistic	neither	optimistic
Physician's statement to patient, *N* (column %)			
pessimistic	78 (37.5)	81 (39.9)	52 (22.9)
neither	38 (18.3)	39 (19.2)	58 (25.6)
optimistic	92 (44.2)	83 (40.9)	117 (51.5)
Total	208 (100.0)	203 (100.0)	227 (100.0)

Note: A likelihood ratio $\chi 2$ test rejects the null hypothesis that there is no relation between what the patient says to the doctor about the prognosis and what the doctor then says to the patient ($p < 0.001$).

Table A2.3. Difference between degree of optimism communicated to a hypothetical patient and to a hypothetical colleague, N (%).

	Physician's statement to colleague				
	pessimistic	neither	optimistic	Total	
Physician's statement to patient, N (%)					
pessimistic	74 (36.5)	6 (3.0)	1 (0.5)	81	(39.9)
neither	34 (16.8)	5 (2.5)	0 (0.0)	39	(19.2)
optimistic	31 (15.3)	29 (14.3)	23 (11.3)	83	(40.9)
Total	139 (68.5)	40 (19.7)	24 (11.8)	203	(100.0)

Note: Subjects (203 internists) received a vignette describing a sixty-six-year-old man with chronic obstructive pulmonary disease and pneumonia necessitating ICU admission who expressed "neither optimism nor pessimism" about his prognosis. Subjects were queried regarding how much prognostic optimism or pessimism they would communicate to the patient and to a colleague. A McNemar $\chi 2$ text rejects the null hypothesis that physicians are as likely to be disproportionately optimistic with patients as compared with colleagues as to be disproportionately pessimistic with colleagues as compared with patients; rather, they are substantially more likely to be disproportionately optimistic with patients ($p < 0.001$).

ments, as well as the tendency of physicians to respond to patient expectations. When the prognosis is both unfavorable and uncertain, as it is in this vignette, optimism is communicated to patients in a way that is recognizant of the patient's expectations. In short, this experiment shows that in their prognostic pronouncements, physicians correct patient pessimism and reinforce patient optimism. Moreover, physicians express substantially more optimism overall to patients than their objective assessment—at least as reflected in their communications to colleagues—would support.

Acknowledgments

I once read an essay by a medical ethicist (whose name I have sadly forgotten) arguing that medical knowledge is not proprietary, but rather is held in trust by physicians. Generations of patients had suffered, and generations of physicians had toiled, to create the knowledge that I was being given. It was mine not to keep, but rather to accept with gratitude, to augment if I could, and to pass on. This fact, the author argued, imposed important, transcendent obligations on physicians. This is how I feel about my work here and about the many individuals who have contributed to it.

I am especially grateful to the numerous physicians who consented to be interviewed; to the hospices that were willing to be visited and have their staff, patients, and physicians interrogated; to the 365 physicians who completed the phone survey eliciting their prognostic estimates; and to the anonymous 697 physicians who returned my lengthy mail survey for no reason other than altruism. For access to additional data, I am grateful to my friend James Tulsky who, along with his collaborators, made available a set of tapes of physicians talking to their patients about advance directives, and to Wendy Levinson, with whom I collaborated to analyze a set of tapes she originally collected of routine discussions between physicians and their patients.

For criticism of several drafts of this book, as well as of raw field notes and interview transcripts, I owe an unrepayable debt to my dear friend, brilliant teacher, treasured mentor, and extraordinary sociologist Renée C. Fox. Her input sharpened and extended the arguments, embellished the prose, and contributed to insights throughout the book. She was usually able to see more in excerpts than I was, even when I had read them a dozen times. "Yes," she would write in the margin in familiar and beautiful ribbonlike, black-ink script, "but you might also wish to note. . . ." This book and the arguments it makes could not have appeared without her.

For additional criticism of either early or partial versions of this manuscript, I have several other friends, colleagues, teachers, and relatives to thank: Paul Beeson, Harold Bershady, Charles Bidwell, Charles Bosk, Alexander Christakis, Chris Feudtner, Arthur Frank, Peter Friedmann, Amy Justice, Robert Klitzman, Elizabeth Lamont, Wendy Levinson,

David Mechanic, Charles Rosenberg, Marta Tienda, Sankey Williams, and especially my dear friend and teacher Paul Allison.

Over the last three years, I have been privileged to work with Jack Iwashyna, a graduate student engaged in M.D./Ph.D. training in medicine and social science at the University of Chicago. First as a student, then as a research assistant, and now as a colleague, Jack has had my highest esteem. He read the entire manuscript, made helpful comments, and collaborated in the analysis of some of the quantitative data. Over the course of these three years, in working on this and several other projects, he has also become a friend. I am very grateful.

For administrative support of the highest caliber, and for good-humored and painstaking attention to detail, I owe substantial thanks to Kimberly Thomas. I thank Tammy Polonsky, Elena Linden, and Jennifer Chertow for help in conducting some of the semistructured interviews, for administration of the hospice phone survey, and for collecting some of the references.

I am grateful to the University of Chicago for providing an extraordinary intellectual environment in which to work—critical, rigorous, synthetic. The Section of General Internal Medicine in the Department of Medicine, and the Department of Sociology, provided supportive and collegial professional homes for me, and I am grateful. I owe thanks as well to my editors at the University of Chicago Press, Doug Mitchell and Joel Score.

Financial support for this work came from several sources. The writing of the book, and some of the data collection, took place while I was partially supported as a Soros Project on Death in America Faculty Scholar at the University of Chicago from 1995 to 1998. The majority of the data collection, and the initial drafting of some of the text, took place while I was supported at the University of Pennsylvania, first as a Robert Wood Johnson Clinical Scholar (from 1991 to 1993) and then as an Agency for Health Care Policy and Research National Research Service Award Fellow (from 1993 to 1995). Part of the cost of the mail survey was defrayed by the Center for Bioethics at the University of Pennsylvania, under the leadership of Arthur Caplan.

I wish also to thank the physicians in my family—my brothers, Dimitri Christakis and Quan-Yang Duh, sister-in-law, Danielle Zerr, and father-in-law, James Zuckerman—for allowing me to engage and enrage them with discussions of prognosis. Katrina Christakis graciously tolerated this.

About my wife, Erika, I have more than the usual sorts of things to say in a place such as this. Of course she read every page several times, put up with my sleepless nights, cared for Sebastian, Lysander, and Eleni at all hours. But her most important contribution was to make use of her remarkable talents as a writer to fix numerous problems in this work. I can trace some of the sections of the book with which I am happiest directly to her suggestions. I hope one day that I will be able to return the favor and edit her prose as she has mine. Her contribution has been remarkable in yet one more way: she makes possible a collaboration in life that is so thoroughgoing that everything I do, and not just this book, is a product of her as well as myself. I am enormously grateful.

Preface

1. See, for example, Aristotle, *Metaphysics,* trans. H. G. Apostle (Bloomington: Indiana University Press, 1966).

2. S. Gilbert, "For Cancer Patients, Hope Can Add to Pain," *New York Times,* 9 June 1998, F7.

3. N. A. Christakis, "Managing Death: The Growing Acceptance of Euthanasia in Contemporary American Society," in R. P. Hamel and E. R. DuBose, eds., *Must We Suffer Our Way to Death? Cultural and Theological Perspectives on Death by Choice* (Dallas: Southern Methodist University Press, 1996), 15–44.

4. Hastings Center, *Guidelines for the Termination of Life-Sustaining Treatment and the Care of the Dying* (Briarcliff Manor, N.Y.: Hastings Center, 1987).

5. *Compassion in Dying v. Washington,* 850 F. Supp. 1454 (W.D. Wash. 1994); Oregon Revised Statute 127,800 to 127,897 (Oregon Death with Dignity Act); M. A. Drickamer, M. A. Lee, and L. Ganzini, "Practical Issues in Physician-Assisted Suicide," *Annals of Internal Medicine* 126 (1997): 146–51; M. A. Lee, H. D. Nelson, B. P. Tilden, et al., "Legalizing Assisted Suicide—Views of Physicians in Oregon," *New England Journal of Medicine* 334 (1996): 310–15.

6. Social Security Act 1861(dd)(3)(A).

7. SUPPORT principal investigators, "A Controlled Trial to Improve Care for Seriously Ill Hospitalized Patients: The Study to Understand Prognoses and Preferences for Outcomes and Risks of Treatments (SUPPORT)," *Journal of the American Medical Association* 274 (1995): 1591–98.

8. See, for example, S. Gilbert, "Study Finds Doctors Refuse Patients' Requests on Death," *New York Times,* 22 November 1995, A1.

9. Regarding these techniques, see, respectively, N. A. Christakis and E. B. Lamont, "The Extent and Determinants of Error in Physicians' Prognoses for Terminally Ill Patients," unpublished manuscript; N. A. Christakis, "Optimal Ways of Predicting Mortality as Assessed by Comparison to the Gold Standard or Observed Mortality," unpublished manuscript; R. M. Poses, C. Bekes, R. L. Winkler, et al., "Are Two (Inexperienced) Heads Better than One (Experienced) Head?" *Archives of Internal Medicine* 150 (1990): 1874–78; and W. A. Knaus, F. E. Harrell Jr., J. Lynn, et al., "The SUPPORT Prognostic Model: Objective Estimates of Survival for Seriously Ill Hospitalized Adults," *Annals of Internal Medicine* 122: 191–203 (1995).

Chapter One

1. R. Hutchison, "Prognosis," *Lancet* 226 (1934): 697–98, 697.

2. P. D. White, "Principles and Practice of Prognosis, with Particular Reference to Heart Disease," *Journal of the American Medical Association* 153 (1953):

75–79, 75. It is my plan, incidentally, to illuminate what the reasons are that it has "rarely been studied."

3. S. W. Fletcher, R. H. Fletcher, and M. A. Greganti, "Clinical Research Trends in General Medical Journals, 1946–1976," in E. B. Roberts, R. I. Levy, S. N. Finkelstein, et al., eds., *Biomedical Innovation* (Cambridge: MIT Press, 1981), 284–300. The category "diagnosis" here includes several of the authors' subcategories. The remaining 26 percent of studies were devoted to issues such as the frequency and manifestations of disease.

4. J. F. Fries and G. B. Ehrlich, *Prognosis: Contemporary Outcomes of Disease* (Bowie, Md.: Charles Press, 1981), 8.

5. N. A. Christakis, *Prognostication and Death in Medical Thought and Practice* (Ann Arbor, Mich.: University Microfilms, 1995), 306ff. The textbook analyzed was J. D. Wilson, E. Braunwald, K. J. Isselbacher, et al., *Harrison's Principles of Internal Medicine*, 12th ed. (New York: McGraw-Hill, 1991).

6. N. A. Christakis, "The Ellipsis of Prognosis in Modern Medical Thought," *Social Science and Medicine* 44 (1997): 301–15; editions of the textbook analyzed included W. Osler, *The Principles and Practice of Medicine*, 1st ed. (New York: D. Appleton Company, 1892); W. Osler and T. McCrae, eds., *The Principles and Practice of Medicine*, 9th ed. (New York: D. Appleton Company, 1924); and H. Christian, ed., *The Principles and Practice of Medicine*, 16th ed. (New York: D. Appleton-Century, 1947). Additional support for this epistemological point can be found elsewhere. For example, regarding the centrality of prognostic concerns in a condition (polio) for which no curative treatment was available, see F. Davis, *Passage through Crisis: Polio Victims and Their Families* (New Brunswick, N.J.: Transaction Publishers, 1991). The Hippocratic medical texts also present prognosis as an active means by which doctors could confront a disease when therapy is limited. See Hippocrates, "Prognosis," in *Hippocratic Writings*, ed. G. E. R. Lloyd, trans. J. Chadwick and W. N. Mann (New York: Penguin, 1978), 170–85.

7. Regarding earlier notions of treatment, see C. E. Rosenberg, "The Therapeutic Revolution: Medicine, Meaning and Social Change in 19th-Century America," in J. W. Leavitt and R. L. Numbers, eds., *Sickness and Health in America* (Madison: University of Wisconsin Press, 1985), 39–52.

8. M. Lerner and O. W. Anderson, *Health Progress in the United States: 1900–1960* (Chicago: University of Chicago Press, 1963); U.S. Bureau of the Census, *Statistical Abstract of the United States, 1976* (Washington, D.C.: Government Printing Office, 1976).

9. Osler and McCrae, *Principles and Practice of Medicine*, 9th ed., 78.

10. In a sense, this transition was presaged by what Michel Foucault has called the "birth of the clinic"; see M. Foucault, *The Birth of the Clinic: An Archaeology of Medical Perception* (New York: Vintage Books, 1975). Fries and Ehrlich, *Prognosis*, 5, also refers to the "unnatural history of disease." See also C. Feudtner, *Bittersweet: The Transformation of Diabetes into a Chronic Illness in Twentieth-Century America* (Ann Arbor, Mich.: University Microfilms, 1995), on the biologically and socially "transmuted" course of a once uniformly and quickly fatal acute disease to a variably and slowly fatal chronic one.

11. The relative salience of prognosis in the "premodern" textbooks is

illustrated not only by the amount of text devoted to the topic, but also by the fact that the section on prognosis *precedes* the sections on diagnosis and therapy.

12. Christakis, "Ellipsis of Prognosis."

13. Foucault, *Birth of the Clinic*, 97.

14. An unexpected and paradoxical corollary of this development, however, is that it becomes possible to define certain features and outcomes of an individual patient's disease as "atypical." This in turn raises new problems of interpretation and meaning for physicians. Whereas typical cases are seen as straightforward, generic, and predictable, atypical cases are complicated, individual, and unpredictable. The prognosis may be presumed in typical cases, but in atypical cases it must be explicitly addressed. Physicians feel less compelled to develop and communicate prognoses if the patient is on a typical course, toward either a good or a bad outcome. When the expected outcome in an individual case deviates from the usual outcome in such cases as a group, physicians feel obliged, to some degree, to prognosticate and to think about what will really happen and why. The notion of typicality and atypicality thus suggests that, whereas in some patients the presentation and course are *generic to the disease,* in some they may be *specific to the individual.* With respect to prognosis, atypical patients are particularly important to physicians, who feel obligated to explore the source of the atypicality. Prognostication is thus paradoxically both confounded and supported by atypicality. On the one hand, atypicality suggests deviation from the prognosis inherent in the diagnosis and therapy, making prognosis more difficult. On the other hand, atypicality provides the basis for, and creates the need for, a physician to formulate a specific prognosis for an individual patient. Atypicality increases the compunction to be explicit about the future. The problem of atypicality is magnified when, because of effective therapy, disease generally has a uniform and favorable outcome. The atypical (in the sense of therapeutically unresponsive) case is a threat not only to the health of the patient, but also to the reputation of the physician. When the physician has powerful therapy, an unfavorable outcome means failure—not just of the therapeutic armamentarium to achieve its objective, but also of physicians to fulfill their social role. Medical advances and discoveries since the turn of the century have held such promise that society has confidently given physicians the duty and the privilege to eradicate disease. In the application of treatment, physicians found a new way to meet their obligation to control disease. This obligation and the relationship between prognosis and therapy were aptly captured by one eminent physician in the mid-1800s, who observed that "the public . . . expect something more of physicians than the power of distinguishing diseases and of predicting their issue. They look to them for the relief of their sufferings, and the cure or removal of their complaints." (See J. Bigelow, *Brief Expositions of Rational Medicine, to Which Is Prefixed the Paradise of Doctors . . .* [Boston: Phillips, Sampson & Co., 1858], iv.) When therapy is unavailable or ineffective, prognosis can come quite forcefully to the foreground. When therapy is available and effective, prognosis often recedes to the background of clinical practice.

15. One of the few clinical books on prognosis with which I am familiar is, in fact, a recently published one in the field of neurology, which opens with the following observation: "Prognosis is a particularly pertinent purpose in neurology.

Although neuroscience has seen stupendous advances in chemistry, physiology, pathology, diagnosis, and therapy, the relative inability of the nervous system to regenerate and recover, its sequestration, and its complexity make the nervous system less amenable to therapeutic strategies that are successful in other organ systems. The neurologist is commonly consulted not only to diagnose, but to prognosticate." See J. M. Gilchrist, ed., *Prognosis in Neurology* (Boston: Butterworth-Heinemann, 1998), xxi.

16. An analogous pattern has been observed, across ethnic groups, with respect to pain; some patients are more interested in relief from their pain ("When will it end?"), others in knowing its origins ("What does it mean?"). See M. Zborowski, "Cultural Components in Responses to Pain," *Journal of Social Issues* 8 (1952): 16–30.

17. Regarding the last item, see, for example, P. G. Filene, *In the Arms of Others: A Cultural History of the Right-to-Die in America* (Chicago: Ivan R. Dee, 1998).

18. Chronic disease currently accounts for 70 to 75 percent of all deaths in the United States and is increasing. See U.S. Bureau of the Census, *Historical Statistics of the United States (1900–1970)* (Washington, D.C.: Government Printing Office, 1975); I. Seeman, *National Mortality Followback Survey: 1986 Summary, United States,* 20(19) (National Center for Health Statistics, Vital and Health Statistics, 1992); United Nations, "World Population Prospects: Estimates and Projections as Assessed in 1982," in *Population Studies,* ST/ESA/SER.A/86 (New York: Department of International Economic and Social Affairs, 1985).

19. Nevertheless, chronicity may also stifle interest in prognosis, insofar as the prospect of curing or eliminating the underlying disease is generally limited. Indeed, Kathy Charmaz argues that chronically ill patients experience time in a foreshortened way, perhaps reducing the importance of prognosis (particularly with regard to long-term sequelae). Nonetheless, patients with chronic disease are keenly concerned with the meaning of time in their lives. Strangely, Charmaz never explicitly considers the role of coping with one's prognosis as such when one is chronically ill. See K. Charmaz, *Good Days, Bad Days: The Self in Chronic Illness and Time* (New Brunswick, N.J.: Rutgers University Press, 1991). It is noteworthy that physicians sometimes avoid chronically ill patients with no prospect for cure; such patients are sometimes described pejoratively as "gomers." See T. Mizrahi, *Getting Rid of Patients: Contradictions in the Socialization of Physicians* (New Brunswick, N.J.: Rutgers University Press, 1986); regarding "gomers," see D. B. Leiderman and J. A. Grisso, "The Gomer Phenomenon," *Journal of Health and Social Behavior* 26 (1985): 222–32.

20. See M. S. Larson, "Proletarianization and Educated Labor," *Theory and Society* 9 (1979): 131–75. This development is consistent with a long-standing trend toward intercalating physicians within institutional structures. See T. Parsons, *The Social System* (New York: Free Press, 1951), e.g. 436; and, generally, P. Starr, *The Social Transformation of American Medicine* (New York: Basic Books, 1982).

21. See N. A. Christakis and J. J. Escarce, "Survival of Medicare Patients after Enrollment in Hospice Programs," *New England Journal of Medicine* 335 (1996): 172–78. See also W. Bulkin and H. Lukashok, "Rx for Dying: The Case for

Hospice," *New England Journal of Medicine* 318 (1988): 376–78. The widespread adoption of the six-month criterion by physicians themselves suggests that bureaucratic, structural circumstances may feed back on the structure of medical knowledge. This criterion is, for example, the standard used in most published studies of "terminal" illness. The six-month standard has also found its way into current proposals to permit physician-assisted suicide—which, incidentally, do not question physicians' ability and willingness to certify that patients have "less than six months to live." Nevertheless, physicians vary in their definition of terminality; see N. A. Christakis and T. J. Iwashyna, "Attitude and Self-Reported Practice Regarding Prognostication in a National Sample of Internists," *Archives of Internal Medicine* 158 (1998): 2389–95.

22. Patients apparently are less attentive to such figures. See, for example, E. C. Schneider and A. M. Epstein, "Use of Public Performance Reports: A Survey of Patients Undergoing Cardiac Surgery," *Journal of the American Medical Association* 279 (1998): 1638–42. Fewer than 1 percent of patients overall knew the success rates of their physicians or hospitals.

23. S. F. Jencks, J. Daley, D. Draper, et al., "Interpreting Hospital Mortality Data: The Role of Clinical Risk Adjustment," *Journal of the American Medical Association* 260 (1988): 3611–16; W. A. Knaus, D. P. Wagner, and E. A. Draper, "The Value of Measuring Severity of Disease in Clinical Research on Acutely Ill Patients," *Journal of Chronic Disease* 37 (1984): 455–63; A. W. Wu, "The Measure and Mismeasure of Hospital Quality: Appropriate Risk-Adjustment Methods in Comparing Hospitals," *Annals of Internal Medicine* 122 (1995): 149–50; S. Greenfield, L. Sullivan, R. Silliman, et al., "Principles and Practice of Case Mix Adjustment: Applications to End-Stage Renal Disease," *American Journal of Kidney Diseases* 24 (1994): 298–307; L. I. Iezzoni, A. S. Ash, G. A. Coffman, and M. A. Moskowitz, "Predicting In-Hospital Mortality: A Comparison of Severity Measurement Approaches," *Medical Care* 30 (1992): 347–59.

24. H. C. Sox, M. A. Blatt, M. C. Higgins, and K. I. Marton, *Medical Decision Making* (Boston: Butterworth Heineman, 1988).

25. A. C. Justice, *The Development, Validation, and Evaluation of Prognostic Systems: An Application to the Acquired Immunodeficiency Syndrome (AIDS)* (Ann Arbor, Mich.: University Microfilms, 1996).

26. Intermediate endpoints have also been used to gauge the benefits of hospitalization. See E. A. Halm, M. J. Fine, T. J. Marrie, et al., "Time to Clinical Stability in Patients Hospitalized with Community-Acquired Pneumonia," *Journal of the American Medical Association* 279 (1998): 1452–57.

27. For example, a standard public policy reference states that "in principle, the procedure followed in a benefit-cost analysis consists of five steps. 1. The project or projects to be analyzed are identified. 2. All the impacts, both favorable and unfavorable, present and future, on all of society are determined. 3. Values, usually in dollars, are assigned to these impacts. Favorable impacts will be registered as benefits, unfavorable ones as costs. 4. The *net benefit* (total benefit minus total cost) is calculated. 5. The choice is made." See E. Stokey and R. Zeckhauser, *A Primer for Policy Analysis* (New York: W. W. Norton, 1978), 136 (emphasis in original). See also Sox, Blatt, Higgins, and Marton, *Medical Decision Making*.

28. The emergence of certain other technologies, specifically designed to predict the outcome of a pregnancy, is also relevant to the increasing salience of prognostication. For example, amniocentesis is applied in an effort to predict which births might produce a "defective" newborn and to afford the opportunity of abortion; it has come to be viewed as routine in many circumstances. See B. K. Rothman, *The Tentative Pregnancy: Prenatal Diagnosis and the Future of Motherhood* (New York: Penguin, 1986). See also D. C. Wertz and J. C. Fletcher, "Fatal Knowledge? Prenatal Diagnosis and Sex Selection," *Hastings Center Report* 19 (1989): 21–27. Prognosis is also the essential aspect of genetic counseling *after* the birth of a child with a manifest birth defect; see C. L. Bosk, *"All God's Mistakes": Genetic Counseling in a Pediatric Hospital* (Chicago: University of Chicago Press, 1992). Other relevant examples of new technologies that provide prognostic information include blood tests for prostate and other cancers, surveillance mammography, HIV testing, and cholesterol screening. With respect to screening for prostate and cervical cancer and of cholesterol, see L. B. Russell, *Educated Guesses: Making Policy about Medical Screening Tests* (Berkeley: University of California Press, 1994).

29. See, for example, B. Kremer, P. Goldberg, S. E. Andrew, et al., "A Worldwide Study of the Huntington's Disease Mutation: The Sensitivity and Specificity of Measuring CAG Repeats," *New England Journal of Medicine* 330 (1994): 1401–6. See also chapter 2 regarding the benefits of testing in terms of the reduction of uncertainty.

30. V. R. Grann, K. S. Panageas, W. Whang, et al., "Decision Analysis of Prophylactic Mastectomy and Oophorectomy in BRCA1-Positive or BRCA2-Positive Patients," *Journal of Clinical Oncology* 16 (1998): 979–85; D. Schrag, K. M. Kuntz, J. E. Garber, and J. C. Weeks, "Decision Analysis—Effects of Prophylactic Mastectomy and Oophorectomy on Life Expectancy among Women with BRCA1 or BRCA2 Mutations," *New England Journal of Medicine* 336 (1997): 1465–71; M. E. Stefanek, "Bilateral Prophylactic Mastectomy: Issues and Concerns," *Journal of the National Cancer Institute* 17 (1995): 37–42. A number of "urban legends" have arisen about this; for example, I have heard what must be apocryphal stories of twelve-year-old girls having mastectomies or women "hysterically" choosing such surgery based on very minimal information. Regarding genetic testing and cancer more generally, see R. M. Lebovitz and S. Albrecht, "Molecular Biology in the Diagnosis and Prognosis of Solid and Lymphoid Tumors," *Cancer Investigation* 10 (1992): 399–416; and, C. Lerman C and R. T. Croyle, "Emotional and Behavioral Responses to Genetic Testing for Susceptibility to Cancer," *Oncology* 10 (1996): 191–95.

31. Regarding emphysema, see E. A. Wulfsberg, D. E. Hoffman, and M. M. Cohen, "Alpha-1 Antitrypsin Deficiency: Impact of Genetic Discovery on Medicine and Society," *Journal of the American Medical Association* 271 (1994): 217–22. Regarding diabetes, see M. Siegler, S. Amiel, and J. Lantos, "Scientific and Ethical Consequences of Disease Prediction," *Diabetologia* 35 (1992): S60—S68. Regarding dementia, see J. C. S. Breitner, "Clinical Genetics and Genetic Counseling in Alzheimer Disease," *Annals of Internal Medicine* 115 (1991): 601–6. Regarding cognitive disability, see R. Plomin and J. C. De Fries, "The Genetics of Cognitive Abilities and Disabilities," *Scientific American* 278, no. 5 (1998): 62–69. Regarding

alcoholism, see A. C. Heath, "Genetic Influences on Drinking Behavior in Humans," in H. Begleiter and B. Kissin, eds., *The Genetics of Alcoholism* (New York: Oxford University Press, 1995), 81–121; and K. A. Quaid, H. Dinwiddie, P. M. Conneally, and J. I. Nurnberger Jr., "Issues in Genetic Testing for Susceptibility to Alcoholism: Lessons from Alzheimer's Disease and Huntington's Disease," *Alcoholism, Clinical & Experimental Research* 20 (1996): 1430–37.

32. S. J. Reiser, *Medicine and the Reign of Technology* (Cambridge: Cambridge University Press, 1978).

33. See R. R. Anspach, *Deciding Who Lives: Fateful Choices in the Intensive-Care Nursery* (Berkeley: University of California Press, 1993), 83, for consideration of this point in the setting of NICUs. In previous generations, physicians had an adage that captured their sense of the relation between diagnosis and therapy: "If a disease is difficult to find, it is easy to treat, and if it is easy to find, it is difficult to treat." Physicians at that time also felt that if a disease was easy to find, then it would be easy to prognosticate about. Nowadays, however, it seems that earlier detection of more and more occult conditions may complicate *both* prognosis and therapy.

34. H. G. Welch and W. Burke, "Uncertainties in Genetic Testing for Chronic Disease," *Journal of the American Medical Association* 280 (1998): 1525–27.

35. For an argument that modern medicine is causing an "epidemic" of iatrogenesis, see I. Illich, *Medical Nemesis: The Expropriation of Health* (New York: Pantheon, 1976).

36. A whole field known as "bioethics" has emerged since the end of the 1960s. See D. J. Rothman, *Strangers at the Bedside: A History of How Law and Bioethics Transformed Medical Decision Making* (New York: Basic Books, 1991); R. C. Fox, "The Entry of U.S. Bioethics into the 1990's: A Sociological Analysis," in E. R. Dubose, R. Hamel, and L. J. O'Connell, eds., *A Matter of Principles? Ferment in U.S. Bioethics* (Valley Forge, Pa.: Trinity Press International, 1994), 21–71; R. C. Fox, "The Evolution of American Bioethics: A Sociological Perspective," in George Weisz, ed., *Social Science Perspectives on Medical Ethics* (Philadelphia: University of Pennsylvania Press, 1991), 201–17. See also E. B. Beresford, "Uncertainty and the Shaping of Medical Decisions," *Hastings Center Report* 21 (1991): 6–11.

37. See R. J. Levine, *Ethics and Regulation of Clinical Research,* 2d ed. (New Haven: Yale University Press, 1986), esp. 103–6, and R. R. Faden and T. L. Beauchamp, *A History and Theory of Informed Consent* (New York: Oxford University Press, 1986).

38. See, for example, R. R. Anspach, "Prognostic Conflict in Life-and-Death Decisions: The Organization as an Ecology of Knowledge," *Journal of Health and Social Behavior* 28 (1987): 215–31; B. W. Levin, "Decision Making about Care of Catastrophically Ill Newborns: The Use of Technological Criteria," in L. M. Whiteford and M. Poland, eds., *New Approaches to Human Reproduction: Social and Ethical Dimensions* (Boulder, Colo.: Westview Press, 1989), 84–97.

39. L. J. Schneiderman, N. S. Jecker, and A. R. Jonsen, "Medical Futility: Its Meaning and Ethical Implications," *Annals of Internal Medicine* 112 (1990): 949–54. See also L. J. Schneiderman and N. S. Jecker, *Wrong Medicine: Doctors, Patients, and Futile Treatment* (Baltimore: Johns Hopkins University Press, 1995).

40. N. S. Jecker and L. J. Schneiderman, "Futility and Rationing," *American Journal of Medicine* 92 (1992): 189–96. See also Fox, "Entry of U.S. Bioethics into the 1990's." Although futility runs counter to the quintessential American medical ethos of limitless medical progress and virtually omnipotent physicians, it is consonant with other important values in medicine, such as nonmalificence and rationality. See N. A. Christakis, "Managing Death: The Growing Acceptance of Euthanasia in Contemporary American Society," in R. P. Hamel and E. R. DuBose, eds., *Must We Suffer Our Way to Death? Cultural and Theological Perspectives on Death by Choice* (Dallas: Southern Methodist University Press, 1996), 15–44.

41. J. M. Teno, D. Murphy, J. Lynn, et al., "Prognosis-Based Futility Guidelines: Does Anyone Win?" *Journal of the American Geriatrics Society* 42 (1994): 1202–7; N. S. Jecker and L. J. Schneiderman, "Medical Futility: The Duty Not to Treat," *Cambridge Quarterly Healthcare Ethics* 2 (1993): 151–59; L. J. Schneiderman and N. S. Jecker, "Futility in Practice," *Archives of Internal Medicine* 153 (1993): 437–41.

42. H. Feifel, ed., *The Meaning of Death* (New York: McGraw-Hill, 1959); E. Kübler-Ross, *On Death and Dying* (New York: Macmillan, 1969).

43. These books include A. Sankar, *Dying at Home: A Family Guide for Caregiving* (Baltimore: Johns Hopkins University Press, 1991); N. L. Mace and P. V. Rabins, *The 36-Hour Day: A Family Guide to Caring for Persons with Alzheimer's Disease, Related Dementing Illnesses, and Memory Loss in Later Life*, rev. ed. (Baltimore: Johns Hopkins University Press, 1991); L. Beresford, *The Hospice Handbook: A Complete Guide* (Boston: Little Brown & Co., 1993); D. Doyle, *Caring for a Dying Relative: A Guide for Families* (Oxford: Oxford University Press, 1994); and M. Lattanzi-Licht, J. J. Mahoney, and G. W. Miller, *The Hospice Movement: In Pursuit of a Peaceful Death* (New York: Fireside Press, 1998).

44. D. Humphry, *Final Exit: The Practicalities of Self-Deliverance and Assisted Suicide for the Dying* (Eugene, Oreg.: Hemlock Society, 1991).

45. Among others, J. Groopman, *The Measure of Our Days: New Beginnings at Life's End* (New York: Viking, 1997); I. Byock, *Dying Well: The Prospect for Growth at the End of Life* (New York: Riverhead Books, 1997); S. B. Nuland, *How We Die: Reflections on Life's Final Chapter* (New York: Alfred A. Knopf, 1994); P. Anderson, *All of Us: Americans Talk about the Meaning of Death* (New York: Delacorte Press, 1996); and M. Webb, *The Good Death: The New American Search to Reshape the End of Life* (New York: Bantam Books, 1997).

46. On the impact of social support on health, see J. S. House, K. R. Landis, and D. Umberson, "Social Relationships and Health," *Science* 241 (1988): 540–45; L. F. Berkman, "The Role of Social Relations in Health Promotion," *Psychosomatic Medicine* 57 (1995): 245–54; L. A. Lillard and L. J. Waite, " 'Til Death Do Us Part': Marital Disruption and Mortality," *American Journal of Sociology* 100 (1995): 1131–56; and L. A. Lillard and C. W. A. Panis, "Marital Status and Mortality: The Role of Health," *Demography* 33 (1996): 313–27. There also appear to be contextual effects on health; that is, different social structures may lead to different health outcomes despite equivalent baseline health status; see, for example, S. A. Robert, "Community-Level Socioeconomic Status Effects on Adult Health," *Journal of Health and Social Behavior* 39 (1998): 18–37. On the impact

of religion, see G. K. Jarvis and H. C. Northcott, "Religion and Differences in Morbidity and Mortality," *Social Science and Medicine* 25 (1987): 813–24; and, for a fascinating illustration, D. P. Phillips and D. G. Smith, "Postponement of Death until Symbolically Meaningful Occasions," *Journal of the American Medical Association* 263 (1990): 1947–51.

47. R. B. Case, A. J. Moss, N. Case, et al., "Living Alone after Myocardial Infarction: Impact on Prognosis," *Journal of the American Medical Association* 267 (1992): 515–19; R. B. Williams, J. C. Barefoot, R. M. Califf, et al., "Prognostic Importance of Social and Economic Resources among Medically Treated Patients with Angiographically Documented Coronary Artery Disease," *Journal of the American Medical Association* 267 (1992): 520–24; L. F. Berkman, L. Leo-Summers, and R. Horwitz, "Emotional Support and Survival after Myocardial Infarction: A Prospective, Population-Based Study of the Elderly," *Annals of Internal Medicine* 117 (1992): 1003–9.

48. Anspach, *Deciding Who Lives*, 65.

49. See, for example, D. Crane, *The Sanctity of Social Life: Physicians' Treatment of Critically Ill Patients* (New Brunswick, N.J.: Transaction Press, 1977). To cite an extreme example, a malformed infant with an uncertain prognosis may not be resuscitated if the "social prognosis" is poor—for instance, if its social circumstances are characterized by poverty, drug abuse, or incompetent parenting. See also N. K. Rhoden, "Treating Baby Doe: The Ethics of Uncertainty," *Hastings Center Report* 16 (1986): 34–42.

50. Specifically, 89 percent of physicians report that "when predicting the likely course of a patient's disease, [they] find it helpful to take into account the patient's social support," 41 percent find it helpful to consider the patient's religion, and 17 percent find it helpful to take the patient's income into account. These data are drawn from the survey described in Christakis and Iwashyna, "Attitude and Self-Reported Practice." The relatively low percentages of physicians admitting to taking religion and income into account are remarkable given the evidence supporting the role of such factors in patient survival, as outlined above.

51. R. A. Pearlman, "Variability in Physician Estimates of Survival for Acute Respiratory Failure in Chronic Obstructive Pulmonary Disease," *Chest* 91 (1987): 515–21.

52. Physicians who have had extended contact with a patient derive important prognostic information from familiarity with changes in the patient's health over time. Such knowledge is often seen as facilitating prognostication by generalist physicians as compared to specialists, but greater contact may in fact compromise the accuracy of the prognosis; see chapter 3.

53. N. A. Christakis and W. Levinson, "Casual Optimism: Prognostication in Routine Medical and Surgical Encounters," unpublished manuscript. Only in the case of sex and race were these associations statistically significant at the customary level ($p < 0.05$). Specifically, 55 percent of the cases in which prognosis was mentioned involved male patients, compared with 35 percent of those where prognosis was not mentioned; 93 percent of the cases where prognosis was mentioned involved white patients, compared with 77 percent of those where prognosis was not mentioned.

54. Davis, *Passage through Crisis*, esp. chap. 3. According to Davis, the *amount* of information communicated and not just its relative optimism or pessimism, may vary according to the social attributes of the person with whom the predictor is interacting—for example, a patient or a member of the patient's family.

55. See, for example, R. F. Antonak, "Prediction of Attitudes toward Disabled Persons: A Multivariate Analysis," *Journal of General Psychology* 104 (1981): 119–23; and S. Dorner, "Adolescents with Spina Bifida: How They See Their Situation," *Archives of Disease in Childhood* 51 (1976): 439–44.

56. Pearlman, "Variability in Physician Estimates."

57. Christakis and Iwashyna, "Attitude and Self-Reported Practice."

58. N. A. Christakis and E. B. Lamont, "The Extent and Determinants of Error in Physicians' Prognoses for Terminally Ill Patients," unpublished manuscript.

59. Christakis and Levinson, "Casual Optimism." This result is not surprising. Surgeons have historically paid close attention to how their interventions might alter the patients' course, for better or for worse; that is, they have compared outcomes observed after surgery with their predictions of what would happen without it. Such comparison is possible partly because of the dramatic and punctuated nature of surgery, where events following it can be—and often are—attributed to the surgery. Indeed, there is a tradition in surgery that any mortality within thirty days of surgery, *whatever* the reason, "even if the patient is hit by a bus in the hospital parking lot after discharge," is to be considered to be a "surgical death." Given this broad commitment to their fiduciary responsibility, as well as their interpretation of the power of their interventions, surgeons are justifiably concerned with the evaluation and anticipation of the consequences of their actions. See C. L. Bosk, *Forgive and Remember: Managing Medical Failure* (Chicago: University of Chicago Press, 1979), and J. Cassell, *Expected Miracles: Surgeons at Work* (Philadelphia: Temple University Press, 1991).

60. Anspach, *Deciding Who Lives*, 69.

61. This observation has also been made by J. H. Guillemin and L. L. Holmstrom, *Mixed Blessings: Intensive Care for Newborns* (New York: Oxford University Press, 1986), and by R. Zussman, *Intensive Care: Medical Ethics and the Medical Profession* (Chicago: University of Chicago Press, 1992), e.g. 120.

62. There is some evidence that this is true; see R. M. Poses, C. Bekes, R. L. Winkler, et al., "Are Two (Inexperienced) Heads Better than One (Experienced) Head?" *Archives of Internal Medicine* 150 (1990): 1874–78.

63. Clinical decisions in general—not just prognostic ones—appear to be increasingly influenced by bureaucratic, institutional, and financial standards. Diagnosis, for example, is structured through the application of the codes used in International Classification of Diseases or Diagnosis Related Groups systems. For a review, see A. R. Feinstein, "ICD, POR, and DRG: Unsolved Scientific Problems in the Nosology of Clinical Medicine," *Archives of Internal Medicine* 148 (1988): 2269–74. Whereas Hippocratic nosology emphasized clinical course and prognosis, including rudimentary notions of acute and chronic disease, in its system of classification, more recent nosologic systems have stressed classification according to diagnosis and have moved toward an etiologic classification

system. As Feinstein observes, "A classification of diseases can . . . be rooted in events of [the] present, past, or future: the current clinical manifestations (such as symptoms or physical signs); the background of etiologic causes and explanations; or the subsequent clinical course and prognosis" (p. 2270). No current nosologic systems of which I am aware are based on prognosis, though there is reason to suppose that such a basis would be clinically useful. Clinical decisions about therapy may also be affected by bureaucratic standards. For example, hospital stays were shortened after the federal government instituted DRG-based reimbursement; that is, ostensibly clinical decisions about how long to hospitalize patients changed in response to new administrative standards. See G. M. Carter, J. P. Newhouse, and D. A. Relles, "How Much Change in the Case Mix Index Is DRG Creep?" *Journal of Health Economics* 9 (1990): 411–28; D. M. Cutler, "The Incidence of Adverse Medical Outcomes under Prospective Payment," *Econometrica* 62 (1995): 29–50. Another example of how reimbursement policy is influencing treatment is the current interest among psychiatrists in "time-limited" or "brief" psychotherapy, the efficacy of which had previously been denied. See S. Stern, "Managed Care, Brief Therapy, and Therapeutic Integrity," *Psychotherapy* 30 (1993): 162–75.

64. Guillemin and Holmstrom, *Mixed Blessings,* 127. See also Anspach, *Deciding Who Lives.* The adequacy of such measures of outcome has sometimes been questioned; see R. J. Mullins, N. C. Mann, J. R. Hedges, et al., "Adequacy of Hospital Discharge Status as a Measure of Outcome among Injured Patients," *Journal of the American Medical Association* 279 (1998): 1727–31.

65. Davis, *Passage through Crisis.*

66. See D. Sudnow, *Passing On: The Social Organization of Dying* (Englewood Cliffs, N.J.: Prentice-Hall, 1967), e.g. 96–98.

67. To the ancient Greeks, prognosis had an additional meaning: the notion of *knowing* ("gnosis") the facts of the case *before* ("pro") actually talking to or examining the patient—that is, the ability of the physician to predict or interpolate facts not actually articulated by the patient. Prognosis is generally not conceived of in this way in modern medicine. See Hippocrates, "Prognosis."

68. Here I am making an analogy to Leon Eisenberg's dichotomy between "disease" and "illness." See L. Eisenberg, "Disease and Illness: Distinctions between Professional and Popular Ideas of Sickness," *Culture, Medicine, and Psychiatry* 1 (1977): 9–23.

69. In this sense, the realized prognosis is analogous to the "definitive diagnosis" provided by pathologists, typically after a postmortem examination.

70. See A. Kleinman, *The Illness Narratives: Suffering, Healing, and the Human Condition* (New York: Basic Books, 1988); R. Dubos, *Mirage of Health: Utopias, Progress, and Biological Change* (New Brunswick, N.J.: Rutgers University Press, 1959); and R. Dubos, *Man Adapting,* enl. ed. (New Haven: Yale University Press, 1965).

71. According to sociologist Everett C. Hughes, relevant attributes of an "ideal patient," one who perfectly fulfills physicians' expectations, include "the nature of the illness and its amenability to treatment; the nature of the interaction between the patient in his role with the physician in his; and finally, the effect of the patient on the physician's career." E. C. Hughes, "The Making of a Physician:

General Statement of Ideas and Problems," *Human Organization* 14 (1956): 21–25, 23. Hughes does not consider the amenability of the illness to prognostication as a relevant feature of an ideal patient, but this certainly could be added to the list.

72. Christakis and Levinson, "Casual Optimism." In this study, we used quantitative and qualitative methods to analyze 125 audiotaped encounters between surgeons or primary care physicians and their established outpatients, noting *any* future-oriented statements that were made. We considered a statement, made by either the doctor or the patient, to be "prognostic" if it involved a more than abstract reference to the future course of the patient's illness and its treatment. We drew a distinction, for example, between individualized predictions about outcome and impersonal discussions of the risks of a disease or therapy; indeed, abstract discussions of risk can be seen as a form of evasion of prognostication, as we shall see. For more on this distinction and our methodology, see appendix 1. Regarding the original data set and its acquisition, see W. Levinson, D. L. Roter, J. P. Mullooly, et al., "Physician-Patient Communication: The Relationship with Malpractice Claims among Primary Care Physicians and Surgeons," *Journal of the American Medical Association* 277 (1997): 553–59.

73. Physicians often feel different about the moral overtones of iatrogenic error. See, for example, N. A. Christakis and D. A. Asch, "Biases in How Physicians Choose to Withdraw Life Support," *Lancet* 324 (1993): 642–46; D. Casarett and L. F. Ross, "Overriding a Patient's Refusal of Treatment after an Iatrogenic Complication," *New England Journal of Medicine* 336 (1997): 1908–10; B. J. Cohen and S. G. Pauker, "How Do Physicians Weigh Iatrogenic Complications?" *Journal of General Internal Medicine* 9 (1994): 20–23.

74. A. McMillan, R. M. Mentnech, J. Lubitz, et al., "Trends and Patterns in Place of Death for Medicare Enrollees," *Health Care Financing Review* 12 (1990): 1–7. Approximately 60 to 65 percent of people die in hospitals, 15 to 20 percent in nursing homes.

75. Center for Evaluative Clinical Sciences, Dartmouth Medical School, *The Dartmouth Atlas of Health Care, 1998*, ed. J. E. Wennberg, M. M. Cooper, and Dartmouth Atlas of Health Care Working Group (Chicago: American Hospital Publishing, 1998), 86; L. C. Hanson, M. Danis, and J. Garrett, "What Is Wrong with End-of-Life Care? Opinions of Bereaved Family Members," *Journal of the American Geriatrics Society* 45 (1997): 1339–44.

76. Seeman, *National Mortality Followback Survey.*

77. C. S. Cleeland, R. Gonin, A. K. Hatfield, et al., "Pain and Its Treatment in Outpatients with Metastatic Cancer," *New England Journal of Medicine* 330 (1994): 592–96; J. Lynn, J. M. Teno, R. S. Phillips, et al., "Perceptions by Family Members of the Dying Experience of Older and Seriously Ill Patients," *Annals of Internal Medicine* 126 (1997): 97–106.

78. Lynn, Teno, Phillips, et al., "Perceptions by Family Members."

79. Lynn, Teno, Phillips, et al., "Perceptions by Family Members"; see also Hanson, Danis, and Garrett, "What Is Wrong with End-of-Life Care?"

80. K. E. Covinsky, L. Goldman, E. F. Cook, et al., "The Impact of Serious Illness on Patients' Families," *Journal of the American Medical Association* 272 (1994): 1839–44; K. E. Covinsky, C. S. Landefeld, J. Teno, et al., "Is Economic

Hardship on the Families of the Seriously Ill Associated with Patient and Surrogate Care Preferences?" *Archives of Internal Medicine* 156 (1996): 1737–41.

81. These figures are based on tables in Seeman, *National Mortality Followback Survey.* See also Center for Evaluative Clinical Sciences, *Dartmouth Atlas of Health Care.*

82. The best data on the experience of death in the United States come from the SUPPORT study, which looked at patients hospitalized with one of nine serious diseases (which together account for about 40 percent of all deaths). Other data, from Britain and from the American National Hospice Study, suggest that many of the physical symptoms that occur in the few days before death may have been present for weeks. Regarding SUPPORT, see Lynn, Teno, Phillips, et al., "Perceptions by Family Members." Regarding British data, see C. Seale and A. Cartwright, *The Year before Death* (Brookfield, Vt.: Ashgate Publishing, 1994). Regarding the hospice study, see J. N. Morris, S. Suissa, S. Sherwood, et al., "Last Days: A Study of the Quality of Life of Terminally Ill Cancer Patients," *Journal of Chronic Disease* 39 (1986): 47–62.

83. E. C. Hughes notes, in his discussion of professions and work, that "one man's routine of work is made of the emergencies of other people." See E. C. Hughes, "Mistakes at Work," in *The Sociological Eye: Selected Papers on Work, Self, and the Study of Society* (Chicago: Aldine-Atherton, 1971), 316–25, 316.

84. See, for example, Cleeland, Gonin, Hatfield, et al., "Pain and Its Treatment"; W. C. Wilson, N. G. Smedira, J. A. McDowell, and J. M. Luce, "Ordering and Administration of Sedatives and Analgesics during the Withholding and Withdrawal of Life Support from Critically Ill Patients," *Journal of the American Medical Association* 267 (1992): 949–53; SUPPORT principal investigators, "A Controlled Trial to Improve Care for Seriously Ill Hospitalized Patients: The Study to Understand Prognoses and Preferences for Outcomes and Risks of Treatments (SUPPORT)," *Journal of the American Medical Association* 274 (1995): 1591–98.

85. N. G. Smedira, B. H. Evans, L. S. Grais, et al., "Withholding and Withdrawal of Life Support from the Critically Ill," *New England Journal of Medicine* 322 (1990): 309–15; Christakis and Asch, "Biases in How Physicians Choose"; D. A. Asch and N. A. Christakis, "Why Do Physicians Prefer to Withdraw Some Forms of Life Support Over Others? Intrinsic Attributes of Life Sustaining Treatments Are Associated with Physicians' Preferences," *Medical Care* 34 (1996): 103–11.

86. N. T. Miyaji, "The Power of Compassion: Truth-Telling among American Doctors in the Care of Dying Patients," *Social Science and Medicine* 36 (1993): 249–64. See also H. G. Prigerson, "Socialization to Dying: Social Determinants of Death Acknowledgment and Treatment among Terminally Ill Geriatric Patients," *Journal of Health and Social Behavior* 33 (1992): 378–95.

87. See, for example, Sudnow, *Passing On;* B. G. Glaser and A. L. Strauss, *Awareness of Dying* (Chicago: Aldine, 1965); B. G. Glaser and A. L. Strauss, *Time for Dying* (Chicago: Aldine, 1968); and T. Walter, *The Revival of Death* (London: Routledge, 1994). Walter is particularly insightful in his characterization of the incipient transition to "neo-modern" death. Regarding change across time, see P. Aries, *The Hour of Our Death* (New York: Alfred A. Knopf, 1981). For

examples of variation across cultures, see P. Metcalf, *A Borneo Journey into Death: Berawan Eschatology from Its Rituals* (Philadelphia: University of Pennsylvania Press, 1982); and J. M. Janzen, *The Quest for Therapy: Medical Pluralism in Lower Zaire* (Berkeley: University of California Press, 1978).

88. Sudnow, *Passing On.*

89. Glaser and Strauss, *Awareness of Dying.*

90. Glaser and Strauss, *Time for Dying.*

91. See, for example, H. O. Mauksch, "The Organizational Context of Dying," in E. Kübler-Ross ed., *Death: The Final Stage of Growth* (Englewood Cliffs, N.J.: Prentice-Hall, 1975), 5–24. That physicians feel guilt when their patients die reflects both irony and arrogance—irony because they are not (ordinarily) truly responsible for the death and arrogance because they believe that they might have prevented it. See also R. C. Fox and J. P. Swazey, *The Courage to Fail: A Social View of Organ Transplants and Dialysis,* 2d rev. ed. (Chicago: University of Chicago Press, 1978). Regarding the explosion of medical technology, see R. Stevens, *In Sickness and in Wealth: American Hospitals in the Twentieth Century* (New York: Basic Books, 1989).

92. R. C. Fox, "Advanced Medical Technology—Social and Ethical Implications," in *Essays in Medical Sociology: Journeys into the Field,* 2d ed. (New Brunswick, N.J.: Transaction Books, 1988), 413–61, 429–30.

93. Illustrative examples include F. M. Hechinger, "They Tortured My Mother: Patronizing Doctors, Agonizing Care," *New York Times,* 24 January 1991, A22; S. Eveloff, "The Prisoner," *American Journal of Medicine* 93 (1992): 313–14; and N. Paradis, "Making a Living Off the Dying," *New York Times,* 25 April 1992, 23.

94. Christakis, "Managing Death." The emergence of interest in euthanasia also reflects a desire for *control* over death and dying.

95. Death in modern hospitals commonly follows a process whereby life support is withdrawn or, more typically, withheld; see Smedira, Evans, Grais, et al., "Withholding and Withdrawal."

96. Walter, *Revival of Death.*

97. The process of developing such measures is discussed in L. I. Iezzoni, *Risk Adjustment for Measuring Health Outcomes* (Chicago: Health Administration Press, 1997). See also J. S. Cowen and M. A. Kelley, "Errors and Bias in Using Predictive Scoring Systems," *Critical Care Clinics* 10 (1994): 53–72; M. Seneff and W. A. Knaus, "Predicting Patient Outcome from Intensive Care: A Guide to APACHE, MPM, SAPS, PRISM, and Other Prognostic Scoring Systems," *Journal of Intensive Care Medicine* 5 (1990): 33–52; and W. A. Knaus, F. E. Harrell Jr., J. Lynn, et al., "The SUPPORT Prognostic Model: Objective Estimates of Survival for Seriously Ill Hospitalized Adults," *Annals of Internal Medicine* 122 (1995): 191–203.

98. See, for example, Aries, *Hour of Our Death,* 10–11.

99. Sudnow, *Passing On,* 92. Regarding the problem of unexpected death, see also Glaser and Strauss, *Awareness of Dying.*

100. People realize, however, that predictions of impending death should be properly timed, as either premature or late announcements can inconvenience patients and their families or embarrass physicians.

101. Advantages from the patient's point of view include the painlessness and abruptness of such a death. Disadvantages include the denial of an opportunity to plan for death, say good-bye to relatives, compose wills, and so forth.

Chapter Two

1. T. Walter, *The Revival of Death* (London: Routledge, 1994); K. A. Steinhauser, E. C. Clipp, M. McNeilly, et al., "In Search of a Good Death: Observations of Patients, Families, and Providers' " unpublished manuscript.

2. See, for example, L. F. Degner, L. J. Kristjanson, D. Bowman, et al., "Information Needs and Decisional Preferences in Women with Breast Cancer," *Journal of the American Medical Association* 277 (1997): 1485–92; B. J. Davison, L. F. Degner, and T. R. Morgan, "Information and Decision-Making Preferences of Men with Prostate Cancer," *Oncology Nursing Forum* 22 (1995): 1401–8; G. J. Meissen, C. A. Mastromauro, D. K. Kiely, et al., "Understanding the Decision to Take the Predictive Test for Huntington Disease," *American Journal of Medical Genetics* 39 (1991): 404–10; A. I. Mushlin, C. Mooney, V. Grow, and C. E. Phelps, "The Value of Diagnostic Information to Patients with Suspected Multiple Sclerosis," *Archives of Neurology* 51 (1994): 67–72. See also C. G. Blanchard, M. S. Labrecque, J. C. Ruckdeschel, and E. B. Blanchard, "Information and Decision-Making Preferences of Hospitalized Adult Cancer Patients," *Social Science and Medicine* 27 (1988): 1139–45; this study of 439 cancer patients showed, among other things, that 92 percent want "all information to be given," even if the news was bad.

3. See, for example, D. J. Murphy, D. Burrows, S. Santilli, et al., "The Influence of the Probability of Survival on Patients' Preferences Regarding Cardiopulmonary Resuscitation," *New England Journal of Medicine* 330 (1994): 545–49; D. Frankl, R. K. Oye, and P. E. Bellamy, "Attitudes of Hospitalized Patients toward Life Support: A Survey of 200 Medical Inpatients," *American Journal of Medicine* 86 (1989): 645–48; J. C. Weeks, E. F. Cook, S. J. O'Day, et al., "Relationship between Cancer Patients' Predictions of Prognosis and Their Treatment Preferences," *Journal of the American Medical Association* 279 (1998): 1709–14; R. S. Schonwetter, R. M. Walker, D. R. Kramer, and B. E. Robinson, "Resuscitation Decision Making in the Elderly: The Value of Outcome Data," *Journal of General Internal Medicine* 8 (1993): 295–300; J. Cohen-Mansfield, J. A. Droge, and N. Billig, "Factors Influencing Hospital Patients' Preferences in the Utilization of Life-Sustaining Treatments," *Gerontologist* 32 (1992): 89–95.

4. See, for example, L. C. Hanson, M. Danis, and J. Garrett, "What Is Wrong with End-of-Life Care? Opinions of Bereaved Family Members," *Journal of the American Geriatrics Society* 45 (1997): 1339–44.

5. N. A. Christakis and T. J. Iwashyna, "Attitude and Self-Reported Practice Regarding Prognostication in a National Sample of Internists," *Archives of Internal Medicine* 158 (1998): 2389–95.

6. N. A. Christakis and W. Levinson, "Casual Optimism: Prognostication in Routine Medical and Surgical Encounters," unpublished manuscript.

7. See chapter 5 for more on the negotiation between physicians and patients regarding prognosis.

8. This point is made both by J. H. Guillemin and L. L. Holmstrom, *Mixed Blessings: Intensive Care for Newborns* (New York: Oxford University Press, 1986), and by R. Zussman, *Intensive Care: Medical Ethics and the Medical Profession* (Chicago: University of Chicago Press, 1992), chap. 9. Regarding "futility," see L. J. Schneiderman and N. S. Jecker, *Wrong Medicine: Doctors, Patients, and Futile Treatment* (Baltimore: Johns Hopkins University Press, 1995).

9. In such circumstances, the prediction may become a "self-fulfilling prophecy," as discussed in chapter 6; see also Guillemin and Holmstrom, *Mixed Blessings,* 117. The opposite can also hold: the assessment that a patient will live may result in redoubled efforts, increased attention to detail in the patient's care, and aggressive intervention.

10. Hastings Center, *Guidelines for the Termination of Life-Sustaining Treatment and the Care of the Dying* (Briarcliff Manor, N.Y.: Hastings Center, 1987).

11. The "burn index" to which this physician refers is B. E. Zawacki, S. P. Azen, S. H. Imbus, and Y. T. Chang, "Multifactorial Probit Analysis of Mortality in Burned Patients," *Annals of Surgery* 189 (1979): 1–5. See also C. M. Ryan, D. A. Schoenfeld, W. P. Thorpe, et al., "Objective Estimates of the Probability of Death from Burn Injuries," *New England Journal of Medicine* 338 (1998): 362–66, and J. R. Saffle, "Predicting Outcomes of Burns," *New England Journal of Medicine* 338 (1998): 387–88.

12. The terms "paralysis" and "aggressiveness" used regarding therapeutic alternatives themselves reflect common parlance in medicine and reflect the underlying attitudes toward these extremes. More neutral terms, for example, might be "minimalism" and "maximalism."

13. B. W. Levin, "Decision Making about Care of Catastrophically Ill Newborns: The Use of Technological Criteria," in L. M. Whiteford and M. Poland, eds., *New Approaches to Human Reproduction: Social and Ethical Dimensions* (Boulder, Colo.: Westview Press, 1989), 84–97; see also B. W. Levin, "International Perspectives on Treatment Choice in Neonatal Intensive Care Units," *Social Science and Medicine* 30 (1990): 901–12, 905. Physicians may also make choices that leave survival uncertain when prognosis is certain but *diagnosis* is uncertain; see N. A. Christakis and D. A. Asch, "Biases in How Physicians Choose to Withdraw Life Support," *Lancet* 324 (1993): 642–46.

14. See Christakis and Asch, "Biases in How Physicians Choose"; D. A. Asch and N. A. Christakis, "Why Do Physicians Prefer to Withdraw Some Forms of Life Support Over Others? Intrinsic Attributes of Life Sustaining Treatments Are Associated with Physicians' Preferences," *Medical Care* 34 (1996): 103–11; D. A. Asch, K. Faber-Langendoen, J. A. Shea, and N. A. Christakis, "The Sequence of Withdrawing Life-Sustaining Treatments from Patients in Four U.S. Hospitals," *American Journal of Medicine,* in press.

15. See C. L. Bosk, "Occupational Rituals in Patient Management," *New England Journal of Medicine* 303 (1980): 71–76; R. C. Fox, "Training for Uncertainty," in *Essays in Medical Sociology: Journeys into the Field,* 2d ed. (New Brunswick, N.J.: Transaction Books, 1988), 19–50; J. P. Kassirer, "Our Stubborn Quest for Diagnostic Certainty: A Cause of Excessive Testing," *New England Journal of Medicine* 320 (1989): 1489–91; and M. S. Gerrity, R. F. DeVellis, and J. A. Earp,

"Physicians' Reactions to Uncertainty in Patient Care: A New Measure and New Insights," *Medical Care* 28 (1990): 724–36.

16. See, for example, Guillemin and Holmstrom, *Mixed Blessings*, 123, and R. R. Anspach, *Deciding Who Lives: Fateful Choices in the Intensive-Care Nursery* (Berkeley: University of California Press, 1993), 76.

17. Zussman, *Intensive Care*, 117. Zussman argues that prognostic certainty depends on diagnostic certainty, but this is only partly true. First, it is often possible to be certain about a prognosis even when the diagnosis is unknown. Second, diagnostic uncertainty is one of many factors that can cause prognostic uncertainty. And third, physicians often inappropriately conflate diagnosis with prognosis, thereby obscuring real distinctions that might be made between diagnostic and prognostic uncertainty.

18. Social Security Act 1861(dd)(3)(A). See also N. A. Christakis and J. J. Escarce, "Survival of Medicare Patients after Enrollment in Hospice Programs," *New England Journal of Medicine* 335 (1996): 172–78, and N. A. Christakis, "Predicting Patient Survival before and after Hospice Enrollment," *Hospice Journal* 13 (1998): 71–87. And see chapter 7.

19. *Compassion in Dying v. Washington* 850 F. Supp. 1454 (W.D. Wash. 1994). Oregon Revised Statute 127,800 to 127,897 (Oregon Death with Dignity Act). See also G. J. Annas, "Death by Prescription: The Oregon Initiative," *New England Journal of Medicine* 331 (1994): 1240–43.

20. M. A. Drickamer, M. A. Lee, and L. Ganzini, "Practical Issues in Physician-Assisted Suicide," *Annals of Internal Medicine* 126 (1997): 146–51; M. A. Lee, H. D. Nelson, B. P. Tilden, et al., "Legalizing Assisted Suicide—Views of Physicians in Oregon," *New England Journal of Medicine* 334 (1996): 310–15; J. M. Teno, D. Murphy, J. Lynn, et al., "Prognosis-Based Futility Guidelines: Does Anyone Win?" *Journal of the American Geriatrics Society* 42 (1994): 1202–7; J. Lynn, F. E. Harrell Jr., F. Cohn, et al., "Defining the 'Terminally Ill': Insights from SUPPORT," *Duquesne Law Review* 35 (1996): 311–36.

21. For example, 42CFR406.13(b) defines ESRD: "End-stage renal disease (ESRD) means that stage of kidney impairment that appears irreversible and permanent and requires a regular course of dialysis or kidney transplantation to maintain life." Determinations of "irreversibility" and "permanence," of course, entail prognostic judgments.

22. D. A. Asch, J. P. Patton, and J. C. Hershey, "Knowing for the Sake of Knowing: The Value of Prognostic Information," *Medical Decision Making* 10 (1990): 47–57. For an example, see Mushlin, Mooney, Grow, and Phelps, "Value of Diagnostic Information."

23. N. A. Christakis, *Prognostication and Death in Medical Thought and Practice* (Ann Arbor, Mich.: University Microfilms, 1995).

24. Christakis and Levinson, "Casual Optimism." Endpoints other than response to treatment included return to work, return of function (e.g., of an injured extremity), future actions the doctor planned to take (such as diagnostic procedures), or side effects.

25. R. K. Merton and E. Barber, "Sociological Ambivalence," in R. K. Merton, ed., *Sociological Ambivalence and Other Essays* (New York: Free Press, 1976), 3–31,

23. Max Weber provides the classic example of such anxiety about the future in his discussion of concern about predestination; M. Weber, *The Protestant Ethic and the Spirit of Capitalism* (London: Unwin Hyman, 1930).

26. There are several examples of the impact of testing on uncertainty, anxiety, and psychological state. Some investigators have shown, for example, that predictive testing for Huntington's disease (an incurable, genetic, progressive, paralyzing neurologic condition) has potential benefits for the psychological health of people who are tested, even if the prognosis is that they will develop the disease, in part because the definite knowledge reduces uncertainty; see S. Wiggins, P. Whyte, M. Huggins, et al., "The Psychological Consequences of Predictive Testing for Huntington's Disease," *New England Journal of Medicine* 327 (1992): 1401–5; and G. J. Meissen, Mastromauro, Kiely, et al., "Understanding the Decision." Other investigators, however, have found that people with positive tests experienced intermittent depression; see C. A. Taylor and R. H. Myers, "Long-Term Impact of Huntington Disease Linkage Testing," *American Journal of Medical Genetics* 70 (1997): 365–70; and G. J. Meissen, R. H. Myers, C. A. Mastromauro, et al., "Predictive Testing for Huntington's Disease with Use of a Linked DNA Marker," *New England Journal of Medicine* 318 (1988): 535–42. See also R. Babul, S. Adam, B. Kremer, et al., "Attitudes toward Direct Predictive Testing for the Huntington Disease Gene: Relevance for Other Adult-Onset Disorders," *Journal of the American Medical Association* 270 (1993): 2321–25. Another example is provided by testing for multiple sclerosis; see P. O'Connor, A. S. Detsky, C. Tansey, et al., "Effect of Diagnostic Testing for Multiple Sclerosis on Patient Health Perceptions," *Archives of Neurology* 51 (1994): 46–51; and Mushlin, Mooney, Grow, and Phelps, "Value of Diagnostic Information." On the relation of anxiety to uncertainty from a psychiatric point of view, see H. W. Krohne, "The Concept of Coping Modes: Relating Cognitive Person Variables to Actual Coping Behavior," *Advances in Behavior Research and Therapy* 11 (1989): 235–47, and R. Ladouceur, F. Talbot, and M. J. Dugas, "Behavioral Expressions of Intolerance of Uncertainty in Worry: Experimental Findings," *Behavior Modification* 21 (1997): 355–71. See also V. Walters and N. Charles, "'I Just Cope from Day to Day': Unpredictability and Anxiety in the Lives of Women," *Social Science & Medicine* 45 (1997): 1729–39.

27. For example, Kathy Charmaz notes that chronically ill patients (with explicitly foreshortened survival horizons) adopt new social personae in their interactions with their families. See K. Charmaz, *Good Days, Bad Days: The Self in Chronic Illness and Time* (New Brunswick, N.J.: Rutgers University Press, 1991).

28. The so-called "sick role," as classically described, includes (1) exemption of the patient from normal social responsibilities, (2) presumption that the patient is not responsible for the illness, (3) presumption that the patient does not wish to be sick, and (4) obligation on the part of the patient to seek competent technical assistance in order to recover. T. Parsons, *The Social System* (New York: Free Press, 1951), esp. 436–37.

29. Evidence that physicians evaluate each other on these grounds is provided in chapter 3 and appendix 2.

30. For example, of the more than thirty physicians interviewed at length

about prognosis, only two were able to give an example of sterling clinical performance on their part that was specifically prognostic in nature.

31. Examples of the form of such conferences may be seen in most issues of the *New England Journal of Medicine.*

32. For an overview of the functioning of such boards, see S. E. Radecki, J. G. Nyquist, J. D. Gates, et al., "Educational Characteristics of Tumor Conferences in Teaching and Non-Teaching Hospitals," *Journal of Cancer Education* 9 (1994): 204–16. The article notes that treatment was discussed in 70 to 90 percent of the cases considered, whereas prognosis was discussed in 26 to 44 percent of cases (p. 212). The latter figures overstate the prominence given to prognosis, given my qualitative data on such meetings, since mentions of prognosis are typically very brief compared with the time devoted to treatment.

33. E. Freidson, *Doctoring Together: A Study of Professional Social Control* (Chicago: University of Chicago Press, 1975), 147.

34. See chapter 6 regarding such "self-negating prophecies."

35. Such mercenary bases for optimism would violate physicians' fiduciary duty to their patients. This tension reflects a broader concern among physicians, who must earn their living from the profession, even while owing a primary allegience to the patient.

36. See Drickamer, Lee, and Ganzini, "Practical Issues"; Lee, Nelson, Tilden, et al., "Legalizing Assisted Suicide."

37. Teno, Murphy, Lynn, et al., "Prognosis-Based Futility Guidelines"; N. S. Jecker and L. J. Schneiderman, "Medical Futility: The Duty Not to Treat," *Cambridge Quarterly Healthcare Ethics* 2 (1993): 151–59; L. J. Schneiderman and N. S. Jecker, "Futility in Practice," *Archives of Internal Medicine* 153 (1993): 437–41.

38. See chapters 3 and 8.

39. B. A. Rich, "Prospective Autonomy and Critical Interests: A Narrative Defense of the Moral Authority of Advance Directives," *Cambridge Quarterly of Healthcare Ethics* 6 (1997): 138–47; S. H. Miles, R. Koepp, and E. P. Weber, "Advance End-of-Life Treatment Planning: A Research Review," *Archives of Internal Medicine* 156 (1996): 1062–68; L. J. Schneiderman, R. Kronick, R. M. Kaplan, et al., "Effects of Offering Advance Directives on Medical Treatments and Costs," *Annals of Internal Medicine* 117 (1992): 599–606.

40. J. A. Tulsky, G. S. Fischer, M. R. Rose, and R. M. Arnold, "Opening the Black Box: How Do Physicians Communicate about Advance Directives," *Annals of Internal Medicine* 129 (1998): 441–49.

41. The foregoing case illustrates another important element to prognostication discussed in chapter 3, namely, the principle of group decision making in prognosis. The requirement that, for such weighty decisions as withdrawal of life support, more than one doctor has to agree serves several purposes, including enhancing the accuracy of the prediction and diffusing responsibility.

42. R. L. Faden and T. L. Beauchamp, *A History and Theory of Informed Consent* (New York: Oxford University Press, 1986), esp. 274–75, 278. See also C. W. Lidz, A. Meisel, E. Zerubavel, et al., *Informed Consent: A Study of Decision Making in Psychiatry* (New York: Guilford Press, 1984).

43. See, for example, N. A. Christakis, "Ethics Are Local: Engaging Cross-cultural Variation in the Ethics for Clinical Research," *Social Science and Medicine*

35 (1992): 1079–91, and G. Weisz, ed., *Social Science Perspectives on Medical Ethics* (Philadelphia: University of Pennsylvania Press, 1990).

44. See Fox, "Training for Uncertainty," in *Essays in Medical Sociology,* 20, and "The Evolution of Medical Uncertainty," 533–71 in the same volume. Most work on uncertainty focuses on the uncertainty inherent in the *current* situation before a physician, for example, with respect to etiology or diagnosis. Uncertainty regarding the future, the use of prognostication as a tool for contending with uncertainty, and the possible uses or advantages of uncertainty itself, have tended to be ignored. F. Davis, *Passage through Crisis: Polio Victims and Their Families* (New Brunswick, N.J.: Transaction Publishers, 1991), is an exception to this.

45. F. Davis, "Uncertainty in Medical Prognosis: Clinical and Functional," in E. Freidson and J. Lorber, eds., *Medical Men and Their Work* (Chicago: Aldine-Atherton, 1972), 239–48.

46. J. Harvey, "Achieving the Indeterminate: Accomplishing Degrees of Certainty in Life and Death Situations," *Sociological Review* 44 (1996): 78–98.

47. Christakis and Levinson, "Casual Optimism." More generally, see J. Katz, *The Silent World of Doctor and Patient* (New York: Free Press, 1984), esp. chap. 7, "Acknowledging Uncertainty: The Confrontation of Knowledge and Ignorance."

48. N. T. Miyaji, "The Power of Compassion: Truth-Telling Among American Doctors in the Care of Dying Patients," *Social Science and Medicine* 36 (1993): 249–64.

49. N. A. Christakis, "The Ellipsis of Prognosis in Modern Medical Thought," *Social Science and Medicine* 44 (1997): 301–15. See also chapter 1.

Chapter Three

1. There is a significant literature on technical aspects of how to evaluate the accuracy of predictions. More sophisticated aspects of prognostic accuracy include whether the physician is able to "discriminate" among patients, that is, whether the doctor is able to recognize if a patient has a higher risk of an outcome such as death than other patients, even if the estimated risk of death in both the patient and the rest of the group do not precisely correspond to the true risk. The presence or absence of such a correspondence is known as "calibration," or "calibration-in-the-large," which is the degree to which the physician's predictions correspond to the overall pattern of mortality in the entire population or group. Thus, if a physician predicts that, overall, 50 percent of patients will die, and 50 percent are observed to die, the physician is said to be "well calibrated." If the 50 percent who live are precisely those the physician predicted would die, the physician would still be considered well calibrated but would be deemed unable to discriminate. Conversely, if a physician predicts probabilities of death of 0 percent, 50 percent, and 100 percent for patient groups in which the actual death rates are 10 percent, 20 percent, and 30 percent, the physician would be deemed to have some discriminating ability but to be poorly calibrated. "Calibration-in-the-small" refers to calibration for subgroups of a population. Physicians may be well calibrated-in-the-large but poorly calibrated-in-the-small; for example, they may tend to overestimate

survival in low-risk patients and underestimate it in high-risk patients. For a comprehensive review of the aspects of prognostic accuracy, see A. C. Justice, *The Development, Validation, and Evaluation of Prognostic Systems: An Application to the Acquired Immunodeficiency Syndrome (AIDS)* (Ann Arbor, Mich.: University Microfilms, 1996), esp. chap. 1; see also A. C. Justice, K. E. Covinsky, and J. A. Berlin, "Assessing the Generalizability of Prognostic Information," *Annals of Internal Medicine* 130 (1999): 515–24.

2. I am aware of fewer than thirty published studies in the peer-reviewed literature that have compared physicians' predictions to observed outcomes for real patients; most of these are cited below. Other studies have compared physicians' predictions to those of computerized or statistical algorithms; for an overview of statistical algorithms and their use, see R. M. Dawes, D. Faust, and P. E. Meehl, "Clinical versus Actuarial Judgment," *Science* 243 (1989): 1668–74; and Justice, *Development, Validation, and Evaluation,* esp. chap. 3.

3. There have also been noteworthy evaluations of prognostic accuracy in certain other clinical circumstances. See D. F. Kong, K. L. Lee, F. E. Harrell, et al., "Clinical Experience and Predicting Survival in Coronary Disease," *Archives of Internal Medicine* 149 (1989): 1177–81; K. L. Lee, D. B. Pryor, F. E. Harrell Jr., et al., "Predicting Outcome in Coronary Disease: Statistical Models Versus Expert Clinicians," *American Journal of Medicine* 80 (1986): 553–60; M. E. Charlson, F. L. Sax, R. MacKenzie, et al., "Assessing Illness Severity: Does Clinical Judgment Work?," *Journal of Chronic Disease* 39 (1986): 439–52; P. Pompei, M. E. Charlson, and R. G. Douglas, Jr., "Clinical Assessments as Predictors of One Year Survival after Hospitalization: Implications for Prognostic Stratification," *Journal of Clinical Epidemiology* 41 (1988): 275–84; R. A. Pearlman, "Variability in Physician Estimates of Survival for Acute Respiratory Failure in Chronic Obstructive Pulmonary Disease," *Chest* 91 (1987): 515–21; G. Durham and J. Durham, "General Practitioners' Ability to Predict Outcome for Elderly Patients Admitted to Acute Medical Beds," *New Zealand Medical Journal* 103 (1990): 585–87; and A. A. Meyer, J. Messick, P. Young, et al., "Prospective Comparison of Clinical Judgment and APACHE II Score in Predicting the Outcome in Critically Ill Surgical Patients," *Journal of Trauma* 32 (1992): 747–54.

4. C. M. Parkes, "Accuracy of Predictions of Survival in Later Stages of Cancer," *British Medical Journal* 2 (1972): 29–31. Parkes considered predictions to be accurate if they were no more than twice and no less than half the actual duration of survival.

5. L. H. Heyse-Moore and V. E. Johnson-Bell, "Can Doctors Accurately Predict the Life Expectancy of Patients with Terminal Cancer?" *Palliative Medicine* 1 (1987): 165–66.

6. One classic study involved only two physicians making predictions for 108 cancer patients admitted to an inpatient hospice. The actual median survival of these patients was 3.5 weeks; the investigators noted that predicted and observed survival bore little correlation. Overall, the two physicians tended to be somewhat "calibrated" in their predictions, though their performance varied according to the method used to elicit the prognosis; when in error, they tended to overestimate survival, by up to a factor of two. See L. E. Forster and J. Lynn, "Predicting Life Span for Applicants to Inpatient Hospice," *Archives of Internal*

Medicine 148 (1988): 2540–43. A study published in 1985, with several health care providers, including three doctors, making 149 predictions regarding 42 cancer patients, again found an optimistic bias: mean predicted survival was just over three times the mean actual survival, and 76 percent of the predictions overestimated survival. See C. Evans and M. McCarthy, "Prognostic Uncertainty in Terminal Care: Can the Karnofsky Index Help?" *Lancet* 1 (1985): 1204–6. A more recent study of 61 patients with advanced cancer admitted to a palliative care unit found that two highly experienced physicians were "not accurate" in estimating survival; this study adopted a very liberal standard for accuracy, but even so 68 percent of their estimates were in error, usually in the optimistic direction. See E. Bruera, M. J. Miller, N. Kuehn, et al., "Estimate of Survival of Patients Admitted to a Palliative Care Unit: A Prospective Study," *Journal of Pain and Symptom Management* 7 (1992): 82–86. Another study, of four Italian physicians predicting survival for 100 cancer outpatients, found that the median predicted survival was six weeks and the observed was five weeks; M. Maltoni, O. Nanni, S. Derni, et al., "Clinical Prediction of Survival Is More Accurate than the Karnofsky Performance Status in Estimating Life Span of Terminally Ill Cancer Patients," *European Journal of Cancer* 30A (1994): 764–66. Finally, a study of thirty patients with one physician predictor found a median predicted survival of about twenty-three days and the median observed survival of about seventeen days; D. Oxenham and M. A. Cornbleet, "Accuracy of Prediction of Survival by Different Professional Goups in a Hospice," *Palliative Medicine* 12 (1998): 117–18.

7. See appendix 1 for more detail; and see N. A. Christakis and E. B. Lamont, "The Extent and Determinants of Error in Physicians' Prognoses for Terminally Ill Patients," unpublished manucript.

8. Regarding cognitive bias toward optimism in areas where one has a personal investment, see N. D. Weinstein, "Optimistic Biases about Personal Risks," *Science* 246 (1989): 1232–33, and R. M. Poses, D. McClish, C. Bekes, et al., "Ego Bias, Reverse Ego Bias, and Physicians' Prognostic Judgments for Critically Ill Patients," *Critical Care Medicine* 19 (1991): 1533–39.

9. M. F. Muers, P. Shevlin, and J. Brown, "Prognosis in Lung Cancer: Physicians' Opinions Compared with Outcome and a Predictive Model," *Thorax* 51 (1996): 894–902.

10. J. M. Addington-Hall, L. D. MacDonald, H. R. Anderson, "Can the Spitzer Quality of Life Index Help to Reduce Prognostic Uncertainty in Terminal Care?" *British Journal of Cancer* 62 (1990): 695–99. Overall, the prognosticators in this study (which included both physicians and nurses) were well calibrated-in-the-large, in that the percentage of patients given a prognosis of less than a year to live (41 percent) closely approximated the percentage who died within a year (38 percent).

11. W. J. Mackillop and C. F. Quirt, "Measuring the Accuracy of Prognostic Judgments in Oncology," *Journal of Clinical Epidemiology* 50 (1997): 21–29.

12. Note that eight of the ten studies of accuracy in cancer patients (the exceptions being the Forster and Lynn study and my own) were conducted outside of the United States, in England, Canada, or Italy. At least with respect to cancer, U.S. physicians may be relatively uninterested in ascertaining their

degree of prognostic accuracy. However, most assessments of prognostic accuracy in ICU settings, as discussed below, have been conducted in the United States.

13. A. S. Detsky, S. C. Stricker, A. G. Mulley, and G. E. Thibault, "Prognosis, Survival, and the Expenditure of Hospital Resources for Patients in an Intensive-Care Unit," *New England Journal of Medicine* 305 (1981): 667–72.

14. W. A. Knaus, D. P. Wagner, and J. Lynn, "Short-Term Mortality Predictions for Critically Ill Hospitalized Adults: Science and Ethics," *Science* 254 (1991): 389–94. See also W. A. Knaus, F. E. Harrell Jr., J. Lynn, et al., "The SUPPORT Prognostic Model: Objective Estimates of Survival for Seriously Ill Hospitalized Adults," *Annals of Internal Medicine* 122 (1995): 191–203, for the final results from the so-called SUPPORT study, which developed quantitative models for the prediction of outcomes of nine severe disease states and evaluated the effect on physicians' practice of giving them this information. See chapter 8 for more on this study.

15. Other studies drawn from this data set have confirmed these findings. See, for example, H. R. Arkes, N. V. Dawson, T. Speroff, et al., "The Covariance Decomposition of the Probability Score and Its Use in Evaluating Prognostic Estimates," *Medical Decision Making* 15 (1995): 120–31.

16. As discussed in chapter 8, providing physicians with objectively computed prognoses and information about patients' preferences did not change physician behavior. See SUPPORT principal investigators, "A Controlled Trial to Improve Care for Seriously Ill Hospitalized Patients: The Study to Understand Prognoses and Preferences for Outcomes and Risks of Treatments (SUPPORT)," *Journal of the American Medical Association* 274 (1995): 1591–98. Other investigators have also documented substantial mismatches between physicians' actions and patients' stated preferences; see J. M. Teno, J. Lynn, R. S. Phillips, et al., "Do Formal Advance Directives Affect Resuscitation Decisions and the Use of Resources for Seriously Ill Patients?," *Journal of Clinical Ethics* 5 (1994): 23–30, and R. B. Hakim, J. M. Teno, F. E. Harrell Jr., et al., "Factors Associated with Do-Not-Resuscitate Orders: Patients' Preferences, Prognoses, and Physicians' Judgments," *Annals of Internal Medicine* 125 (1996): 284–93.

17. These studies typically involved several hundred patients but fewer than ten doctors. See J. A. Kruse, M. C. Thill-Baharozian, and R. W. Carlson, "Comparison of Clinical Assessment with APACHE II for Predicting Mortality Risk in Patients Admitted to a Medical Intensive Care Unit," *Journal of the American Medical Association* 260 (1988): 1739–42; D. McClish and S. H. Powell, "How Well Can Physicians Estimate Mortality in a Medical Intensive Care Unit?" *Medical Decision Making* 9 (1989): 125–32; R. M. Poses, C. Bekes, F. J. Copare, and W. E. Scott, "The Answer to "What Are My Chances, Doctor?" Depends on Whom Is Asked: Prognostic Disagreement and Inaccuracy for Critically Ill Patients," *Critical Care Medicine* 17 (1989): 827–33; and R. M. Poses, C. Bekes, R. L. Winkler, et al., "Are Two (Inexperienced) Heads Better than One (Experienced) Head?" *Archives of Internal Medicine* 150 (1990): 1874–78.

18. H. S. Perkins, A. R. Jonsen, and W. V. Epstein, "Providers as Predictors: Using Outcome Predictions in Intensive Care," *Critical Care Medicine* 14 (1986): 105–10.

19. See, for example, N. V. Dawson, T. Speroff, A. Connors, et al., "Use of the Mean Probability Score: Comparison of the SUPPORT Prognostic Model with Physicians' Subjective Estimates of Survival," *Medical Decision Making* 12 (1992): 336 (abstract). A study of non-ICU patients similarly found no effect of measured physician variables; see Kong, Lee, Harrell, et al., "Clinical Experience." Another paper found that while nurses were not as accurate as doctors, among the 57 doctors whose predictions in 366 cases were evaluated, level of training was *not* associated with accuracy; see Kruse, Thill-Baharozian, and Carlson, "Comparison of Clinical Assessment." Regarding this last point, a few studies have compared the accuracy of physicians' and nurses' prognostic performance in hospice or cancer patients; nurses have proven sometimes more accurate and sometime less accurate than physicians. See L. E. Forster and J. Lynn, "Predicting Life Span for Applicants to Inpatient Hospice," *Archives of Internal Medicine* 148 (1988): 2540–43; Parkes, "Accuracy of Predictions"; Addington-Hall, MacDonald, and Anderson, "Can the Spitzer Quality of Life Index Help"; and Oxenham and Cornbleet, "Accuracy of Prediction."

20. A. F. Connors, N. V. Dawson, T. Speroff, et al., "Physicians' Confidence in Their Estimates of the Probability of Survival: Relationship to Accuracy," *Medical Decision Making* 12 (1992): 336.

21. Poses, Bekes, Copare, and Scott, "Answer to 'What Are My Chances, Doctor?'" This study, involving 256 patients referred to ICUs, found that referring primary physicians who had known their patients longest were more optimistic in estimating survival than the ICU attendings. For example, for the patients whose probability of survival the primary physicians estimated to be 50 percent, the actual rate of survival was about 30 percent; by contrast, for those whose probability of survival was estimated by the ICU attending to be 50 percent, the actual survival rate was about 52 percent. Using a very similar data set, however, these authors also found that, at least for ICU patients and over a two-day period, greater knowledge of the patient's current clinical problems did *not* enhance the accuracy of survival estimates; see R. M. Poses, M. C. Bekes, F. J. Copare, and W. E. Scott, "What Difference Do Two Days Make? The Inertia of Physicians' Sequential Prognostic Judgments for Critically Ill Patients," *Medical Decision Making* 10 (1990): 6–14.

22. See chapter 7 for more detail.

23. More accurately, physicians would be even less able to discriminate survivors from nonsurvivors at any given distant time point, though they might well be better calibrated.

24. It seems likely, however, that people estimate their own long-term prospects for survival and act accordingly, for example with respect to insurance purchases.

25. N. A. Christakis and T. J. Iwashyna, "Attitude and Self-Reported Practice Regarding Prognostication in a National Sample of Internists," *Archives of Internal Medicine* 158 (1998): 2389–95.

26. There was no association between holding this belief and physician attributes such as age, sex, specialty, board certification status, or finding prognostication to be difficult or stressful.

27. E. C. Hughes, "Mistakes at Work," in E. C. Hughes, ed., *The Sociological*

Eye: Selected Papers on Work, Self, and the Study of Society (Chicago: Aldine-Atherton, 1971), 316–25.

28. For more on the results, see appendix 2; for methodologic details regarding the survey itself, see appendix 1.

29. This is known technically as a "loss function" for prediction; see A. Zellner, "Bayesian Estimation and Prediction Using Asymmetric Loss Functions," *Journal of the American Statistical Association* 81 (1986): 446–51; M. Cain and C. Janssen, "Bayesian Valuation with an Elicited Nonsymmetric Loss Function," in D. A. Berry, K. M. Chaloner, and J. K. Geweke, eds., *Bayesian Analysis in Statistics and Econometrics* (New York: John Wiley & Sons, 1996), 165–78.

30. Poses, Bekes, Winkler, et al., "Are Two (Inexperienced) Heads Better." In a sense, the "signal" is enhanced and the "noise" averaged out.

31. See, for example, R. R. Anspach, "Prognostic Conflict in Life-and-Death Decisions: The Organization as an Ecology of Knowledge," *Journal of Health and Social Behavior* 28 (1987): 215–31. Uncertainty can also provide a vehicle for a bond between the patient and the doctor; see chapter 3.

32. Christakis and Iwashyna, "Attitude and Self-Reported Practice." The need for explanation even when the outcome is unexpectedly favorable is an illustration of what sociologist Renée Fox has termed the "crisis of good fortune"; see R. C. Fox, *Experiment Perilous* (Boston: Free Press, 1959).

33. Part of the explanation for this may also be the historicizing examined in chapter 1.

34. Hughes, "Mistakes at Work," 317. For Hughes, "fateful" mistakes are *consequential* and *meaningful*.

35. While lawsuits related to errors in diagnosis or therapy are common, suits over mistakes in prognostication appear extremely rare. I could not find any such cases for which the defendant was a physician. A few cases were identified, however, in which a prognosis rendered at the time of some initial hearing, typically in a worker's compensation case, was subsequently found to be discordant with the observed prognosis. See, for example, *Gleason v. Guzman* 623 P.2d 378 (Colo. 1981); *Schoenfeld v. Buker* 114 N.W.2d 560, 262 Minn. 122 (Minn. 1962); *U.S. Fidelity & Guaranty Company v. Wilson* 120 S.E.2d 198, 103 (Ga. App. 674, 1961); and *Raines v. State Compensation Commissioner* 108 S.E.2d 519, 144 (W.Va. 430, 1959). It seems the public understands that knowledge of the future is provisional and is tolerant of mistakes in this area, especially since it is difficult to know when a mistake has occurred. This state of affairs is fostered by the language of predictions, which, as we will see, is often deliberately ambiguous. Moreover, suits may be based on improper treatment or failure to treat, thus obscuring the fact that these errors may in fact have been due to errors in prognostication. As compared with misprognosis, errors attributable to "nonprognosis," that is, a failure to communicate a prognosis altogether, can be causes for lawsuits; see G. J. Annas, "Informed Consent, Cancer, and Truth in Prognosis," *New England Journal of Medicine* 330 (1994): 223–25.

36. The solution to the problem may be to reset a priori expectations through better, more "accurate," prognostication. In this vein, Joan Cassell argues that, since the expectation cannot logically be justified, it is inappropriate for either patients or surgeons to expect "miracles" in surgery; see J. Cassell, *Expected*

Miracles: Surgeons at Work (Philadelphia: Temple University Press, 1991). With respect to mistakes in general, see C. L. Bosk, *Forgive and Remember: Managing Medical Failure* (Chicago: University of Chicago Press, 1979).

37. Studies documenting the frequency of "adverse events" include L. B. Andrews, C. Stocking, T. Krizek, et al., "An Alternative Strategy for Studying Adverse Events in Medical Care," *Lancet* 349 (1997): 311; T. A. Brennan, et al., "Incidence of Adverse Events and Negligence and Hospitalized Patients: Results from the Harvard Medical Practice Study I," *New England Journal of Medicine* 324 (1991): 370–76; and L. L. Leape, et al., "The Nature of Adverse Events in Hospitalized Patients: Results from the Harvard Medical Practice Study II," *New England Journal of Medicine* 324 (1991): 377–84. For a critical care–oriented typology of forms of iatrogenesis with some reference to the evolution of medical recognition of the phenomenon, see M. G. McKenney and J. M. Civetta, "Iatrogenesis," in J. M. Civetta, R. W. Taylor, and R. R. Kirby, eds., *Critical Care*, 3d ed. (Philadelphia: Lippencott-Raven, 1997). For a stinging critique of the medical profession on this point, see I. Illich, *Medical Nemesis: The Expropriation of Health* (New York: Pantheon, 1976).

38. An analogous function is played by what Renée Fox has characterized as a "game of chance" wherein the realization of the role of chance relieves physicians of the responsibility for outcomes. See Fox, *Experiment Perilous*.

39. See, for example, D. A. Matthews and C. Clark, *The Faith Factor: Proof of the Healing Power of Prayer* (New York: Viking, 1998), e.g. 17–18.

40. In discussing prognosis, physicians also sometimes allude to the "sinfulness" of prediction, the "martyrdom" of patients, the "grace" of the unexpected, and so forth.

41. The passage alluded to is in *Hamlet*, act 1, scene 5: "There are more things in heaven and earth, Horatio, than are dreamt of in your philosophy."

Chapter Four

1. N. A. Christakis and T. J. Iwashyna, "Attitude and Self-Reported Practice Regarding Prognostication in a National Sample of Internists," *Archives of Internal Medicine* 158 (1998): 2389–95. Physicians who find it difficult to make predictions were 2.7 times as likely those who do not to report that they find it stressful to make predictions ($p < 0.001$).

2. R. C. Fox, "Training for Uncertainty," in *Essays in Medical Sociology: Journeys into the Field*, 2d ed. (New Brunswick, N.J.: Transaction Books, 1988), 19–50.

3. Christakis and Iwashyna, "Attitude and Self-Reported Practice"; indeed, physicians who believe that their patients have such high expectations were 2.3 times as likely as other physicians to find prognosis stressful ($p < 0.001$).

4. A parallel division of labor between doctors and nurses in ICUs has been described by Renée Anspach; R. R. Anspach, *Deciding Who Lives: Fateful Choices in the Intensive-Care Nursery* (Berkeley: University of California Press, 1993).

5. Christakis and Iwashyna, "Attitude and Self-Reported Practice."

6. They were 1.6 times more likely to find prognosis stressful than physicians reporting adequate training ($p < 0.001$).

7. The fact that this (fatal) complication was deemed relevant to the prognosis is in keeping with the meaning of "complications" for prognostication discussed in N. A. Christakis, "The Ellipsis of Prognosis in Modern Medical Thought," *Social Science and Medicine* 44 (1997): 301–15.

8. Finding prognosis stressful is independent of physicians' demographic and other attributes, of the number of times in the preceding year a physician has been asked "How long do I have to live?," and of the number of times a physician has withdrawn life support. Christakis and Iwashyna, "Attitude and Self-Reported Practice."

9. T. Parsons, *The Social System* (New York: Free Press, 1951), esp. 298–325. By "role," I mean, following Talcott Parsons's definition, a "processual aspect" of an actor's participation in a social system, that is, a set of normative constraints on action dictated by the collectivity. A role involves the specification of how its incumbent should act towards others, and how others may expect the incumbent to act. See Parsons, *Social System*, esp. 25–40, 447–54, and 466–69. By "strain," I mean the unsettling difficulties encountered by an actor in fulfilling role obligations. An example distinct from those considered here is when a physician finds performing an abortion objectionable but is in a role that would seem to require it; see J. B. Imber, *Abortion and the Private Practice of Medicine* (New Haven: Yale University Press, 1986).

10. Such conflicts may lead to syncretic syntheses, as with the notion of "detached concern." See H. I. Lief and R. C. Fox, "The Medical Student's Training for 'Detached Concern,'" in H. I. Lief, V. Lief, and N. R. Lief, eds., *The Psychological Basis of Medical Practice* (New York: Harper & Row, 1963), 12–35. The tension between treating patients as independent, autonomous agents and as vulnerable people deserving treatment under a more fiduciary rubric is commonly discussed in the bioethics literature. See, in general, R. J. Levine, *Ethics and Regulation of Clinical Research*, 2d ed. (New Haven: Yale University Press, 1986).

11. R. K. Merton and E. Barber, "Sociological Ambivalence," in R. K. Merton, ed., *Sociological Ambivalence and Other Essays* (New York: Free Press, 1976), 3–31, 8. Emphasis in the original has been suppressed. Merton does not appear to consider the kind of ambivalence we will consider here, even in his essay "The Ambivalence of Physicians," 65–72 in the same volume. Incidentally, there are still other types of sociological ambivalence unrelated to the type considered by Merton (as he notes); see, for example, E. C. Hughes, "Dilemmas and Contradictions of Status," *American Journal of Sociology* 50 (1945): 353–59.

12. The best medical example I am aware of regarding such a syncretic melding or dynamic equilibrium is the notion of "detached concern" developed by Lief and Fox. Here, it is not as if physicians oscillate between detachment and concern, nor as if detached concern is some simple sum of the two. Rather, the two extremes fuse to form an altogether new and different attitude and value. See Lief and Fox, "Medical Student's Training."

13. See Parsons, *Social System*, esp. 304. These three ways of coping (avoidance, ambiguity, and optimism/pessimism) are, I believe, prototypic responses to role strain and not limited to physicians engaged in prognostication. What I mean is that ambivalence in a social role can result in avoidance, submersion,

and syncresis as well as oscillation. I consider ambiguity in chapter 5 and the ritualization of optimism and pessimism in chapter 7.

14. Both professional *attitudes* (which are relatively specific) and *values* (which are more general) are intrinsic to a individuals. In contrast, I take professional *norms* to be extrinsic to individual practitioners, though internalized by them.

15. Christakis and Iwashyna, "Attitude and Self-Reported Practice." See also M. Amir, "Considerations Guiding Physicians When Informing Cancer Patients," *Social Science and Medicine* 24 (1987): 741–48.

16. Another physician admonished: "When the doctor has made a prognosis, the question whether he should communicate it to the patient or his friends is often a difficult one. Perhaps it is judicious never to give a forecast unless it is asked for, and even then to speak cautiously but with as much hopefulness as circumstances allow." See R. Hutchison, "Prognosis," *Lancet* 226 (1934): 697–98, 698. The use by physicians of a strategy of countering "undue" pessimism with optimism (and optimism with pessimism) is discussed in chapter 5.

17. Older physicians are somewhat more likely to believe that prognoses should not be volunteered. In our survey, 40 percent of internists less than fifty years old thought that they should wait to be asked before making a prognosis, compared to 52 percent of those fifty or older, a difference that is statistically significant. For details regarding this survey, see appendix 1.

18. A. Girgis and R. W. Sanson-Fisher, "Breaking Bad News: Consensus Guidelines for Medical Practitioners," *Journal of Clinical Oncology* 13 (1995): 2449–56, 2453.

19. Another physician writing about prognosis observed, "One of the first rules of communicating with incurable patients is [to] never give them a specific estimate of survival." Instead, doctors were admonished to ask why the patient wants to know, since the physician might be better able to answer specific queries such as whether the patient could "plan his summer vacation." See R. J. Miller, "Predicting Survival in Advanced Cancer Patients," *Henry Ford Hospital Medical Journal* 39 (1991): 81–84.

20. For some examples of what physicians think of colleagues who behave this way, see chapter 5.

21. Regarding textbooks, see chapter 1 and Christakis, "Ellipsis of Prognosis." With respect to journals, a computer search of the English-language medical literature revealed that, between 1995 and 1997, 173,459 articles mentioned treatment, 47,038 mentioned diagnosis, and 10,309 mentioned prognosis. Christakis and Iwashyna, "Attitude and Self-Reported Practice," considers medical education. Incidentally, in the course of an analysis I conducted of twenty-four reports recommending reform of the American system of medical education, I noted that prognosis was virtually unmentioned, whereas diagnosis and therapy were regularly discussed. See N. A. Christakis, "The Similarity and Frequency of Proposals to Reform U.S. Medical Education: Constant Concerns," *Journal of the American Medical Association* 274 (1995): 706–11.

22. Lief and Fox, "Medical Student's Training." See also F. W. Hafferty, *Into the Valley: Death and the Socialization of Medical Students* (New Haven: Yale University Press, 1991).

23. Regarding such avoidance in the physician-patient encounter, see J. Katz, *The Silent World of Doctor and Patient* (New York: Free Press, 1984).

24. J. H. Brunvand, *The Vanishing Hitchhiker: American Urban Legends and Their Meanings* (New York: W. W. Norton, 1981), 11.

25. This is also an example of "positive self-negating prophecy," as discussed in chapter 6.

26. One author writing about the "limits of prognostication" coincidentally cited a paper of mine which noted that 15 percent of hospice patients outlived the six-month prognosis required for hospice admission. The author noted with intentional irony that "Christakis and Escarce do not report what percentage of the doctors had died during this time." See E. Chevlen, "The Limits of Prognostication," *Duquesne Law Review* 35 (1996): 336–54, 351. The paper of mine he refers to is N. A. Christakis and J. J. Escarce, "Survival of Medicare Patients after Enrollment in Hospice Programs," *New England Journal of Medicine* 335 (1996): 172–78.

27. C. L. Bosk, *Forgive and Remember: Managing Medical Failure* (Chicago: University of Chicago Press, 1979), esp. 103–10.

28. R. C. Fox, *Experiment Perilous* (Boston: Free Press, 1959), esp. 76–82.

29. For an example, involving the development of psychosis following successful cardiac surgery, see Fox, *Experiment Perilous*.

30. Parsons, *Social System*, 449.

31. M. B. Scott and S. M. Lyman, "Accounts," *American Sociological Review* 33 (1968): 46–62.

32. For example, Hippocrates explicitly identifies the role of prognosis in preserving professional reputation by avoiding assumption of responsibility for fatal cases. See Hippocrates, "Prognosis," in *Hippocratic Writings*, ed. G. E. R. Lloyd (New York: Penguin Books, 1983), 170–85. To give a modern example, some observers expressed the concern that hospitals might respond to federal guidelines mandating hospital disclosure of mortality rates for certain conditions or procedures by refusing patients they felt were too sick to survive simply in order to improve their statistics. Similarly, there was a concern that, with the development of prospective payment, patients with poor prognoses would either be excluded entirely or dumped "quicker and sicker." On the degree of empirical support for the latter concern, see J. Kosecoff, K. L. Kahn, W. H. Rogers, et al., "Prospective Payment System and Impairment at Discharge: The 'Quicker-and-Sicker' Story Revisited," *Journal of the American Medical Association* 264 (1990): 1980–83. Insurance companies, of course, have always behaved this way, in essence prognosticating about applicants partly in order to exclude people at high risk of disease. For an introduction to the practice of "adverse selection," see K. Polzer, "The Role of Risk Adjustment in National Health Reform," *Academic Medicine* 69 (1994): 445–51.

Chapter Five

1. With respect to doctor-patient communication in general, see M. Lipkin Jr., S. M. Putnam, and A. Lazare, eds., *The Medical Interview: Clinical Care, Education, and Research* (New York: Springer-Verlag, 1995). With respect to communication of problematic information, good examples of prescriptive analyses

include R. Buckman, *How to Break Bad News: A Guide for Health Care Professionals* (Baltimore: Johns Hopkins University Press, 1992); T. B. Brewin, "Three Ways of Giving Bad News," *Lancet* 337 (1991): 1207–9; J. A. Billings, "Sharing Bad News," *Outpatient Management of Advanced Cancer* (Philadelphia: Lippincott, 1985); and J. T. Placek and T. L. Eberhardt, "Breaking Bad News: A Review of the Literature," *Journal of the American Medical Association* 276 (1996): 496–502.

2. A noteworthy exception is N. T. Miyaji, "The Power of Compassion: Truth-Telling among American Doctors in the Care of Dying Patients," *Social Science and Medicine* 36 (1993): 249–64. Other descriptive studies include S. E. Lind, M. Good, S. Seidel, et al., "Telling the Diagnosis of Cancer," *Journal of Clinical Oncology* 7 (1989): 583–89; M. Good, B. J. Good, C. Schaffer, and S. E. Lind, "American Oncology and the Discourse on Hope," *Culture, Medicine, and Psychiatry* 14 (1990): 59–79; C. Seale, "Communication and Awareness about Death: A Study of a Random Sample of Dying People," *Social Science and Medicine* 32 (1991): 943–52; A. Chan and R. K. Woodruff, "Communicating with Patients with Advanced Cancer," *Journal of Palliative Care* 13 (1997): 29–33; A. Surbone and M. Zwitter, eds., *Communication with the Cancer Patient: Information and Truth, Annals of the New York Academy of Sciences*, vol. 809 (New York: New York Academy of Sciences, 1997).

3. Buckman, *How to Break Bad News*, 15; emphasis added.

4. However, it is possible to imagine bad news about nonmortal concerns, such as disability, congenital anomalies, unpleasant treatments, or medical error. Regarding communication about certain other types of bad news, see, for example, C. L. Bosk, *"All God's Mistakes": Genetic Counseling in a Pediatric Hospital* (Chicago: University of Chicago Press, 1992), and B. L. Svarstad and H. Lipton, "Informing Parents about Mental Retardation: A Study of Professional Communication and Parent Acceptance," *Social Science and Medicine* 11 (1977): 645–51.

5. Buckman, *How to Break Bad News*, 82. The reference to a "warning shot" is typical of the militaristic imagery that accompanies physicians' discussions of prognosis and pervades medicine more generally, as discussed below.

6. Lind, Good, Seidel, et al., "Telling the Diagnosis," found that about 20 percent of patients studied were given bad diagnostic-prognostic news while still recovering from anesthesia related to their surgery, as in the foregoing case!

7. See B. G. Glaser and A. L. Strauss, *Awareness of Dying* (Chicago: Aldine, 1965), esp. 147. More generally, see D. W. Maynard, "On 'Realization' in Everyday Life: The Forecasting of Bad News as a Social Relation," *American Sociological Review* 61 (1996): 109–31. Maynard considers why foreshadowing bad news is superior to "being blunt" or "stalling." However, he overlooks some alternatives considered below, such as "optimistic presentation," "statistical prognostication," and "negotiation."

8. For a classic examination of the use of military metaphors with respect to cancer, see S. Sontag, *Illness as Metaphor* (New York: Vintage Books, 1977), chap. 8. With respect to immunology, see E. Martin, *Flexible Bodies: The Role of Immunity in American Culture from the Days of Polio to the Age of AIDS* (Boston: Beacon Press, 1994), esp. chap. 1, "The Body at War: Media Views of the Immune System."

9. One study of thirty-two physicians found that in communicating prognoses to seriously ill, dying patients, 66 percent of physicians were "optimistic," 3 percent were "pessimistic," and 31 percent "shared their uncertainty" with patients. See Miyaji, "Power of Compassion."

10. Statistics were mentioned during 15 percent of prognostic discussions in *routine* clinical encounters; surgeons were more likely to use statistics than primary care physicians (20.8 percent versus 4.0 percent, $p < 0.05$). Doctors were more likely to use statistics in their prognostic statements when the patient was college educated (21.3 percent versus 3.8 percent, $p = 0.05$) or had a high income (23.5 percent versus 8.1 percent, $p = 0.07$), a practice explicitly acknowledged by many informants. See N. A. Christakis and W. Levinson, "Casual Optimism: Prognostication in Routine Medical and Surgical Encounters," unpublished manuscript. My impression that the use of statistics is somewhat higher in serious prognosis (for example, in situations involving intensive care or withdrawal of life support) is confirmed by at least one study of physicians' ideals regarding the care of dying patients: Miyaji found that 25 percent of physicians reported using statistics in telling prognoses all of the time, 38 percent some of the time, and 38 percent never; see Miyaji, "Power of Compassion."

11. Kathy Charmaz considers chronically ill patients' use of reference groups (and reference time periods) to gauge their illness; see K. Charmaz, *Good Days, Bad Days: The Self in Chronic Illness and Time* (New Brunswick, N.J.: Rutgers University Press, 1991).

12. Miyaji, "Power of Compassion," 254.

13. Such a conception of ethical behavior, which privileges the *motives* of the individual actor, is somewhat at odds with contemporary American rule-based conceptualizations of medical ethics. Still, it is in keeping with other systems of medical ethics, such as the Chinese one, that emphasize the virtue of the physician as the key component of ethical behavior. See, in passing, N. A. Christakis, "Ethics Are Local: Engaging Cross-cultural Variation in the Ethics for Clinical Research," *Social Science and Medicine* 35 (1992): 1079–91.

14. Some patients and their families have criticized contemporary practice, calling for the return of some withholding of the truth; see, for example, M. W. Lear, "Should Doctors Tell the Truth: The Case against Terminal Candor," *New York Times Magazine*, 24 January 1993, 17. This ethos of silence remains prevalent in Europe, China, Japan, Latin America, and other parts of the world; for an overview of the practices in many countries, see Surbone and Zwitter, *Communication with the Cancer Patients*. Regarding ethnic variation in patients' preferences regarding communication of prognoses in the United States, see L. J. Blackhall, S. T. Murphy, G. Frank, et al., "Ethnicity and Attitudes toward Patient Autonomy," *Journal of the American Medical Association* 274 (1995): 820–25. See also B. Freedman, "Offering Truth: One Ethical Approach to the Uninformed Cancer Patient," *Archives of Internal Medicine* 153 (1993): 572–76. It is worth noting, however, that even a hundred years ago, some elite American physicians deplored lying about prognosis; see, for example, R. C. Cabot, "The Use of Truth and Falsehood in Medicine: An Experimental Study," *American Medicine*, 28 February 1903, 344–349, esp. 346ff.

15. K. Mannheim, *Ideology and Utopia* (London: Routledge & Kegan Paul, 1936), 49.

16. Mannheim, *Ideology and Utopia*, 176. As such, they may be self-fulfilling prophecies, as discussed in chapter 6.

17. I use "impersonal" to describe prognosis in two ways. First, physicians discuss prognosis in detached ways, often devoid of individual particularity or emotion. Second, here, I use the term when physicians are discussing prognosis with disinterested parties, such as other clinicians who might or might not be involved in the patient's care.

18. N. A. Christakis, "Discrepancy between Objective Estimates of Prognosis and Those Communicated to Terminally Ill Outpatients," unpublished manuscript. Since Medicare regulations require development of a prognosis prior to hospice referral, the marginal effort required of the physician in these cases was simply to *communicate*, and not to develop, the prognosis.

19. N. A. Christakis, *Prognostication and Death in Medical Thought and Practice* (Ann Arbor, Mich.: University Microfilms, 1995). Some of these results are reviewed below in this chapter and in appendix 2.

20. N. A. Christakis and T. J. Iwashyna, "Attitude and Self-Reported Practice Regarding Prognostication in a National Sample of Internists," *Archives of Internal Medicine* 158 (1998): 2389–95.

21. These experiments were of a similar design but involved different vignettes and prompts than those discussed in chapters 3 and 6. See appendix 2 and Christakis, *Prognostication and Death*.

22. I assume here that the ("impersonal") prognoses physicians share with colleagues approximate their best belief about patients' true prospects more closely than the ("personal") prognoses shared with patients. While it is possible that physicians have *three* prognostic assessments—their true belief, the belief they share with colleagues, and the belief they share with patients—interview and observational data suggest that there is little or no difference between the first two. Such a difference, if it were to exist, might be motivated by a desire to somehow manage the expectations of one's colleagues regarding one's competence, or to "show off."

23. Most, but not all, studies show that pessimism in patients is associated with worse outcomes and so would call for a worse articulated prognosis. Regarding the tendency of outcomes to be related to expectations, see, for example, M. E. Seligman, *Helplessness: On Development, Depression, and Death* (New York: W. H. Freeman, 1975), and J. D. Frank and J. B. Frank, *Persuasion and Healing: A Comparative Study of Psychotherapy* (Baltimore: Johns Hopkins University Press, 1961). Regarding the possibly *beneficial* effect of negative emotions on outcome, however, see L. R. Derogatis, M. D. Abeloff, and N. Melisaratos, "Psychological Coping Mechanisms and Survival Time in Metastatic Breast Cancer," *Journal of the American Medical Association* 242 (1979): 1504–8.

24. Regarding such bargaining, see, for example, Buckman, *How to Break Bad News*; E. Kübler-Ross, *On Death and Dying* (New York: Macmillan, 1969); and D. E. Hayes-Bautista, "Modifying the Treatment: Patient Compliance, Patient Control, and Medical Care," *Social Science and Medicine* 10 (1976): 233–38. More often, such bargaining takes place between the patients and either themselves or God.

25. Here I mean something different from a mathematically formalized notion of ambiguity that analogizes it to physicians' lack of "confidence" in their decisions or in their probability estimates; see S. P. Curley, M. J. Young, and J. F. Yates, "Characterizing Physicians' Perceptions of Ambiguity," *Medical Decision Making* 9 (1989): 116–24.

26. M. Good, "Cultural Studies of Biomedicine: An Agenda for Research," *Social Science and Medicine* 41 (1995): 461–73. See also Surbone and Zwitter, *Communication with the Cancer Patients,* and Blackhall, Murphy, Frank, et al., "Ethnicity and Attitudes."

27. Regarding detachment, see H. I. Lief and R. C. Fox, "The Medical Student's Training for 'Detached Concern,'" in H. I. Lief, V. Lief, and N. R. Lief, eds., *The Psychological Basis of Medical Practice* (New York: Harper & Row, 1963), 12–35. Regarding "gaze," see M. Foucault, *The Birth of the Clinic: An Archaeology of Medical Perception* (New York: Vintage Books, 1975). And out of an enormous literature regarding physician's power, see I. Illich, *Medical Nemesis: The Expropriation of Health* (New York: Pantheon, 1976).

28. T. Parsons, *The Social System* (New York: Free Press, 1951), esp. 436–47.

29. This expectation can be so omnipresent as to become oppressive; patients with serious illness sometimes come to resent the overwhelming demand that they have hope or think positively about the future. See, for example, Sontag, *Illness as Metaphor.*

30. D. N. Levine, *The Flight from Ambiguity* (Chicago: University of Chicago Press, 1985), 21. Of course, sometimes the ambiguity in the situation is real and not merely "articulated." Regarding one aspect of ambiguity from the *patient's* perspective, see J. Comaroff and P. Maguire, "Ambiguity and the Search for Meaning: Childhood Leukemia in the Modern Clinical Context," *Social Science and Medicine* 15B (1981): 115–23.

Chapter Six

1. R. K. Merton, "The Self-Fulfilling Prophecy," in *Social Theory and Social Structure* (New York: Free Press, 1968), 475–90. See also R. K. Merton, "The Thomas Theorem and the Matthew Effect," *Social Forces* 74 (1995): 379–422. The original reference is W. I. Thomas and D. Thomas, *The Child in America: Behavior Problems and Programs* (New York: Alfred A. Knopf, 1928), 572. For a broader consideration of the self-fulfilling prophecy, see R. L. Henshel, "The Boundary of the Self-Fulfilling Prophecy and the Dilemma of Social Prediction," *British Journal of Sociology* 33 (1982): 511–28.

2. Regarding the issue of indeterminism more generally, see K. Popper, *The Open Universe: An Argument for Indeterminism* (London: Routledge, 1982).

3. Self-fulfilling prophecy, and concern for the future more generally, manifests itself not only in medical care, but in disparate areas of social life—from education to criminal justice (where people labeled as poor students or good students, or as lawbreakers or upstanding citizens may fulfill such expectations) to business. See, for example, W. E. Wilkins, "The Concept of a Self-Fulfilling Prophecy," *Sociology of Education* 49 (1976): 175–83; S. S. Wineburg and L. S. Shulman, "The Self-Fulfilling Prophecy: Its Genesis and Development in American Education," in J. Clark, C. Modgil, and S. Modgil, eds., *Robert K. Merton:*

Consensus and Controversy (Bristol, Pa.: Falmer Press, Taylor & Francis, 1990), 261–81; R. A. Farrell and V. L. Swigert, "Prior Offense Record as a Self-Fulfilling Prophecy," *Law and Society Review* 12 (1978): 437–53. Regarding prediction in criminology more generally, see D. P. Farrington and R. Tarling, eds., *Prediction in Criminology* (Albany: State University of New York Press, 1985). Regarding self-fulfilling prophecy in business, see A. S. King, "Self-Fulfilling Prophecies in Organizational Change," *Social Science Quarterly* 54 (1973): 384–93. For an argument that entire civilations can rise and fall according to the images of the future that they fashion for themselves, see Fred Polak's magisterial *The Image of the Future* (New York: Oceana Publications, 1961).

4. This occurs when a patient (literally) renounces the physician's prognosis and tries (successfully) to prove it wrong. Such behavior is analogous to the self-glorification that takes place in many social groups in the face of persistent belittlement; that is, negative statements from without may engender a compensatory positive belief from within (see Merton, "Self-Fulfilling Prophecy," 485). Merton touches on the problem of what he calls "self-defeating predictions" in R. K. Merton, "The Unanticipated Consequences of Purposive Social Action," *American Sociological Review* 1 (1936): 894–904; however, Merton is primarily concerned with how such predictions might result in "unanticipated" effects and he does not appear to discuss the possibility that one of the causes of unanticipated consequences may be an erroneous (meaning unduly favorable) prediction to begin with.

5. Some nonmedical examples of the four types follow. (1) Positive self-fulfilling prophecy: a prediction that real estate prices in a neighborhood will rise causes people to buy neighborhood property, which causes prices to rise. (2) Negative self-fulfilling prophecy: a prediction that a bank will fail causes a run on the bank, which causes the bank to fail. (3) Positive self-negating prophecy: a prediction that a sports team will lose a game causes the team to practice harder, which causes the team to win. (4) Negative self-negating prophecy: a prediction that a class will be oversubscribed causes students not to enroll, which causes the class to be undersubscribed.

6. Each of these mechanisms is "social" in that it is influenced by, or reflects the action of, social forces. All three involve the social interaction of a physician and a patient and the modification of the socially defined functions and roles of each. Moreover, all three involve the intermediation of socially patterned and culturally specific "explanatory models" about illness. Regarding these models, see, for example, A. Kleinman, *Patients and Healers in the Context of Culture: An Exploration of the Borderland between Anthropology, Medicine, and Psychiatry* (Berkeley: University of California Press, 1980), and A. Kleinman, *The Illness Narratives: Suffering, Healing, and the Human Condition* (New York: Basic Books, 1988).

7. T. Parsons, *The Social System* (New York: Free Press, 1951), esp. 437ff.

8. Thus, there is a connection between the clinical course the patient experiences and fulfillment of a social role. This connection finds an analogy in the work of sociologist Diana Crane, which showed that a key determinant of physicians' decisions to withdraw life support was the capacity of the patient to interact socially; in other words, fulfillment of a social role (e.g., having the

capacity to interact with others) was instrumental to the choice of treatment and thus to the course of the illness. See D. Crane, *The Sanctity of Social Life: Physicians' Treatment of Critically Ill Patients* (New Brunswick, N.J.: Transaction Press, 1977).

9. For examples of this perspective on the discipline and control of the patient and the patient's body, see A. Petersen and R. Bunton, eds., *Foucault: Health and Medicine* (London: Routledge, 1997). Works by Michel Foucault setting forth the relevant ideas include *Discipline and Punish: The Birth of the Prison* (New York: Vintage Books, 1979), *The Birth of the Clinic: An Archaeology of Medical Perception* (New York: Vintage Books, 1975), *The History of Sexuality,* vol. 1 (New York: Random House, 1978), and *Madness and Civilization: A History of Insanity in the Age of Reason* (New York: Random House, 1965).

10. R. C. Fox, *Experiment Perilous* (Boston: Free Press, 1959), 143ff.

11. Articles addressing some of these effects include D. V. Nelson, L. C. Friedman, P. E. Baer, et al., "Attitudes to Cancer: Psychometric Properties of Fighting Spirit and Denial," *Journal of Behavioral Medicine* 12 (1989): 341–55; M. F. Scheier and C. S. Carver, "Dispositional Optimism and Physical Well-Being: The Influence of Generalized Outcome Expectancies on Health," *Journal of Personality* 55 (1987): 169–210; D. S. Brody, S. M. Miller, C. E. Lerman, et al., "Patient Perception of Involvement in Medical Care: Relationship to Illness Attitudes and Outcomes," *Journal of General Internal Medicine* 4 (1989): 506–11; B. Olsson, B. Olsson, and G. Tibblin, "Effect of Patients' Expectations on Recovery from Acute Tonsillitis," *Family Practice* 6 (1989): 188–92; S. J. Almada, A. B. Zonderman, R. B. Shekelle, et al., "Neuroticism and Cynicism and Risk of Death in Middle-Aged Men: The Western Electric Study," *Psychosomatic Medicine* 53 (1991): 165–75; R. Anda, D. Williamson, D. Jones, et al., "Depressed Affect, Hopelessness, and the Risk of Ischemic Heart Disease in a Cohort of U.S. Adults," *Epidemiology* 4 (1993): 285–94; M. E. Lancman, J. J. Asconapé, W. J. Craven, et al., "Predictive Value of Induction of Psychogenic Seizures by Suggestion," *Annals of Neurology* 35 (1994): 359–61; T. J. Luparello, H. A. Lyons, E. R. Bleecker, and E. R. McFadden Jr., "Influences of Suggestion on Airway Reactivity in Asthmatic Subjects," *Psychosomatic Medicine* 30 (1968): 819–25; T. J. Luparello, N. Leist, C. H. Lourie, and P. Sweet, "The Interaction of Psychologic Stimuli and Pharmacologic Agents on Airway Reactivity in Asthmatic Subjects," *Psychosomatic Medicine* 32 (1970): 509–13; A. Schweiger and A. Parducci, "Nocebo: The Psychologic Induction of Pain," *Pavlovian Journal of Biological Science* 16 (1981): 140–43; R. A. Sternbach, "The Effects of Instructional Sets on Autonomic Responsivity," *Psychophysiology* 1 (1964): 67–72; A. D. Weisman and T. P. Hackett, "Predilection to Death: Death and Dying as a Psychiatric Problem," *Psychosomatic Medicine* 23 (1961): 232–56; T. S. Walczak, D. T. Williams, and W. Berten, "Utility and Reliability of Placebo Infusion in the Evaluation of Patients with Seizures," *Neurology* 44 (1994): 394–99; W. B. Cannon, "Voodoo Death," *American Anthropologist* 44 (1942): 169–81; D. Lester, "Voodoo Death: Some New Thoughts on an Old Phenomenon," *American Anthropologist* 74 (1972): 386–90; G. Lewis, "Fear of Sorcery and the Problem of Death by Suggestion," *Social Science and Medicine* 24 (1987): 997–1010; and G. L. Engel, "Sudden and Rapid Death during Psychological Stress: Folklore or Folk Wisdom?" *Annals of Internal Medicine* 74 (1971): 771–82.

12. Note that the physician's prediction can also affect the behavior of other health professionals. The notion of "laying crepe" is discussed in chapter 7.

13. See chapter 1 and Crane, *Sanctity of Social Life.*

14. A study of 1,065 critically ill patients in France found that giving the responsible physicians some objective estimates of the patient's prospects for survival meaningfully increased the likelihood that treatment would be withdrawn or withheld (in one subgroup of patients, from 11 percent absent the estimates to 36 percent when the estimates were given); see W. A. Knaus, A. Rauss, A. Alperovitch, et al., "Do Objective Estimates of Chances for Survival Influence Decisions to Withhold or Withdraw Treatment," *Medical Decision Making* 10 (1990): 163–71. Similar results were obtained in a trial giving prognostic information to neurosurgeons caring for 1,025 patients in England; see L. S. Murray, G. M. Teasdale, G. D. Murray, et al., "Does Prediction of Outcome Alter Patient Management?," *Lancet* 341 (1993): 1487–91. Finally, see SUPPORT principal investigators, "A Controlled Trial to Improve Care for Seriously Ill Hospitalized Patients: The Study to Understand Prognoses and Preferences for Outcomes and Risks of Treatments (SUPPORT)," *Journal of the American Medical Association* 274 (1995): 1591–98, and the discussion of this study in chapter 8.

15. See, for example, A. K. Shapiro, "Iatroplacebogenics," *International Pharmacopsychiatry* 2 (1969): 215–48.

16. For a useful introduction to the enormous literature on the placebo effect, see A. Harrington, ed., *The Placebo Effect* (Cambridge: Harvard University Press, 1997).

17. R. A. Hahn, "The Nocebo Phenomenon: Scope and Foundations," in Harrington, *Placebo Effect,* 56–76.

18. Cannon, "Voodoo Death."

19. Hahn, "Nocebo Phenomenon," esp. 69.

20. For example, fainting among women in Victorian England was a biological response that was recognized by lay people and physicians as an illness and at times engendered by prescribed circumstances. On the prescriptive nature of disease nosologies, see B. Ehrenreich and D. English, *For Her Own Good: 150 Years of the Experts' Advice to Women* (New York: Anchor Books, 1978).

21. I address the role of prognosis in previous generations in chapter 1 and in N. A. Christakis, "The Ellipsis of Prognosis in Modern Medical Thought," *Social Science and Medicine* 44 (1997): 301–15.

22. The statement that the patient "would weep from his wounds" is an example of the religious metaphors sometimes (implicitly or explicitly) invoked by physicians in discussions of prognosis, as discussed in chapter 3. Also noteworthy in this case is the sad symmetry between the statements that the physician "hates" the patient and that the family "hates" the physician; it seems likely, however, that this expressed hatred is not personal as such.

23. For methodological details and specific findings, see appendices 1 and 2.

24. Indeed, Kathy Charmaz has argued that a fundamental mechanism for coping with chronic disease is to emphasize stability and lack of novel events—a one-day-at-a-time strategy. See K. Charmaz, *Good Days, Bad Days: The Self in Chronic Illness and Time* (New Brunswick, N.J.: Rutgers University Press, 1991).

25. In interpreting the observed differences in physicians' beliefs in these

two experiments, it is of course appropriate to bear in mind that the clinical cases in the two experiments differ in details other than the survival horizon of the patients, for example, in the gender of the patients and in their diagnoses. These differences, however, do not appear to be central enough to undermine the comparison. Moreover, qualitative results based on interviews with physicians support the general conclusion that prognoses are viewed as especially effective when they deviate from prior expectations.

26. These results also are consistent with the behaviors of physicians with respect to the predictions they offer (documented in chapter 3). For chronically ill patients, physicians tended to overestimate survival, consistent with avoidance of negative self-fulfilling prophecy; for acutely ill patients, they tended to underestimate survival, consistent with avoidance of positive self-fulfilling prophecy. While the former behavior seems justifiable, the latter raises the unlikely possibility that physicians' concern with self-fulfilling prophecy precludes even favorable predictions. Of course, the avoidance of favorable predictions has numerous other explanations, as we have seen.

27. See appendix 2 for quantitative details.

28. The relation between belief in positive self-fulfilling prophecy and age could represent either a change with age or a cohort effect, whereby people entering medicine in different eras have different attitudes; it is not possible to distinguish the two with data such as these. See J. Hobcraft, J. Menken, and S. Preston, "Age, Period, and Cohort Effects in Demography: A Review," in W. M. Mason and S. E. Fienberg, eds., *Cohort Analysis in Social Research* (New York: Springer-Verlag, 1985), 89–136.

29. Multiple logistic regression models that assessed the robustness of these bivariate associations, while adjusting for other demographic and situational attributes of respondents, revealed that only age, optimism, and experience with requests for prognostic information were independently significant. Whether the respondent was a specialist or a generalist was not found to be associated with belief in positive self-fulfilling prophecy. This suggests that the difference between specialists' and generalists' belief was attributable to the extent to which they were called upon to render prognostic assessments. Conversely, this suggests that specialization alone cannot account for the effect of frequent demand for prognostic information upon belief in the self-fulfilling prophecy. (A logistic regression model with two independent variables, namely, generalist/specialist status and experience with requests for prognostic information, and with belief in either positive or negative self-fulfilling prophecy as the dependent variable, yields the same result.)

30. Part of the "danger" also arises from the notion that the self-fulfilling nature of prediction may itself unsettle the "natural" order of things. The sense that the future depends on present actions makes the actors feel considerable responsibility while simultaneously rendering the future unnatural and therefore dangerous. See M. Douglas, *Purity and Danger: An Analysis of the Concepts of Pollution and Taboo* (London: Routledge, 1966). Douglas notes, for example, at p. 114, that she is attempting to define "a particular class of dangers which are not powers vested in humans, but which can be released by human action. The power which presents a danger for careless humans is very evidently a power

inhering in the structure of ideas, a power by which the structure is expected to protect itself."

31. According to sociologist Marcel Mauss: "In medical practices, words, incantations, ritual and astrological observances are magical; this is the realm of the occult and of the spirits, a world of ideas which imbues ritual movements and gestures with a special kind of effectiveness, quite different from their mechanical effectiveness. It is not really believed that the gestures themselves bring about the result. The effect derives from something else, and usually this is not of the same order." M. Mauss, *A General Theory of Magic*, trans. R. Brain (New York: Norton, 1972), 20.

32. Mauss, *General Theory of Magic*, 59. This tradition is even today more widespread than is appreciated; see S. J. Reiser, "Words as Scalpels: Transmitting Evidence in the Clinical Dialogue," *Annals of Internal Medicine* 92 (1980): 837–42. For a historical perspective on the notion that a prediction can have a magical effect, see K. Thomas, *Religion and the Decline of Magic* (New York: Scribner's, 1971), esp. chap. 5, "Prayer and Prophecy," and chap. 13, "Ancient Prophecies."

33. Parsons, *Social System*, 469.

34. R. C. Fox, "The Human Condition of Health Professionals," in *Essays in Medical Sociology: Journeys into the Field* (New Brunswick, N.J.: Transaction Books, 1988), 572–87, 581.

35. R. C. Fox, *The Sociology of Medicine* (Englewood Cliffs, N.J.: Prentice Hall, 1989), 198.

36. Fox, "Human Condition," 581.

37. See R. G. Collingwood, "On the So-Called Idea of Causation," in H. Morris, ed., *Freedom and Responsibility: Readings in Philosophy and Law* (Stanford: Stanford University Press, 1961), 303–13, and R. A. Shweder, N. C. Much, M. Mahapatra, and L. Park, "The 'Big Three' of Morality (Autonomy, Community, Divinity) and the 'Big Three' Explanations of Suffering," in A. M. Brandt and P. Rozin, eds., *Morality and Health* (New York: Routledge, 1997), 119–69.

38. Shweder, Much, Mahapatra, and Park, " 'Big Three' of Morality," 125.

39. This is also an example of the "crisis of good fortune" explored in Fox, *Experiment Perilous*, and discussed in chapter 4.

40. As discussed in chapter 5, physicians are more likely to share predictions with patients' families than with patients and more likely to err optimistically with patients.

41. This term, first used by Bronislaw Malinowski (*Magic, Science and Religion* [Boston: Beacon Press, 1948], 70), has previously been applied to medicine by Talcott Parsons and Renée Fox. I will explore the ritualization of optimism, and its intriguing counterpart, the ritualization of pessimism, in the next chapter.

Chapter Seven

1. R. C. Fox, "The Human Condition of Health Professionals," in *Essays in Medical Sociology: Journeys into the Field* (New Brunswick, N.J.: Transaction Books, 1988), 572–87, 574.

2. C. Geertz, "Religion as a Cultural System," in *The Interpretation of Cultures* (New York: Basic Books, 1973), 87–125, 112.

3. B. Malinowski, *Magic, Science and Religion* (Boston: Beacon Press, 1948), 12.

4. Malinowski, *Magic, Science and Religion,* 70.

5. See, for example, M. F. Scheier and C. S. Carver, "Dispositional Optimism and Physical Well-Being: The Influence of Generalized Outcome Expectancies on Health," *Journal of Personality* 55 (1987): 169–210; C. Peterson and M. E. P. Seligman, "Explanatory Style and Illness," *Journal of Personality* 55 (1987): 237–65. Physicians' *belief* that optimism is beneficial for patients, regardless of whether it really *is*, is discussed in chapter 5.

6. M. Good, B. J. Good, C. Schaffer, and S. E. Lind, "American Oncology and the Discourse on Hope," *Culture, Medicine, and Psychiatry* 14 (1990): 59–79.

7. This propensity is somewhat heterogeneously distributed. After adjusting for other measured attributes and attitudes of physicians, older physicians have a greater tendency to shade their predictions toward optimism, while those experiencing more situations calling for prognoses have a lesser tendency; on the other hand, this propensity is independent of gender, specialization, or self-identification as an optimist. See N. A. Christakis and T. J. Iwashyna, "Attitude and Self-Reported Practice Regarding Prognostication in a National Sample of Internists," *Archives of Internal Medicine* 158 (1998): 2389–95, and N. A. Christakis, *Prognostication and Death in Medical Thought and Practice* (Ann Arbor, Mich.: University Microfilms, 1995). Of course, it is often the case, especially in routine medical encounters, that optimism is appropriate, as when the patient's condition is objectively self-limited, curable, or minor. And, indeed, in routine clinical encounters, when they do express a prognosis, physicians tend to express a favorable one. See N. A. Christakis and W. Levinson, "Casual Optimism: Prognostication in Routine Medical and Surgical Encounters," unpublished manuscript.

8. Christakis, *Prognostication and Death.*

9. Although certain cancers (e.g., chronic lymphocytic leukemia, indolent prostate cancer) can arguably be termed "chronic," it requires a major leap to consider the type and stage of cancer in this patient to be a chronic condition.

10. See, for example, A. Wagg, M. Kinirons, and K. Stewart, "Cardiopulmonary Resuscitation: Doctors and Nurses Expect Too Much," *Journal of the Royal College of Physicians of London* 29 (1995): 20–24.

11. This belief is very homogeneously distributed and, except for age, no measured attribute was associated with it in a statistically significant fashion. Older physicians are less likely to express pessimism. See Christakis and Iwashyna, "Attitude and Self-Reported Practice."

12. Such mistakes, in the opinion of physicians, typically call for explanations. Physicians may thus protect themselves by erring on the side of pessimism when there is uncertainty associated with the prognosis, a preference discussed at greater length in chapter 3.

13. See M. Siegler, "Pascal's Wager and the Hanging of Crepe," *New England Journal of Medicine* 293 (1975): 853–57.

14. Robert Zussman argues that DNR orders may be seen as rituals that serve a symbolic function. See R. Zussman, *Intensive Care: Medical Ethics and the Medical Profession* (Chicago: University of Chicago Press, 1992), chap. 12, "The 'Do Not Resuscitate' Order as Ritual."

15. Regarding one source of patients' misperceptions about CPR, see S. J. Diem, J. D. Lantos, and J. A. Tulsky, "Cardiopulmonary Resuscitation on Television: Miracles and Misinformation," *New England Journal of Medicine* 334 (1996): 1578–82.

16. Complete uncertainty is not essential for these behavioral strategies to be expressed. Physicians may demonstrate ritualized pessimism when the prognosis is relatively certain, especially if the prognosis is unfavorable and considered immutable. On the other hand, physicians may demonstrate ritualized optimism in such circumstances as well.

17. The importance of age is seen also in neonatal intensive care units, where it seems these very young patients are treated aggressively precisely because of ritualized optimism; that is, they are considered to have a better prognosis than they do. See J. H. Guillemin and L. L. Holmstrom, *Mixed Blessings: Intensive Care for Newborns* (New York: Oxford University Press, 1986), esp. 125ff.

18. R. K. Merton and E. Barber, "Sociological Ambivalence," in R. K. Merton, ed., *Sociological Ambivalence and Other Essays* (New York: Free Press, 1976), 3–31, 19. See also chapter 4.

19. T. J. Scheff, "Decision Rules, Types of Error, and Their Consequences in Medical Diagnosis," *Behavioral Science* 8 (1963): 97–107. In current epidemiological parlance, physicians have a relatively high "sensitivity" and a low "specificity" for disease.

20. See chapter 2 on the role of prognosis in the process of differential diagnosis.

21. C. M. Moinpour and L. Polissar, "Factors Affecting Place of Death of Hospice and Non-Hospice Cancer Patients," *American Journal of Public Health* 79 (1989): 1549–51; V. Mor and J. Hiris, "Determinants of Site of Death among Hospice Cancer Patients," *Journal of Health and Social Behavior* 24 (1983): 375–85. About 80 percent of patients have hospice care provided in their home; see National Hospice Organization, "1992 Stats Show Continued Growth in Programs and Patients," *NHO Newsline* 3 (1993): 1–2.

22. D. Greer, V. Mor, J. Morris, et al., "An Alternative in Terminal Care: Results of the National Hospice Study," *Journal of Chronic Diseases* 39 (1986): 9–26.

23. V. Mor, D. S. Greer, and R. Kastenbaum, *The Hospice Experiment* (Baltimore: Johns Hopkins Press, 1988); D. Kidder, "The Effects of Hospice Coverage on Medicare Expenditures," *Health Services Research* 27 (1992): 195–217; V. Mor and D. Kidder, "Cost Savings in Hospice: Final Result of the National Hospice Study," *Health Services Research* 20 (1985): 407–21.

24. N. J. Dawson, "Need Satisfaction in Terminal Care Settings," *Social Science and Medicine* 32 (1991): 83–87; R. L. Kane, S. J. Klei, L. Bernstein, et al., "Hospice Role in Alleviating the Emotional Stress of Terminal Patients and Their Families," *Medical Care* 23 (1985): 189–97; K. A. Wallston, C. Burger, R. A. Smith, and R. J. Baugher, "Comparing the Quality of Death for Hospice and Non-Hospice Cancer Patients," *Medical Care* 26 (1988): 177–82.

25. See F. A. Davis, "Medicare Hospice Benefit: Early Program Experience," *Health Care Financing Review* 9 (1988): 99–111; and W. Bulkin and H. Lukashok, "Rx for Dying: The Case for Hospice," *New England Journal of Medicine* 318 (1988):

376–78. The 1997 figures are unpublished data provided by the Health Care Financing Administration.

26. Social Security Act 1861(dd)(3)(A). This definition of "terminal illness" is explicitly prognostic, though, in principle, it need not be. For example, the regulations could have specified that certain diseases or stages of diseases, or certain levels of patient function (e.g., being bedridden nearly all day), would qualify as "terminal."

27. N. A. Christakis and J. J. Escarce, "Survival of Medicare Patients after Enrollment in Hospice Programs," *New England Journal of Medicine* 335 (1996): 172–78.

28. Two randomized controlled trials, however, have failed to reveal any shortening of life associated with hospice use. See R. L. Kane, J. Wales, L. Bernstein, et al., "A Randomised Trial of Hospice Care," *Lancet* 1 (1984): 890–94, and J. M. Addington-Hall, L. D. MacDonald, H. R. Anderson, et al., "Randomised Controlled Trial of Effects of Coordinating Care for Terminally Ill Cancer Patients," *British Medical Journal* 305 (1992): 1317–22.

29. Christakis and Escarce, "Survival of Medicare Patients."

30. H. Brody, and J. Lynn, "The Physician's Responsibility under the New Medicare Reimbursement for Hospice Care," *New England Journal of Medicine* 310 (1984): 920–22, 921. See also R. A. Pearlman, "Inaccurate Predictions of Life Expectancy: Dilemmas and Opportunities," *Archives of Internal Medicine* 148 (1988): 2537–38, and J. F. Potter, "A Challenge for the Hospice Movement," *New England Journal of Medicine* 302 (1980): 53–55. The six-month standard may be difficult for physicians to interpret or apply; see J. Lynn, J. M. Teno, and F. M. Harrell, "Accurate Prognostication of Death: Opportunities and Challenges for Clinicians," *Western Journal of Medicine* 163 (1995): 250–57.

Chapter Eight

1. The argument here, that "more" knowledge is optimally necessary for "more" action, stands in opposition to the notion that with perfect knowledge, no action is necessary or desired. As expressed by Friedrich Nietzsche, "Understanding kills action." See F. Nietzsche, *The Birth of Tragedy* (New York: Doubleday Anchor Books, 1956), 51. In essence, Nietzsche argues that when someone realizes that "no action of theirs can work any change in the eternal condition of things," the motivation to act falls away. Nevertheless, as compared with the abstract human, the real human *must* act, and knowledge is generally a useful predicate for action. Moreover, most social action is not (consciously) concerned with working a change in the "eternal condition of things" but has a more immediate and concrete purpose.

2. Conversely and symmetrically, foresight by individuals facilitates their interaction with others and so stabilizes collective behavior. See C. W. Mills, "Situated Actions and Vocabularies of Motive," *American Sociological Review* 5 (1944): 904–13.

3. This is not restricted to medicine. Foretelling the future is often a deliberate means of affecting social phenomena; for example, the leaders of doomsday movements articulate particular images of the future and motivate groups of followers to behave in concerted and typically extraordinary ways. For a

nonmedical illustration, see L. Festinger, H. W. Riecken, and S. Schachter, *When Prophecy Fails: A Social and Psychological Study of a Modern Group That Predicted the Destruction of the World* (New York: Harper and Row, 1964). See also W. A. Sherden, *The Fortune Sellers: The Big Business of Buying and Selling Predictions* (New York: John Wiley & Sons, 1998), and P. Boyer, *When Time Shall Be No More: Prophecy Belief in Modern American Culture* (Cambridge: Harvard University Press, 1992).

4. There is, nevertheless, often an implicit or explicit agreement regarding the area about which a predictor may foretell the future. One does not ordinarily ask one's physician to predict the direction of one's stock portfolio, and solicited or unsolicited predictions in this area would be regarded as quite peculiar. Moreover, such predictions by a physician would not be perceived as either an appropriate or obligatory basis for action by the patient.

5. Physicians are perceived to be better predictors of the outcome of illness than are other professionals (such as nurses). Nevertheless, studies that have, albeit peripherally, compared physicians' and nurses' predictions have failed to find a consistent difference between these two professional groups. See chapter 3. Regarding professional authority, see also E. Freidson, *Profession of Medicine: A Study of the Sociology of Applied Knowledge* (Chicago: University of Chicago Press, 1970).

6. Hippocrates, "Prognosis," in *Hippocratic Writings,* ed. G. E. R. Lloyd, trans. J. Chadwick and W. N. Mann (New York: Penguin, 1978), 170–85, 170.

7. L. Edelstein, "Hippocratic Prognosis," in O. Temkin and C. L. Temkin, eds., *Ancient Medicine: Selected Papers by Ludwig Edelstein* (Baltimore: Johns Hopkins University Press, 1967), 65–110, esp. 77ff.

8. These are "differentiated" roles subject to what Parsons has called "the double contingency of interaction"; see T. Parsons, *The Social System* (New York: Free Press, 1951), esp. 25ff. and 114. The physician and the patient do not just differ in their roles, however, they also differ in their *status*. The difference between "role" and "status" may be appreciated by noting that the former is a "processual aspect" and the latter a "positional aspect" in the social system. I believe that the prophet/supplicant relationship is as archetypical as other, classically described relationships, such as merchant/customer, bureaucrat/client, expert/layperson, and so forth.

9. See B. Malinowski, *Magic, Science and Religion* (Boston: Beacon Press, 1948), esp. 59–61. Malinowski argues that the fountainhead of magic in society is emotional wishes that are unfulfillable or unfulfilled. Incidentally, this is somewhat analogous to Freud's reasoning about the origin of dreams in individuals; see S. Freud, *The Interpretation of Dreams*, trans. J. Strachey (New York: Avon Books, 1965).

10. M. Weber, *The Sociology of Religion* (Boston: Beacon Press, 1993), 58–59.

11. The function of prophecy in providing meaning is manifest, for example, in ancient Greek plays, where the inexorable fulfillment of prophecy provides the backdrop against which the tragic hero lives out his fateful life. Indeed, the order represented by the oracular prediction is the source of the play's dramatic power; the hero must fail because he undermines that sacred order. See R. W. Bushnell, *Prophesying Tragedy: Sign and Voice in Sophocles' Theban Plays* (Ithaca,

N.Y.: Cornell University Press, 1988), esp. 18. See also J. J. O'Hara, *Death and the Optimistic Prophecy in Vergil's Aeneid* (Princeton, N.J.: Princeton University Press, 1990).

12. A. Kleinman, *The Illness Narratives: Suffering, Healing, and the Human Condition* (New York: Basic Books, 1988), 48.

13. A. Kleinman, " 'Everything That Really Matters': Social Suffering, Subjectivity, and the Remaking of Human Experience in a Disordering World," *Harvard Theological Review* 1997; 90: 315–335, 320; see also A. Kleinman, *Writing at the Margin: Discourse between Anthropology and Medicine* (Berkeley: University of California Press, 1996).

14. A prognosis provides a reference for patients as they move forward into their illness. This is analogous to hospitalization which, with its daily rhythms and prescribed patters of care, with its occupational division of labor and caretakers matched to patients' needs, imposes an order on an uncertain illness trajectory—if not on the disease physiology, then on its management. That is, there is a performative and prescriptive element to the prognosis that physicians articulate.

15. See H. Jonas, *The Gnostic Religion: The Message of the Alien God and the Beginnings of Christianity,* 2d ed. (Boston: Beacon Press, 1958), 336.

16. This concern has ancient roots in the Judaic tradition. See "Prophets and Prophecy," *Encyclopedia Judaica* (New York: Macmillan, 1971), 13: 1150–81.

17. See chapter 2 on physicians' possibly self-interested use of prognosis.

18. SUPPORT principal investigators, "A Controlled Trial to Improve Care for Seriously Ill Hospitalized Patients," *Journal of the American Medical Association* 274 (1995): 1591–98. While the number of patients in this study was very large, the physicians themselves were drawn from only twenty-seven group practices in five specialties (internal medicine, intensive care, oncology, surgery, and cardiology) at the five hospitals.

19. For example, approximately 50 percent of the hospitalized patients in this study had very significant pain prior to their deaths, a totally correctable and needless deficit in care. See J. Lynn, J. M. Teno, R. S. Phillips, et al., "Perceptions by Family Members of the Dying Experience of Older and Seriously Ill Patients," *Annals of Internal Medicine* 126 (1997): 97–106. See also chapter 1.

20. SUPPORT principal investigators, "Controlled Trial," 1592.

21. Technically, they were well calibrated-in-the-large and, for most subgroups, well calibrated-in-the-small. However, discrimination was moderate. See W. A. Knaus, F. E. Harrell Jr., J. Lynn, et al., "The SUPPORT Prognostic Model: Objective Estimates of Survival for Seriously Ill Hospitalized Adults," *Annals of Internal Medicine* 122 (1995): 191–203.

22. J. C. Weeks, E. F. Cook, S. J. O'Day, et al., "Relationship between Cancer Patients' Predictions of Prognosis and Their Treatment Preferences," *Journal of the American Medical Association* 279 (1998): 1709–14.

23. Similar findings about patients' mistaken impressions of their prognosis were noted in another study of one hundred lung cancer patients; see W. J. Mackillop, W. E. Stewart, A. D. Ginsburg, and S. S. Stewart, "Cancer Patients' Perceptions of Their Disease and Its Treatment," *British Journal of Cancer* 58 (1988): 355–58. See also C. F. Quirt, W. J. Mackillop, A. D. Ginsburg, et al.,

"Do Doctors Know When Their Patients Don't? A Survey of Doctor-Patient Communication in Lung Cancer," *Lung Cancer* 18 (1997): 1–20.

24. Weeks, Cook, O'Day, et al., "Relationship between Cancer Patients' Predictions," 1714.

25. Of course, we have just seen data indicating that patients sometimes claim to remember discussions of prognosis that doctors do not remember.

26. See, for example, Mackillop, Stewart, Ginsburg, and Stewart, "Cancer Patients' Perceptions"; L. A. Siminoff, J. H. Fetting, and M. D. Abeloff, "Doctor-Patient Communication about Breast Cancer Adjuvant Therapy," *Journal of Clinical Oncology* 7 (1989): 1192–1200; P. Mosconi, B. E. Meyerowitz, M. C. Liberati, and A. Liberati, "Disclosure of Breast Cancer Diagnosis: Patient and Physician Reports," *Annals of Oncology* 2 (1991): 273–280 (regarding Italian patients); and B. Pfefferbaum, P. M. Levenson, and J. van Eys, "Comparison of Physician and Patient Perceptions of Communications Issues," *Southern Medical Journal* 75 (1982): 1080–83. We should not be suprised about the discordance here; indeed, physicans often are unaware of patients' end-of-life preferences and values; see M. Danis, M. S. Gerrity, L. I. Southerland, and D. L. Patrick, "A Comparison of Patient, Family, and Physician Assessments of the Value of Medical Intensive Care," *Critical Care Medicine* 16 (1988): 594–600; R. F. Uhlmann, R. A. Pearlman, and K. C. Cain, "Understanding of Elderly Patients' Resuscitation Preferences by Physicians and Nurses," *Western Journal of Medicine* 150 (1989): 705–7; and A. B. Seckler, D. E. Meier, M. Mulvihill, and B. E. Paris, "Substituted Judgement: How Accurate Are Proxy Predictions?" *Annals of Internal Medicine* 115 (1991): 92–98.

27. Quirt, Mackillop, Ginsburg, et al., "Do Doctors Know." See also P. M. Ravdin, I. A. Siminoff, and J. A. Harvey, "Survey of Breast Cancer Patients Concerning Their Knowledge and Expectations of Adjuvant Therapy," *Journal of Clinical Oncology* 16 (1998): 515–21; and the discussion of discrepant communication above in chapter 5.

28. Siminoff, Fetting, and Abeloff, "Doctor-Patient Communication." Some investigators, incidentally, have shown benefits from giving patients audiotapes of consultations, perhaps because this decreases discrepancies in recall; see P. McHugh, S. Lewis, S. Ford, et al., "The Efficacy of Audiotapes in Promoting Psychological Well-Being in Cancer Patients: A Randomised, Controlled Trial," *British Journal of Cancer* 71 (1995): 388–92.

29. SUPPORT principal investigators, "Controlled Trial," 1597.

30. See, for example, L. F. Degner, L. J. Kristjanson, D. Bowman, et al., "Information Needs and Decisional Preferences in Women with Breast Cancer," *Journal of the American Medical Association* 277 (1997): 1485–92. See also chapter 2.

31. For a good argument about this, from the clinical literature, see A. Girgis and R. W. Sanson-Fisher, "Breaking Bad News: Consensus Guidelines for Medical Practitioners," *Journal of Clinical Oncology* 13 (1995): 2449–56. For an illustration of the variation in patient preferences, see J. McIntosh, "Patients' Awareness and Desire for Information about Diagnosed but Undisclosed Malignant Disease," *Lancet* 2 (1976): 300–303.

32. The implications of some of these questions are examined in D. Callahan, *The Troubled Dream of Life: In Search of a Peaceful Death* (New York: Simon & Schuster, 1993).

33. A corollary of this asymmetry in power between patient and physician is that prognostication is open to manipulation by the physician for self-serving ends. For example, a physician could make dire predictions to oblige the patient to adopt an expensive therapeutic plan that benefits the physician but that the patient might not otherwise choose; alternatively, the physician might paint a rosy picture to keep the patient as a client. Sometimes self-interest is implicit and does not reflect nefarious motives, but in any case physicians are not supposed to use prognosis to achieve their own ends at the expense of the patient. The possibility of such manipulation, however, adds to the perception that prognosis, like medical care generally, should be governed by ethical precepts.

34. Indeed, as we saw in chapter 3, there are public, occupational rituals for evaluating mistakes in diagnosis and therapy but not for evaluating mistakes in prognosis. There are, it is worth noting, no particular incentives or professional rewards for doing long-term follow-up studies and checking results against past predictions. For an illustration from the field of neonatology, see J. H. Guillemin and L. L. Holmstrom, *Mixed Blessings: Intensive Care for Newborns* (New York: Oxford University Press, 1986), 129. See R. R. Anspach, *Deciding Who Lives: Fateful Choices in the Intensive-Care Nursery* (Berkeley: University of California Press, 1993), 238, for the same observation in a different neonatal intensive care unit.

35. Regarding clinical prognostic information, see, for example, J. F. Fries and G. B. Ehrlich, *Prognosis: Contemporary Outcomes of Disease* (Bowie, Md.: Charles Press, 1981), and J. M. Gilchrist, ed., *Prognosis in* Neurology (Boston: Butterworth-Heinemann, 1998). Regarding formulating and using prognostic information, see A. C. Justice, K. E. Covinsky, and J. A. Berlin, "Assessing the Generalizability of Prognostic Information," *Annals of Internal* Medicine 130 (1999): 515–24; N. A. Christakis and G. A. Sachs, "The Role of Prognosis in Clinical Decision Making," *Journal of General Internal Medicine* 11 (1996): 422–25; C. M. Watts and W. A. Knaus, "The Case for Using Objective Scoring Systems to Predict Intensive Care Unit Outcome, *Critical Care Clinics* 10 (1994): 73–89; M. Seneff and W. A. Knaus, "Predicting Patient Outcome from Intensive Care: A Guide to APACHE, MPM, SAPS, PRISM, and Other Prognostic Scoring Systems," *Journal of Intensive Care Medicine* 5 (1990): 33–52; J. E. Zimmerman, D. P. Wagner, E. A. Draper, and W. A. Knaus, "Improving Intensive Care Unit Discharge Decisions: Supplementing Physician Judgment with Predictions of Next Day Risk of Life Support," *Critical Care Medicine* 22 (1994): 1371–84; A. Laupacis, G. Wells, W. S. Richardson, and P. Tuswell, "User's Guide to the Medical Literature V: How to Use an Article about Prognosis," *Journal of the American Medical Association* 272 (1994): 234–37; and J. H. Wasson, H. C. Sox, R. K. Neff, and L. Goldman, "Clinical Prediction Rules: Applications and Methodologic Standards," *New England Journal of Medicine* 313 (1985): 793–99. In evaluating published prognostic studies, physicians should at a minimum direct attention to the representativeness of the sample, the length of follow-up, the relevance of the outcomes examined, the objectiveness of the outcomes studied, the appropriateness of adjustment for other important prognostic factors such as comorbid conditions or psychosocial factors, and how well the predictions perform in independent samples of patients.

36. N. A. Christakis and E. B. Lamont, "The Extent and Determinants of Error in Physicians' Prognoses for Terminally Ill Patients," unpublished manuscript. See also R. M. Poses, C. Bekes, F. J. Copare, and W. E. Scott, "The Answer to 'What Are My Chances, Doctor?' Depends on Whom Is Asked: Prognostic Disagreement and Inaccuracy for Critically Ill Patients," *Critical Care Medicine* 17 (1989): 827–33.

37. N. A. Christakis, "Optimal Ways of Predicting Mortality as Assessed by Comparison to the Gold Standard of Observed Mortality," unpublished manuscript. In other words, physicians are more accurate if they predict that a patient has "a 50 percent chance of living three months" than if they predict "the patient will live about three months."

38. See, for example, R. M. Poses, C. Bekes, R. L. Winkler, et al., "Are Two (Inexperienced) Heads Better than One (Experienced) Head?" *Archives of Internal Medicine* 150 (1990): 1874–78.

39. Knaus, Harrell, Lynn, et al., "SUPPORT Prognostic Model." See also Watts and Knaus, "Case for Using Objective Scoring Systems."

40. See, for example, R. Buckman, *How to Break Bad News: A Guide for Health Care Professionals* (Baltimore: Johns Hopkins University Press, 1992). Additional resources are discussed in chapter 5.

41. A. R. Feinstein, "An Additional Basic Science for Clinical Medicine I: The Constraining Fundamental Paradigms," *Annals of Internal Medicine* 99 (1983): 393–97, 394.

42. One description of the content and form of the most widespread licensing exam—the Federated Licensing Examination Program (FLEX)—is replete with mentions of how students will be evaluated with respect to "diagnosis and management" but ignores prognosis; see A. LaDuca, D. D. Taylor, and I. K. Hill, "The Design of a New Physician Licensure Examination," *Evaluation and the Health Professions* 7 (1984): 115–40.

43. J. H. Glick, B. A. Chabner, and J. A. Benson Jr., "Evaluation of Clinical Competence in Medical Oncology Training Programs," *Journal of Clinical Oncology* 6 (1988): 1516–19, 1517.

44. There may eventually be tables specifying percentage risks, with confidence intervals, for numerous conditions, given particular combinations of genes and family history: "Oh, you are a fifty-year-old woman with this gene and this family history? Then your risk of developing breast cancer in the next ten years is between 25 and 35 percent."

45. H. G. Welch and W. Burke, "Uncertainties in Genetic Testing for Chronic Disease," *Journal of the American Medical Association* 280 (1998): 1525–27.

46. J. A. Billings and J. D. Stoeckle, *The Clinical Encounter: A Guide to the Medical Interview and Case Presentation* (Chicago: Year Book Medical Publishers, 1989). Regarding the notion of a patient's "story" more broadly and metaphysically, see A. W. Frank, *The Wounded Storyteller: Body, Illness, and Ethics* (Chicago: University of Chicago Press, 1995).

47. With respect to different ways of communicating mathematically equivalent quantitative information, see, out of a large literature on this topic, N. D. Weinstein, K. Kolb, and B. D. Goldstein, "Using Time Intervals between

Expected Events to Communicate Risk Magnitudes," *Risk Analysis* 16 (1996): 305–8, and J. F. Steiner, "Talking about Treatment: The Language of Populations and the Language of Individuals," *Annals of Internal Medicine* 130 (1999): 618–21.

Appendix One

1. N. A. Christakis and T. J. Iwashyna, "Attitude and Self-Reported Practice Regarding Prognostication in a National Sample of Internists," *Archives of Internal Medicine* 158 (1998): 2389–95.

2. American Medical Association, Department of Data Services, *Physicians' Characteristics and Distribution in the U.S.* (Chicago: American Medical Association, 1994).

3. D. A. Asch, M. K. Jedrziewski, and N. A. Christakis, "Response Rates to Mail Surveys Published in Medical Journals," *Journal of Clinical Epidemiology* 50 (1997): 1129–36.

4. L. A. Aday, *Designing and Conducting Health Surveys* (San Francisco: Jossey-Bass, 1989).

5. E. S. Tambor, G. A. Chase, and R. R. Faden, "Improving Response Rates through Incentive and Follow-up: The Effect on a Survey of Physicians' Knowledge of Genetics," *American Journal of Public Health* 83 (1993): 1599–1603.

6. For additional discussion of this point, see Tambor, Chase, and Faden, "Improving Response Rates," and K. Sheikh and S. Mattingly, "Investigating Non-response Bias in Mail Surveys," *Journal of Epidemiology and Community Health* 35 (1981): 293–96.

7. An early version of the interview schedule is available in N. A. Christakis, *Prognostication and Death in Medical Thought and Practice* (Ann Arbor, Mich.: University Microfilms, 1995).

8. N. A. Christakis, "The Ellipsis of Prognosis in Modern Medical Thought," *Social Science and Medicine* 44 (1997): 301–15.

9. Christakis, *Prognostication and Death.*

10. For a recent analysis of the coverage in four widely used contemporary textbooks on end-of-life care more generally, see A. T. Carron, J. Lynn, and P. Keaney, "End-of-Life Care in Medical Textbooks," *Annals of Internal Medicine* 130 (1999): 82–86. This paper also examines the prognostic aspects of end-of-life care and finds that the textbooks do indeed provide some prognostic information for most of the twelve diseases considered. But, the authors note, "the threshold for each designation was low" and "text that contained any statement about clinical signs that helped to anticipate death would receive [the maximum rating]" (p. 83).

11. J. A. Tulsky, G. S. Fischer, M. R. Rose, and R. M. Arnold, "Opening the Black Box: How Do Physicians Communicate about Advance Directives?" *Annals of Internal Medicine* 129 (1998): 441–49.

12. Regarding the original data set and its acquisition, see W. Levinson, D. L. Roter, J. P. Mullooly, et al., "Physician-Patient Communication: The Relationship with Malpractice Claims among Primary Care Physicians and Surgeons," *Journal of the American Medical Association* 277 (1997): 553–59; and W. Levinson, V. T. Dull,

D. L. Roter, et al., "Recruiting Physicians for Office-Based Research," *Medical Care* 36 (1998): 934–37.

13. N. A. Christakis and W. Levinson, "Casual Optimism: Prognostication in Routine Medical and Surgical Practice," unpublished manuscript.

Appendix Two

1. For details regarding the workings of this method see P. H. Rossi, "Vignette Analysis: Uncovering the Normative Structure of Complex Judgments," in R. K. Merton, J. S. Coleman, and P. H. Rossi, eds., *Qualitative and Quantitative Social Research: Papers in Honor of Paul F. Lazarsfeld* (New York: Free Press, 1979); P. H. Rossi and A. B. Anderson, "The Factorial Survey Approach: An Introduction," in P. H. Rossi and S. L. Nock, eds., *Measuring Social Judgments: The Factorial Survey Approach* (Beverly Hills, Calif.: Sage, 1982). For other illustrations of this method, see N. A. Christakis and D. A. Asch, "Biases in How Physicians Choose to Withdraw Life Support," *Lancet* 324 (1993): 642–46, and J. A. Kelly, J. S. St. Lawrence, S. Smith Jr., et al., "Stigmatization of AIDS Patients by Physicians," *American Journal of Public Health* 77 (1987): 789–91.

2. The magnitude of the possible error in this experiment (twenty-four months versus two months) substantially exceeded the error generally seen in the studies reviewed in chapter 3, though such errors do occur. That is, the extent of the possible prognostic error was particularly pronounced here. However, the plausibility of the two survival outcomes was evaluated as part of the survey, using question 1 in each of the vignettes (figs. A2.1, A2.2). The proportion of physicians who felt that the two outcomes were "unusual" in this case was the same: comparing versions NU and NF of the vignette, 30.2 percent thought that the long survival was unusual, 33.0 percent that the short survival was unusual (p = n.s.).

3. Again, the clinical details were carefully chosen so that two different survival outcomes were plausible. As with the first vignette, this was evaluated formally. The results suggest that both outcomes are indeed plausible, though death was considered to be more likely. Comparing responses to versions NU and NF of the vignette, 29.0 percent of physicians thought death was unusual and 44.3 percent thought recovery was unusual; this difference was statistically significant (p = 0.03 by Fischer's exact test).

4. That is, they include answers of "4" or "5" on the Likert scale. Analyses that made use of all the information provided by the five-point scale were also performed, but in no case did such analyses contradict the simplified findings presented here.

5. The effect of accuracy *independent* of the choice to make a prediction in the first place is seen by comparing version FU with UU and version UF with FF.

6. A statistical test of the global hypothesis that articulating a favorable prediction (comparison of versions NF and FF) *and* that articulating an unfavorable prediction (comparison of versions NU and UU) increases confidence—that is, a test of the benefits of articulating predictions overall—supports the hypothesis that physicians believe that there is an association between patient confidence and articulating a prognosis (p < 0.05). The benefits of articulating a prognosis

accrue especially when the outcome is favorable (that is, the difference between NF and FF is significant whereas the difference between NU and UU is not).

7. The data also hint that physicians believe patients lose confidence in a physician in part because of the nature of the outcome, regardless of whether the physician predicted it accurately or not. In other words, physicians may believe that patients will inevitably judge them adversely if outcomes are unfavorable, at least in cases of acute illness. This impact of outcome, independent of prediction, may be seen, for example, by comparing versions NU and NF in figure A2.4, though this difference did not reach statistial significance at the customary level of $p < 0.05$.

8. These patterns of responses, wherein an unduly unfavorable prediction is deemed more of a threat to patient and colleague confidence, are one way that the ritualization of optimism (discussed in chapter 7) and the avoidance or prognostication (discussed in chapter 4) are sustained: namely, through both colleague and patient approval and disapproval. This behavior is also consistent with a belief in the negative self-fulfilling prophecy (discussed in chapter 6).

9. See chapter 7 for discussion of some of the reasons militating towards pessimism.

10. Specifically, a test of the global hypothesis that the proportion in NU differs from the proportion in UU *and* that the proportion in NF differs from the proportion in FF supports the hypothesis that physicians believe there is an association between the prediction and the outcome ($p < 0.001$).

11. The observation that physicians believe in the ability of a prediction to bring about a corresponding outcome is secondarily supported by a comparison of version UU with UF and version FF with FU. Comparing UU with UF reveals that physicians are much more likely to believe that making an unfavorable prediction will cause an unfavorable outcome than that it will cause a favorable outcome (which is logically the only alternative). Similarly, comparing FF with FU reveals that physicians are much more likely to believe that making a favorable prediction will cause a favorable outcome than that it will cause an unfavorable outcome.

12. The difference was more pronounced when the entire five-point range of the Likert response scale was used.

13. Again, the observation that physicians believe in the ability of a prediction to bring about a corresponding outcome is further supported by a comparison of version UU with UF and version FF with FU. Comparing UU with UF reveals that physicians are much more likely to believe that making an unfavorable prediction will cause an unfavorable outcome than that it will cause a favorable outcome. Similarly, comparing FF with FU reveals that physicians are much more likely to believe that making a favorable prediction will cause a favorable outcome than that it will cause an unfavorable outcome.

14. The difference was more pronounced when the entire five-point range of the Likert response scale was used.

15. N. A. Christakis, *Prognostication and Death in Medical Thought and Practice* (Ann Arbor, Mich.: University Microfilms, 1995).

16. Permitted answers ranged along a five-point Likert-type scale. Analyses making use of all the information provided by a five-point scale did not con-

tradict the findings presented here, based on a simplified scale of "optimism," "pessimism," or "neither."

17. I am assuming that the prognoses physicians share with colleagues approximate their best belief about patients' true prospects more closely than the prognoses they share with patients. Indeed, interview and observational data suggest that there is little or no difference between their true belief and the belief they share with colleagues.

18. The findings are very similar in the other situations, where patients expressed various levels of optimism or pessimism about their prognosis.

Bibliography

Aday, L. A. *Designing and Conducting Health Surveys.* San Francisco: Jossey-Bass, 1989.

Addington-Hall, J. M., L. D. MacDonald, and H. R. Anderson. "Can the Spitzer Quality of Life Index Help to Reduce Prognostic Uncertainty in Terminal Care?" *British Journal of Cancer* 62 (1990): 695–99.

Addington-Hall, J. M., L. D. MacDonald, H. R. Anderson, J. Chamberlain, P. Freeling, J. M. Bland, and J. Raftery. "Randomised Controlled Trial of Effects of Coordinating Care for Terminally Ill Cancer Patients." *British Medical Journal* 305 (1992): 1317–22.

Almada, S. J., A. B. Zonderman, R. B. Shekelle, A. R. Dyer, M. L. Daviglus, P. T. Costa, and J. Stamler. "Neuroticism and Cynicism and Risk of Death in Middle-Aged Men: The Western Electric Study." *Psychosomatic Medicine* 53 (1991): 165–75.

American Medical Association, Department of Data Services. *Physicians' Characteristics and Distribution in the U.S.* Chicago: American Medical Association, 1994.

Amir, M. "Considerations Guiding Physicians When Informing Cancer Patients." *Social Science and Medicine* 24 (1987): 741–48.

Anda, R., D. Williamson, D. Jones, C. Macera, E. Eaker, A. Glassman, and J. Marks. "Depressed Affect, Hopelessness, and the Risk of Ischemic Heart Disease in a Cohort of U.S. Adults." *Epidemiology* 4 (1993): 285–94.

Anderson, P. *All of Us: Americans Talk about the Meaning of Death.* New York: Delacorte Press, 1996.

Andrews, L. B., C. Stocking, T. Krizek, L. Gottlieb, C. Krizek, T. Vargish, and M. Siegler. "An Alternative Strategy for Studying Adverse Events in Medical Care." *Lancet* 349 (1997): 309–13.

Annas, G. J. "Death by Prescription: The Oregon Initiative." *New England Journal of Medicine* 331 (1994): 1240–43.

———. "Informed Consent, Cancer, and Truth in Prognosis." *New England Journal of Medicine* 330 (1994): 223–25.

Anspach, R. R. *Deciding Who Lives: Fateful Choices in the Intensive-Care Nursery.* Berkeley: University of California Press, 1993.

———. "Prognostic Conflict in Life-and-Death Decisions: The Organization as an Ecology of Knowledge." *Journal of Health and Social Behavior* 28 (1987): 215–31.

Antonak, R. F. "Prediction of Attitudes toward Disabled Persons: A Multivariate Analysis." *Journal of General Psychology* 104 (1981): 119–23.

Aries, P. *The Hour of Our Death.* New York: Alfred A. Knopf, 1981.

Aristotle. *Metaphysics.* Translated by H. G. Apostle. Bloomington: Indiana University Press, 1966.

Arkes, H. R., N. V. Dawson, T. Speroff, F. E. Harrell Jr., C. Alzola, R. Phillips, N. Desbiens, R. Oye, W. Knaus, and A. F. Connors Jr. "The Covariance Decomposition of the Probability Score and Its Use in Evaluating Prognostic Estimates." *Medical Decision Making* 15 (1995): 120–31.

Asch, D. A., and N. A. Christakis. "Why Do Physicians Prefer to Withdraw Some Forms of Life Support over Others? Intrinsic Attributes of Life Sustaining Treatments Are Associated with Physicians' Preferences." *Medical Care* 34 (1996): 103–11.

Asch, D. A., K. Faber-Langendoen, J. A. Shea, and N. A. Christakis. "The Sequence of Withdrawing Life-Sustaining Treatments from Patients in Four U.S. Hospitals." *American Journal of Medicine,* in press.

Asch, D. A., M. K. Jedrziewski, and N. A. Christakis. "Response Rates to Mail Surveys Published in Medical Journals." *Journal of Clinical Epidemiology* 50 (1997): 1129–36.

Asch, D. A., J. P. Patton, and J. C. Hershey. "Knowing for the Sake of Knowing: The Value of Prognostic Information." *Medical Decision Making* 10 (1990): 47–57.

Babul, R., S. Adam, B. Kremer, S. Dufrasne, S. Wiggins, M. Huggins, J. Theilmann, M. Bloch, and M. R. Hayden. "Attitudes toward Direct Predictive Testing for the Huntington Disease Gene: Relevance for Other Adult-Onset Disorders." *Journal of the American Medical Association* 270 (1993): 2321–25.

Beresford, E. B. "Uncertainty and the Shaping of Medical Decisions." *Hastings Center Report* 21 (1991): 6–11.

Beresford, L. *The Hospice Handbook: A Complete Guide.* Boston: Little Brown & Co., 1993.

Berger, J., and J. Mohr. *A Fortunate Man: The Story of a Country Doctor.* New York: Pantheon, 1967.

Berkman, L. F. "The Role of Social Relations in Health Promotion." *Psychosomatic Medicine* 57 (1995): 245–54.

Berkman, L. F., L. Leo-Summers, and R. Horwitz. "Emotional Support and Survival after Myocardial Infarction: A Prospective, Population-Based Study of the Elderly." *Annals of Internal Medicine* 117 (1992): 1003–9.

Bigelow, J. *Brief Expositions of Rational Medicine, to Which Is Prefixed the Paradise of Doctors . . .* Boston: Phillips, Sampson & Co., 1858.

Billings, J. A. "Sharing Bad News." In *Outpatient Management of Advanced Cancer.* Philadelphia: Lippincott, 1985.

Billings, J. A., and J. D. Stoeckle. *The Clinical Encounter: A Guide to the Medical Interview and Case Presentation.* Chicago: Year Book Medical Publishers, 1989.

Blackhall, L. J., S. T. Murphy, G. Frank, V. Michel, and S. Azen. "Ethnicity and Attitudes toward Patient Autonomy." *Journal of the American Medical Association* 274 (1995): 820–25.

Blanchard, C. G., M. S. Labrecque, J. C. Ruckdeschel, and E. B. Blanchard. "Information and Decision-Making Preferences of Hospitalized Adult Cancer Patients." *Social Science and Medicine* 27 (1988): 1139–45.

Bosk, C. L. *"All God's Mistakes": Genetic Counseling in a Pediatric Hospital.* Chicago: University of Chicago Press, 1992.

————. *Forgive and Remember: Managing Medical Failure.* Chicago: University of Chicago Press, 1979.

————. "Occupational Rituals in Patient Management." *New England Journal of Medicine* 303 (1980): 71–76.

Boudon, R., and F. Bourricaud. "Social Symbolism." In *A Critical Dictionary of Sociology,* edited by R. Boudon and F. Bourricaud, 346–55. Chicago: University of Chicago Press, 1989.

Boyer, P. *When Time Shall Be No More: Prophecy Belief in Modern American Culture.* Cambridge: Harvard University Press, 1992.

Breitner, J. C. S. "Clinical Genetics and Genetic Counseling in Alzheimer Disease." *Annals of Internal Medicine* 115 (1991): 601–6.

Brennan, T. A., L. L. Leape, N. M. Laird, L. Hebert, A. R. Localio, A. G. Lawthers, J. F. Newhouse, P. C. Weiler, and H. H. Hiatt. "Incidence of Adverse Events and Negligence and Hospitalized Patients: Results from the Harvard Medical Practice Study I." *New England Journal of Medicine* 324 (1991): 370–76.

Brewin, T. B. "Three Ways of Giving Bad News." *Lancet* 337 (1991): 1207–9.

Brody, D. S., S. M. Miller, C. E. Lerman, D. G. Smith, and G. C. Caputo. "Patient Perception of Involvement in Medical Care: Relationship to Illness Attitudes and Outcomes." *Journal of General Internal Medicine* 4 (1989): 506–11.

Brody, H., and J. Lynn. "The Physician's Responsibility under the New Medicare Reimbursement for Hospice Care." *New England Journal of Medicine* 310 (1984): 920–22.

Brody, H., and D. B. Waters. "Diagnosis Is Treatment." *Journal of Family Practice* 10 (1980): 445–49.

Bruera, E., M. J. Miller, N. Kuehn, T. MacEachern, and J. Hanson. "Estimate of Survival of Patients Admitted to a Palliative Care Unit: A Prospective Study." *Journal of Pain and Symptom Management* 7 (1992): 82–86.

Brunvand, J. H. *The Vanishing Hitchhiker: American Urban Legends and Their Meanings.* New York: W. W. Norton, 1981.

Buckman, R. *How to Break Bad News: A Guide for Health Care Professionals.* Baltimore: Johns Hopkins University Press, 1992.

Bulkin, W., and H. Lukashok. "Rx for Dying: The Case for Hospice." *New England Journal of Medicine* 318 (1988): 376–78.

Bushnell, R. W. *Prophesying Tragedy: Sign and Voice in Sophocles' Theban Plays.* Ithaca, N.Y.: Cornell University Press, 1988.

Byock, I. *Dying Well: The Prospect for Growth at the End of Life.* New York: Riverhead Books, 1997.

Cabot, R. C. "The Use of Truth and Falsehood in Medicine: An Experimental Study." *American Medicine,* 28 February 1903, 344–49.

Cain, M., and C. Janssen. "Bayesian Valuation with an Elicited Nonsymmetric Loss Function." In *Bayesian Analysis in Statistics and Econometrics,* edited by D. A. Berry, K. M. Chaloner, and J. K. Geweke, 165–78. New York: John Wiley & Sons, 1996.

Callahan, D. *The Troubled Dream of Life: In Search of a Peaceful Death.* New York: Simon & Schuster, 1993.

Cannon, W. B. "Voodoo Death." *American Anthropologist* 44 (1942): 169–81.

Carron, A. T., J. Lynn, and P. Keaney. "End-of-Life Care in Medical Textbooks." *Annals of Internal Medicine* 130 (1999): 82–86.

Carter, G. M., J. P. Newhouse, and D. A. Relles. "How Much Change in the Case Mix Index Is DRG Creep?" *Journal of Health Economics* 9 (1990): 411–28.

Casarett, D., and L. F. Ross. "Overriding a Patient's Refusal of Treatment after an Iatrogenic Complication." *New England Journal of Medicine* 336 (1997): 1908–10.

Case, R. B., A. J. Moss, N. Case, M. McDermott, and S. Eberly. "Living Alone after Myocardial Infarction: Impact on Prognosis." *Journal of the American Medical Association* 267 (1992): 515–19.

Cassell, J. *Expected Miracles: Surgeons at Work.* Philadelphia: Temple University Press, 1991.

Center for Evaluative Clinical Sciences, Dartmouth Medical School. *The Dartmouth Atlas of Health Care, 1998.* Edited by J. E. Wennberg, M. M. Cooper, and Dartmouth Atlas of Health Care Working Group. Chicago: American Hospital Publishing, 1998.

Chan, A., and R. K. Woodruff. "Communicating with Patients with Advanced Cancer." *Journal of Palliative Care* 13 (1997): 29–33.

Charlson, M. E., F. L. Sax, R. MacKenzie, S. D. Fields, R. L. Braham, and R. G. Douglas Jr. "Assessing Illness Severity: Does Clinical Judgment Work?" *Journal of Chronic Disease* 39 (1986): 439–52.

Charmaz, K. *Good Days, Bad Days: The Self in Chronic Illness and Time.* New Brunswick, N.J.: Rutgers University Press, 1991.

Chevlen, E. "The Limits of Prognostication." *Duquesne Law Review* 35 (1996): 336–54.

Christakis, N. A. "Asymmetry in Bayesian Loss Functions in Physician Survival Estimates in a Novel Data Set." Unpublished manuscript.

———. "Discrepancy between Objective Estimates of Prognosis and Those Communicated to Terminally Ill Outpatients." Unpublished manuscript.

———. "The Ellipsis of Prognosis in Modern Medical Thought." *Social Science and Medicine* 44 (1997): 301–15.

———. "Ethics Are Local: Engaging Cross-cultural Variation in the Ethics for Clinical Research." *Social Science and Medicine* 35 (1992): 1079–91.

———. "Managing Death: The Growing Acceptance of Euthanasia in Contemporary American Society." In *Must We Suffer Our Way to Death? Cultural and Theological Perspectives on Death by Choice,* edited by R. P. Hamel and E. R. DuBose, 15–44. Dallas: Southern Methodist University Press, 1996.

———. "Optimal Ways of Predicting Mortality as Assessed by Comparison to the Gold Standard of Observed Mortality." Unpublished manuscript.

———. "Predicting Patient Survival before and after Hospice Enrollment." *Hospice Journal* 13 (1998): 71–87.

———. *Prognostication and Death in Medical Thought and Practice.* Ann Arbor, Mich.: University Microfilms, 1995.

———. "The Similarity and Frequency of Proposals to Reform U.S. Medical Education: Constant Concerns." *Journal of the American Medical Association* 274 (1995): 706–11.

————. "A Simple Mathematical Model of Physicians' Hospice Referral Decisions." Unpublished manuscript.

Christakis, N. A., and D. A. Asch. "Biases in How Physicians Choose to Withdraw Life Support." *Lancet* 324 (1993): 642–46.

Christakis, N. A., and J. J. Escarce. "Survival of Medicare Patients after Enrollment in Hospice Programs." *New England Journal of Medicine* 335 (1996): 172–78.

Christakis, N. A., and T. J. Iwashyna. "Attitude and Self-Reported Practice Regarding Prognostication in a National Sample of Internists." *Archives of Internal Medicine* 158 (1998): 2389–95.

Christakis, N. A., and E. B. Lamont. "The Extent and Determinants of Error in Physicians' Prognoses for Terminally Ill Patients." Unpublished manuscript.

Christakis, N. A., and R. J. Levine. "Multinational Research." In *Encyclopedia of Bioethics,* edited by W. T. Reich, 1780–87. New York: Macmillan, 1995.

Christakis, N. A., and W. Levinson. "Casual Optimism: Prognostication in Routine Medical and Surgical Encounters." Unpublished manuscript.

Christakis, N. A., and G. A. Sachs. "The Role of Prognosis in Clinical Decision Making." *Journal of General Internal Medicine* 11 (1996): 422–25.

Christian, H., ed. *The Principles and Practice of Medicine.* 16th ed. New York: D. Appleton-Century, 1947.

Cleeland, C. S., R. Gonin, A. K. Hatfield, J. H. Edmonson, R. H. Blum, J. A. Stewart, and K. J. Pandya. "Pain and Its Treatment in Outpatients with Metastatic Cancer." *New England Journal of Medicine* 330 (1994): 592–96.

Cohen, B. J., and S. G. Pauker. "How Do Physicians Weigh Iatrogenic Complications?" *Journal of General Internal Medicine* 9 (1994): 20–23.

Cohen-Mansfield, J., J. A. Droge, and N. Billig. "Factors Influencing Hospital Patients' Preferences in the Utilization of Life-Sustaining Treatments." *Gerontologist* 32 (1992): 89–95.

Collingwood, R. G. "On the So-Called Idea of Causation." In *Freedom and Responsibility: Readings in Philosophy and Law,* edited by H. Morris, 303–13. Stanford: Stanford University Press, 1961.

Comaroff, J., and P. Maguire. "Ambiguity and the Search for Meaning: Childhood Leukemia in the Modern Clinical Context." *Social Science and Medicine* 15B (1981): 115–23.

Commission on Chronic Illness. *Chronic Illness in a Large City: The Baltimore Study.* Vol. 4. Cambridge: Harvard University Press, 1957.

Compassion in Dying v. Washington, 850 F. Supp. 1454 (W.D. Wash. 1994), Oregon Revised Statute 127,800–127,897 (Oregon Death with Dignity Act).

Connors, A. F., N. V. Dawson, T. Speroff, H. Arkes, W. A. Knaus, F. E. Harrell, J. Lynn, J. Teno, L. Goldman, R. Califf, W. Fulkerson, R. Oye, P. Bellamy, N. Desbiens, and the SUPPORT investigators. "Physicians' Confidence in Their Estimates of the Probability of Survival: Relationship to Accuracy." *Medical Decision Making* 12 (1992): 336.

Covinsky, K. E., L. Goldman, E. F. Cook, R. Oye, N. Desbiens, D. Reding, W. Fulkerson, A. F. Connors, J. Lynn, and R. S. Phillips. "The Impact of Serious Illness on Patients' Families." *Journal of the American Medical Association* 272 (1994): 1839–44.

Covinsky, K. E., C. S. Landefeld, J. Teno, A. F. Connors, N. Dawson, S. Youngner, N. Desbiens, J. Lynn, W. Fulkerson, D. Reding, R. Oye, and R. S. Phillips. "Is Economic Hardship on the Families of the Seriously Ill Associated with Patient and Surrogate Care Preferences?" *Archives of Internal Medicine* 156 (1996): 1737–41.

Cowen, J. S., and M. A. Kelley. "Errors and Bias in Using Predictive Scoring Systems." *Critical Care Clinics* 10 (1994): 53–72.

Crane, D. *The Sanctity of Social Life: Physicians' Treatment of Critically Ill Patients.* New Brunswick, N.J.: Transaction Press, 1975.

Curley, S. P., M. J. Young, and J. F. Yates. "Characterizing Physicians' Perceptions of Ambiguity." *Medical Decision Making* 9 (1989): 116–24.

Cutler, D. M. "The Incidence of Adverse Medical Outcomes under Prospective Payment." *Econometrica* 62 (1995): 29–50.

Danis, M., M. S. Gerrity, L. I. Southerland, and D. L. Patrick. "A Comparison of Patient, Family, and Physician Assessments of the Value of Medical Intensive Care." *Critical Care Medicine* 16 (1988): 594–600.

Davis, F. *Passage through Crisis: Polio Victims and Their Families.* New Brunswick, N.J.: Transaction Publishers, 1991.

———. "Uncertainty in Medical Prognosis, Clinical and Functional." In *Medical Men and Their Work,* edited by E. Freidson and J. Lorber, 239–48. Chicago: Aldine-Atherton, 1972.

Davis, F. A. "Medicare Hospice Benefit: Early Program Experience." *Health Care Financing Review* 9 (1988): 99–111.

Davison, B. J., L. F. Degner, and T. R. Morgan. "Information and Decision-Making Preferences of Men with Prostate Cancer." *Oncology Nursing Forum* 22 (1995): 1401–8.

Dawes, R. M., D. Faust, and P. E. Meehl. "Clinical versus Actuarial Judgment." *Science* 243 (1989): 1668–74.

Dawson, N. J. "Need Satisfaction in Terminal Care Settings." *Social Science and Medicine* 32 (1991): 83–87.

Dawson, N. V., T. Speroff, A. Connors, H. Arkes, W. A. Knaus, F. E. Harrell, J. Lynn, J. Teno, L. Goldman, R. Califf, W. Fulkerson, R. Ove, P. Bellamy, N. Desbiens, and the SUPPORT investigators. "Use of the Mean Probability Score: Comparison of the SUPPORT Prognostic Model with Physicians' Subjective Estimates of Survival." *Medical Decision Making* 12 (1992): 336.

Degner, L. F., L. J. Kristjanson, D. Bowman, J. A. Sloan, K. C. Carriere, J. O'Neil, B. Bilodeau, P. Watson, and B. Mueller. "Information Needs and Decisional Preferences in Women with Breast Cancer." *Journal of the American Medical Association* 277 (1997): 1485–92.

Derogatis, L. R., M. D. Abeloff, and N. Melisaratos. "Psychological Coping Mechanisms and Survival Time in Metastatic Breast Cancer." *Journal of the American Medical Association* 242 (1979): 1504–8.

Detsky, A. S., S. C. Stricker, A. G. Mulley, and G. E. Thibault. "Prognosis, Survival, and the Expenditure of Hospital Resources for Patients in an Intensive-Care Unit." *New England Journal of Medicine* 305 (1981): 667–72.

Diem, S. J., J. D. Lantos, and J. A. Tulsky. "Cardiopulmonary Resuscitation on

Television: Miracles and Misinformation." *New England Journal of Medicine* 334 (1996): 1578–82.

Dorner, S. "Adolescents with Spina Bifida: How They See Their Situation." *Archives of Disease in Childhood* 51 (1976): 439–44.

Douglas, M. *Purity and Danger: An Analysis of the Concepts of Pollution and Taboo.* London: Routledge, 1966.

Doyle, D. *Caring for a Dying Relative: A Guide for Families.* Oxford: Oxford University Press, 1994.

Drickamer, M. A., M. A. Lee, and L. Ganzini. "Practical Issues in Physician-Assisted Suicide." *Annals of Internal Medicine* 126 (1997): 146–51.

Dubos, R. *Man Adapting.* Enl. ed. New Haven: Yale University Press, 1965.

———. *Mirage of Health: Utopias, Progress, and Biological Change.* New Brunswick, N.J.: Rutgers University Press, 1959.

Durham, G., and J. Durham. "General Practitioners' Ability to Predict Outcome for Elderly Patients Admitted to Acute Medical Beds." *New Zealand Medical Journal* 103 (1990): 585–87.

Edelstein, L. "Hippocratic Prognosis." In *Ancient Medicine: Selected Papers by Ludwig Edelstein,* edited by O. Temkin and C. L. Temkin, 65–110. Baltimore: Johns Hopkins University Press, 1967.

Ehrenreich, B., and D. English. *For Her Own Good: 150 Years of the Experts' Advice to Women.* New York: Anchor Books, 1978.

Eisenberg, L. "Disease and Illness: Distinctions between Professional and Popular Ideas of Sickness." *Culture, Medicine, and Psychiatry* 1 (1977): 9–23.

Engel, G. L. "Sudden and Rapid Death during Psychological Stress: Folklore or Folk Wisdom?" *Annals of Internal Medicine* 74 (1971): 771–82.

Evans, C., and M. McCarthy. "Prognostic Uncertainty in Terminal Care: Can the Karnofsky Index Help?" *Lancet* 1 (1985): 1204–6.

Evans-Pritchard, E. E. *Witchcraft, Oracles, and Magic among the Azande.* Oxford: Clarendon Press, 1937.

Eveloff, S. "The Prisoner." *American Journal of Medicine* 93 (1992): 313–14.

Faden, R. L., and T. L. Beauchamp. *A History and Theory of Informed Consent.* New York: Oxford University Press, 1986.

Farrell, R. A., and V. L. Swigert. "Prior Offense Record as a Self-Fulfilling Prophecy." *Law and Society Review* 12 (1978): 437–53.

Farrington, D. P., and R. Tarling, eds. *Prediction in Criminology.* Albany: State University of New York Press, 1985.

Feifel, H., ed. *The Meaning of Death.* New York: McGraw-Hill, 1959.

Feinstein, A. R. "An Additional Basic Science for Clinical Medicine: I. The Constraining Fundamental Paradigms." *Annals of Internal Medicine* 99 (1983): 393–97.

———. "ICD, POR, and DRG: Unsolved Scientific Problems in the Nosology of Clinical Medicine." *Archives of Internal Medicine* 148 (1988): 2269–74.

Festinger, L., H. W. Riecken, and S. Schachter. *When Prophecy Fails: A Social and Psychological Study of a Modern Group That Predicted the Destruction of the World.* New York: Harper & Row, 1964.

Feudtner, C. *Bittersweet: The Transformation of Diabetes into a Chronic Illness in Twentieth-Century America.* Ann Arbor, Mich.: University Microfilms, 1995.

Filene, P. G. *In the Arms of Others: A Cultural History of the Right-to-Die in America.* Chicago: Ivan R. Dee, 1998.

Fletcher, S. W., R. H. Fletcher, and M. A. Greganti. "Clinical Research Trends in General Medical Journals, 1946–1976." In *Biomedical Innovation,* edited by E. B. Roberts, R. I. Levy, S. N. Finkelstein, J. Moskowitz, and E. J. Sondik, 284–300. Cambridge: MIT Press, 1981.

Ford, S., L. Fallowfield, and S. Lewis. "Doctor-Patient Interactions in Oncology." *Social Science and Medicine* 42 (1996): 1511–19.

Forster, L. E., and J. Lynn. "Predicting Life Span for Applicants to Inpatient Hospice." *Archives of Internal Medicine* 148 (1988): 2540–43.

Foucault, M. *The Birth of the Clinic: An Archaeology of Medical Perception.* New York: Vintage Books, 1975.

———. *Discipline and Punish: The Birth of the Prison.* New York: Vintage Books, 1979.

———. *The History of Sexuality.* Vol. 1. New York: Random House, 1978.

———. *Madness and Civilization: A History of Insanity in the Age of Reason.* New York: Random House, 1965.

Fox, R. C. "The Entry of U.S. Bioethics into the 1990's: A Sociological Analysis." In *A Matter of Principles? Ferment in U.S. Bioethics,* edited by E. R. Dubose, R. Hamel, and L. J. O'Connell, 21–71. Valley Forge, Pa.: Trinity Press International, 1994.

———. *Essays in Medical Sociology: Journeys into the Field.* 2d ed. New Brunswick, N.J.: Transaction Books, 1988. Esp. "Training for Uncertainty," 19–50; "The Autopsy: Its Place in the Attitude-Learning of Second-Year Medical Students," 51–77; "Is There a 'New' Medical Student?: A Comparative View of Medical Socialization in the 1950's and the 1970's," 78–101; "Advanced Medical Technology—Social and Ethical Implications," 413–61; "The Evolution of Medical Uncertainty," 533–71; and "The Human Condition of Health Professionals," 572–87.

———. "The Evolution of American Bioethics: A Sociological Perspective." In *Social Science Perspectives on Medical Ethics,* edited by G. Weisz, 201–17. Philadelphia: University of Pennsylvania Press, 1991.

———. *Experiment Perilous.* Boston: Free Press, 1959.

———. *The Sociology of Medicine.* Englewood Cliffs, N.J.: Prentice-Hall, 1989.

Fox, R. C., and J. P. Swazey. *The Courage to Fail: A Social View of Organ Transplants and Dialysis.* 2d rev. ed. Chicago: University of Chicago Press, 1978.

Frank, A. W. *The Wounded Storyteller: Body, Illness, and Ethics.* Chicago: University of Chicago Press, 1995.

Frank, J. D., and J. B. Frank. *Persuasion and Healing: A Comparative Study of Psychotherapy.* Baltimore: Johns Hopkins University Press, 1961.

Frankl, D., R. K. Oye, and P. E. Bellamy. "Attitudes of Hospitalized Patients toward Life Support: A Survey of 200 Medical Inpatients." *American Journal of Medicine* 86 (1989): 645–48.

Freedman, B. "Offering Truth: One Ethical Approach to the Uninformed Cancer Patient." *Archives of Internal Medicine* 153 (1993): 572–76.

Freidson, E. *Doctoring Together: A Study of Professional Social Control.* Chicago: University of Chicago Press, 1975.

————. *Profession of Medicine: A Study of the Sociology of Applied Knowledge.* Chicago: University of Chicago Press, 1970.

Freud, S. *The Interpretation of Dreams.* Translated by J. Strachey. New York: Avon Books, 1965.

Fries, J. F., and G. B. Ehrlich. *Prognosis: Contemporary Outcomes of Disease.* Bowie, Md.: Charles Press, 1981.

Fye, W. B. "Active Euthanasia: An Historical Survey of Its Conceptual Origins and Introduction into Medical Thought." *Bulletin of the History of Medicine* 52 (1978): 492–502.

Geertz, C. "Religion as a Cultural System." In *The Interpretation of Cultures,* 87–125. New York: Basic Books, 1973.

Gerrity, M. S., R. F. DeVellis, and J. A. Earp. "Physicians' Reactions to Uncertainty in Patient Care: A New Measure and New Insights." *Medical Care* 28 (1990): 724–36.

Gilbert, S. "For Cancer Patients, Hope Can Add to Pain," *New York Times,* 9 June 1998, F7.

————. "Study Finds Doctors Refuse Patients' Requests on Death." *New York Times,* 22 November 1995, A1.

Gilchrist, J. M., ed. *Prognosis in Neurology.* Boston: Butterworth-Heinemann, 1998.

Girgis, A., and R. W. Sanson-Fisher. "Breaking Bad News: Consensus Guidelines for Medical Practitioners." *Journal of Clinical Oncology* 13 (1995): 2449–56.

Glaser, B. G., and A. L. Strauss. *Awareness of Dying.* Chicago: Aldine, 1965.

————. *Time for Dying.* Chicago: Aldine, 1968.

Gleason v. Guzman, 623 P.2d 378 (Colo. 1981).

Glick, J. H., B. A. Chabner, and J. A. Benson Jr. "Evaluation of Clinical Competence in Medical Oncology Training Programs." *Journal of Clinical Oncology* 6 (1988): 1516–19.

Good, M. "Cultural Studies of Biomedicine: An Agenda for Research." *Social Science and Medicine* 41 (1995): 461–73.

Good, M., B. J. Good, C. Schaffer, and S. E. Lind. "American Oncology and the Discourse on Hope." *Culture, Medicine, and Psychiatry* 14 (1990): 59–79.

Grann, V. R., K. S. Panageas, W. Whang, K. H. Antman, and A. I. Neugut. "Decision Analysis of Prophylactic Mastectomy and Oophorectomy in BRCA1-Positive or BRCA2-Positive Patients." *Journal of Clinical Oncology* 16 (1998): 979–85.

Greenfield, S., L. Sullivan, R. Silliman, K. Dukes, and S. Kaplan. "Principles and Practice of Case Mix Adjustment: Applications to End-Stage Renal Disease." *American Journal of Kidney Diseases* 24 (1994): 298–307.

Greer, D., V. Mor, J. Morris, S. Sherwood, D. Kidder, and H. Birnbaum. "An Alternative in Terminal Care: Results of the National Hospice Study." *Journal of Chronic Diseases* 39 (1986): 9–26.

Groopman, J. *The Measure of Our Days: New Beginnings at Life's End.* New York: Viking, 1997.

Guillemin, J. H., and L. L. Holmstrom. *Mixed Blessings: Intensive Care for Newborns.* New York: Oxford University Press, 1986.

Hack, T. F., L. F. Degner, and D. G. Dyck. "Relationship between Preferences for Decisional Control and Illness Information among Women with Breast Cancer: A Quantitative and Qualitative Analysis." *Social Science and Medicine* 39 (1994): 279–89.

Hafferty, F. W. *Into the Valley: Death and the Socialization of Medical Students.* New Haven: Yale University Press, 1991.

Hahn, R. A. "The Nocebo Phenomenon: Scope and Foundations." In *The Placebo Effect*, edited by A. Harrington, 56–76. Cambridge: Harvard University Press, 1997.

Hakim, R. B., J. M. Teno, F. E. Harrell Jr., W. A. Knaus, N. Wenger, R. S. Phillips, P. Layde, R. Califf, A. F. Connors Jr., and J. Lynn. "Factors Associated with Do-Not- Resuscitate Orders: Patients' Preferences, Prognoses, and Physicians' Judgments." *Annals of Internal Medicine* 125 (1996): 284–93.

Halm, E. A., M. J. Fine, T. J. Marrie, C. M. Coley, W. N. Kapoor, D. S. Obrosky, and D. E. Singer. "Time to Clinical Stability in Patients Hospitalized with Community-Acquired Pneumonia." *Journal of the American Medical Association* 279 (1998): 1452–57.

Hamel, M. B., L. Goldman, J. Teno, J. Lynn, R. B. Davis, F. E. Harrell Jr., A. F. Connors Jr., R. Califf, P. Kussin, P. Bellamy, H. Vidaillet, and R. S. Phillips. "Identification of Comatose Patients at High Risk for Death or Severe Disability." *Journal of the American Medical Association* 273 (1995): 1842–48.

Hanson, L. C., M. Danis, and J. Garrett. "What Is Wrong with End-of-Life Care? Opinions of Bereaved Family Members." *Journal of the American Geriatrics Society* 45 (1997): 1339–44.

Harrington, A., ed. *The Placebo Effect.* Cambridge: Harvard University Press, 1997.

Harvey, J. "Achieving the Indeterminate: Accomplishing Degrees of Certainty in Life and Death Situations." *Sociological Review* 44 (1996): 78–98.

Hastings Center. *Guidelines for the Termination of Life-Sustaining Treatment and the Care of the Dying.* Briarcliff Manor, N.Y.: Hastings Center, 1987.

Hayes-Bautista, D. E. "Modifying the Treatment: Patient Compliance, Patient Control, and Medical Care." *Social Science and Medicine* 10 (1976): 233–38.

Heath, A. C. "Genetic Influences on Drinking Behavior in Humans." In *The Genetics of Alcoholism*, edited by H. Begleiter and B. Kissin, 82–121. New York: Oxford University Press, 1995.

Hechinger, F. M. "They Tortured My Mother: Patronizing Doctors, Agonizing Care." *New York Times*, 24 January 1991, A22.

Henshel, R. L. "The Boundary of the Self-Fulfilling Prophecy and the Dilemma of Social Prediction." *British Journal of Sociology* 33 (1982): 511–28.

Heyse-Moore, L. H., and V. E. Johnson-Bell. "Can Doctors Accurately Predict the Life Expectancy of Patients with Terminal Cancer?" *Palliative Medicine* 1 (1987): 165–66.

Hippocrates. "Prognosis." In *Hippocratic Writings*, edited by G. E. R. Lloyd, translated by J. Chadwick and W. N. Mann, 170–85. New York: Penguin, 1978.

Hobcraft, J., J. Menken, and S. Preston. "Age, Period, and Cohort Effects in Demography: A Review." In *Cohort Analysis in Social Research*, edited by W. M. Mason and S. E. Fienberg, 89–136. New York: Springer-Verlag, 1985.

Hofmann, J. C., N. S. Wenger, R. B. Davis, J. Teno, A. F. Connors Jr., N. Desbiens, J. Lynn, and R. S. Phillips. "Patient Preferences for Communication with Physicians about End-of-Life Decisions." *Annals of Internal Medicine* 127 (1997): 1–12.

House, J. S., K. R. Landis, and D. Umberson. "Social Relationships and Health." *Science* 241 (1988): 540–45.

Hughes, E. C. "Dilemmas and Contradictions of Status." *American Journal of Sociology* 50 (1945): 353–59.

———. "The Making of a Physician: General Statement of Ideas and Problems." *Human Organization* 14 (1956): 21–25.

———. "Mistakes at Work." In *The Sociological Eye: Selected Papers on Work, Self, and the Study of Society,* edited by E. C. Hughes, 316–25. Chicago: Aldine-Atherton, 1971.

Humphry, D. *Final Exit: The Practicalities of Self-Deliverance and Assisted Suicide for the Dying.* Eugene, Oreg.: Hemlock Society, 1991.

Hutchison, R. "Prognosis." *Lancet* 226 (1934): 697–98.

Iezzoni, L. I. *Risk Adjustment for Measuring Health Outcomes.* Chicago: Health Administration Press, 1997.

Iezzoni, L. I., A. S. Ash, G. A. Coffman, and M. A. Moskowitz. "Predicting In-Hospital Mortality: A Comparison of Severity Measurement Approaches." *Medical Care* 30 (1992): 347–59.

Illich, I. *Medical Nemesis: The Expropriation of Health.* New York: Pantheon, 1976.

Imber, J. B. *Abortion and the Private Practice of Medicine.* New Haven: Yale University Press, 1986.

Janzen, J. M. *The Quest for Therapy: Medical Pluralism in Lower Zaire.* Berkeley: University of California Press, 1978.

Jarvis, G. K., and H. C. Northcott. "Religion and Differences in Morbidity and Mortality." *Social Science and Medicine* 25 (1987): 813–24.

Jecker, N. S., and L. J. Schneiderman. "Futility and Rationing." *American Journal of Medicine* 92 (1992): 189–96.

———. "Medical Futility: The Duty Not to Treat." *Cambridge Quarterly Healthcare Ethics* 2 (1993): 151–59.

Jencks, S. F., J. Daley, D. Draper, N. Thomas, G. Lenhart, and J. Walker. "Interpreting Hospital Mortality Data: The Role of Clinical Risk Adjustment." *Journal of the American Medical Association* 260 (1988): 3611–16.

Jewett, D. L., G. Fein, and M. H. Greenberg. "A Double-Blind Study of Symptom Provocation to Determine Food Sensitivity." *New England Journal of Medicine* 323 (1990): 429–33.

Jonas, H. *The Gnostic Religion: The Message of the Alien God and the Beginnings of Christianity.* 2d ed. Boston: Beacon Press, 1958.

Justice, A. C. *The Development, Validation, and Evaluation of Prognostic Systems: An Application to the Acquired Immunodeficiency Syndrome (AIDS).* Ann Arbor, Mich.: University Microfilms, 1996.

Justice, A. C., K. E. Covinsky, and J. A. Berlin. "Assessing the Generalizability of Prognostic Information." *Annals of Internal Medicine* 130 (1999): 515–24.

Kane, R. L., S. J. Klei, L. Bernstein, R. Rothenberg, and J. Wales. "Hospice Role

in Alleviating the Emotional Stress of Terminal Patients and Their Families."
Medical Care 23 (1985): 189–97.

Kane, R. L., J. Wales, L Bernstein, A. Leibowitz, and S. Kaplan. "A Randomised Trial of Hospice Care." *Lancet* 1 (1984): 890–94.

Kassirer, J. P. "Our Stubborn Quest for Diagnostic Certainty: A Cause of Excessive Testing." *New England Journal of Medicine* 320 (1989): 1489–91.

Katz, J. *The Silent World of Doctor and Patient.* New York: Free Press, 1984.

Kelly, J. A., J. S. St. Lawrence, S. Smith Jr., H. V. Hood, and D. J. Cook. "Stigmatization of AIDS Patients by Physicians." *American Journal of Public Health* 77 (1987): 789–91.

Kidder, D. "The Effects of Hospice Coverage on Medicare Expenditures." *Health Services Research* 27 (1992): 195–217.

King, A. S. "Self-Fulfilling Prophecies in Organizational Change." *Social Science Quarterly* 54 (1973): 384–93.

Kleinman, A. " 'Everything That Really Matters': Social Suffering, Subjectivity, and the Remaking of Human Experience in a Disordering World." *Harvard Theological Review* 90 (1997): 315–35.

——. *The Illness Narratives: Suffering, Healing, and the Human Condition.* New York: Basic Books, 1988.

——. *Patients and Healers in the Context of Culture: An Exploration of the Borderland between Anthropology, Medicine, and Psychiatry.* Berkeley: University of California Press, 1980.

——. *Writing at the Margin: Discourse between Anthropology and Medicine.* Berkeley: University of California Press, 1996.

Knaus, W. A., F. E. Harrell Jr., J. Lynn, L. Goldman, R. S. Phillips, A. F. Connors Jr., N. V. Dawson, W. J. Fulkerson Jr., R. M. Califf, N. Desbiens, P. Layde, R. K. Oye, P. E. Bellamy, R. B. Hakim, and D. P. Wagner. "The SUPPORT Prognostic Model: Objective Estimates of Survival for Seriously Ill Hospitalized Adults." *Annals of Internal Medicine* 122 (1995): 191–203.

Knaus, W. A., A. Rauss, A. Alperovitch, J. Le Gall, P. Loirat, E. Patois, S. E. Marcus, and the French Multicentric Group of ICU Research. "Do Objective Estimates of Chances for Survival Influence Decisions to Withhold or Withdraw Treatment." *Medical Decision Making* 10 (1990): 163–71.

Knaus, W. A., D. P. Wagner, and E. A. Draper. "The Value of Measuring Severity of Disease in Clinical Research on Acutely Ill Patients." *Journal of Chronic Disease* 37 (1984): 455–63.

Knaus, W. A., D. P. Wagner, and J. Lynn. "Short-Term Mortality Predictions for Critically Ill Hospitalized Adults: Science and Ethics." *Science* 254 (1991): 389–94.

Kong, D. F., K. L. Lee, F. E. Harrell, J. M. Boswick, D. B. Mark, M. A. Hlatky, R. M. Califf, and D. B. Pryor. "Clinical Experience and Predicting Survival in Coronary Disease." *Archives of Internal Medicine* 149 (1989): 1177–81.

Korenman, S., N. Goldman, and H. Fu. "Misclassification Bias in Estimates of Bereavement Effects." *American Journal of Epidemiology* 145 (1997): 995–1002.

Kosecoff, J., K. L. Kahn, W. H. Rogers, E. J. Reinisch, M. J. Sherwood, L. V. Rubenstein, D. Draper, C. P. Roth, C. Chew, and R. H. Brook. "Prospective Payment

System and Impairment at Discharge: The 'Quicker-and-Sicker' Story Revisited." *Journal of the American Medical Association* 264 (1990): 1980–83.

Kremer, B., P. Goldberg, S. E. Andrew, J. Theilmann, H. Telenius, J. Zeisler, F. Squitieri, B. Lin, A. Bassett, E. Almqvist, and T. D. Bird. "A Worldwide Study of the Huntington's Disease Mutation: The Sensitivity and Specificity of Measuring CAG Repeats." *New England Journal of Medicine* 330 (1994): 1401–6.

Krohne, H. W. "The Concept of Coping Modes: Relating Cognitive Person Variables to Actual Coping Behavior." *Advances in Behavior Research and Therapy* 11 (1989): 235–47.

Kruse, J. A., M. C. Thill-Baharozian, and R. W. Carlson. "Comparison of Clinical Assessment with APACHE II for Predicting Mortality Risk in Patients Admitted to a Medical Intensive Care Unit." *Journal of the American Medical Association* 260 (1988): 1739–42.

Kübler-Ross, E. *On Death and Dying.* New York: Macmillan, 1969.

Ladouceur, R., F. Talbot, and M. J. Dugas. "Behavioral Expressions of Intolerance of Uncertainty in Worry: Experimental Findings." *Behavior Modification* 21 (1997): 355–71.

LaDuca, A., D. D. Taylor, and I. K. Hill. "The Design of a New Physician Licensure Examination." *Evaluation and the Health Professions* 7 (1984): 115–40.

Lancman, M. E., J. J. Asconapé, W. J. Craven, G. Howard, and J. K. Penry. "Predictive Value of Induction of Psychogenic Seizures by Suggestion." *Annals of Neurology* 35 (1994): 359–61.

Larson, M. S. "Proletarianization and Educated Labor." *Theory and Society* 9 (1979): 131–75.

Lattanzi-Licht, M., J. J. Mahoney, and G. W. Miller. *The Hospice Movement: In Pursuit of a Peaceful Death.* New York: Fireside Press, 1998.

Laupacis, A., G. Wells, W. S. Richardson, and P. Tugwell. "Users' Guides to the Medical Literature V: How to Use an Article about Prognosis." *Journal of the American Medical Association* 272 (1994): 234–37.

Leape, L. L., T. A. Brennan, N. M. Laird, A. G. Lawthers, A. R. Localio, B. A. Barnes, L. Hebert, J. P. Newhouse, P. C. Weiler, and H. Hiatt. "The Nature of Adverse Events in Hospitalized Patients: Results from the Harvard Medical Practice Study II." *New England Journal of Medicine* 324 (1991): 377–84.

Lear, M. W. "Should Doctors Tell the Truth: The Case against Terminal Candor." *New York Times Magazine,* 24 January 1993, 17.

Lebovitz, R. M., and S. Albrecht. "Molecular Biology in the Diagnosis and Prognosis of Solid and Lymphoid Tumors." *Cancer Investigation* 10 (1992): 399–416.

Lee, K. L., D. B. Pryor, F. E. Harrell Jr., R. M. Califf, V. S. Behar, W. L. Floyd, J. J. Morris, R. A. Waugh, R. E. Whalen, and R. A. Rosati. "Predicting Outcome in Coronary Disease: Statistical Models Versus Expert Clinicians." *American Journal of Medicine* 80 (1986): 553–60.

Lee, M. A., H. D. Nelson, B. P. Tilden, L. Ganzini, T. A. Schmidt, and S. W. Tolle. "Legalizing Assisted Suicide—Views of Physicians in Oregon." *New England Journal of Medicine* 334 (1996): 310–15.

Leiderman, D. B., and J. A. Grisso. "The Gomer Phenomenon." *Journal of Health and Social Behavior* 26 (1985): 222–32.

Lerman, C., and R. T. Croyle. "Emotional and Behavioral Responses to Genetic Testing for Susceptibility to Cancer." *Oncology* 10 (1996): 191–95.

Lerner, M., and O. W. Anderson. *Health Progress in the United States: 1900–1960.* Chicago: University of Chicago Press, 1963.

Lester, D. "Voodoo Death: Some New Thoughts on an Old Phenomenon." *American Anthropologist* 74 (1972): 386–90.

Levin, B. W. "Decision Making about Care of Catastrophically Ill Newborns: The Use of Technological Criteria." In *New Approaches to Human Reproduction: Social and Ethical Dimensions,* edited by L. M. Whiteford and M. Poland, 84–97. Boulder, Colo.: Westview Press, 1989.

———. "International Perspectives on Treatment Choice in Neonatal Intensive Care Units." *Social Science and Medicine* 30 (1990): 901–12.

Levine, D. N. *The Flight from Ambiguity.* Chicago: University of Chicago Press, 1985.

Levine, R. J. *Ethics and Regulation of Clinical Research.* 2d ed. New Haven: Yale University Press, 1986.

Levinson, W., V. T. Dull, D. L. Roter, N. Chaumeton, and R. M. Frankel. "Recruiting Physicians for Office-Based Research." *Medical Care* 36 (1998): 934–37.

Levinson, W., D. L. Roter, J. P. Mullooly, V. T. Dull, and R. M. Frankel. "Physician-Patient Communication: The Relationship with Malpractice Claims among Primary Care Physicians and Surgeons." *Journal of the American Medical Association* 277 (1997): 553–59.

Lewis, G. "Fear of Sorcery and the Problem of Death by Suggestion." *Social Science and Medicine* 24 (1987): 997–1010.

Lidz, C. W., A. Meisel, E. Zerubavel, M. Carter, R. M. Sestak, and L. H. Roth. *Informed Consent: A Study of Decision Making in Psychiatry.* New York: Guilford Press, 1984.

Lief, H. I., and R. C. Fox. "The Medical Student's Training for 'Detached Concern.' " In *The Psychological Basis of Medical Practice,* edited by H. I. Lief, V. Lief, and N. R. Lief, 12–35. New York: Harper & Row, 1963.

Light, J. M., K. M. Irvine, and L. Kjerulf. "Estimating Genetic and Environmental Effects of Alcohol Use and Dependence from a National Survey: A 'Quasi-Adoption' Study." *Journal of Studies on Alcohol* 57 (1996): 507–20.

Lillard, L. A., and C. W. A. Panis. "Marital Status and Mortality: The Role of Health." *Demography* 33 (1996): 313–27.

Lillard, L. A., and L. J. Waite. " 'Til Death Do Us Part': Marital Disruption and Mortality." *American Journal of Sociology* 100 (1995): 1131–56.

Lind, S. E., M. Good, S. Seidel, T. Csordas, and B. J. Good. "Telling the Diagnosis of Cancer." *Journal of Clinical Oncology* 7 (1989): 583–89.

Lipkin, M., Jr., S. M. Putnam, and A. Lazare, eds. *The Medical Interview: Clinical Care, Education, and Research.* New York: Springer-Verlag, 1995.

Luparello, T. J., N. Leist, C. H. Lourie, and P. Sweet. "The Interaction of Psychologic Stimuli and Pharmacologic Agents on Airway Reactivity in Asthmatic Subjects." *Psychosomatic Medicine* 32 (1970): 509–13.

Luparello, T. J., H. A. Lyons, E. R. Bleecker, and E. R. McFadden Jr. "Influences of Suggestion on Airway Reactivity in Asthmatic Subjects." *Psychosomatic Medicine* 30 (1968): 819–25.

Lynn, J., F. E. Harrell Jr., F. Cohn, M. B. Hamel, N. Dawson, and A. W. Wu. "Defining the 'Terminally Ill': Insights from SUPPORT." *Duquesne Law Review* 35 (1996): 311–36.

Lynn, J., J. M. Teno, and F. E. Harrell. "Accurate Prognostication of Death: Opportunities and Challenges for Clinicians." *Western Journal of Medicine* 163 (1995): 250–57.

Lynn, J., J. M. Teno, R. S. Phillips, A. W. Wu, N. Desbiens, J. Harrold, M. T. Claessens, N. Wenger, B. Kreling, and A. F. Connors Jr. "Perceptions by Family Members of the Dying Experience of Older and Seriously Ill Patients." *Annals of Internal Medicine* 126 (1997): 97–106.

Mace, N. L., and P. V. Rabins. *The 36-Hour Day: A Family Guide to Caring for Persons with Alzheimer's Disease, Related Dementing Illnesses, and Memory Loss in Later Life.* Rev. ed. Baltimore: Johns Hopkins University Press, 1991.

Mackillop, W. J., and C. F. Quirt. "Measuring the Accuracy of Prognostic Judgments in Oncology." *Journal of Clinical Epidemiology* 50 (1997): 21–29.

Mackillop, W. J., W. E. Stewart, A. D. Ginsburg, and S. S. Stewart. "Cancer Patients' Perceptions of Their Disease and Its Treatment." *British Journal of Cancer* 58 (1988): 355–58.

Malinowski, B. *Magic, Science and Religion.* Boston: Beacon Press, 1948.

Maltoni, M., O. Nanni, S. Derni, M. P. Innocenti, L. Fabbri, N. Riva, R. Maltoni, and D. Amadori. "Clinical Prediction of Survival Is More Accurate than the Karnofsy Performance Status in Estimating Life Span of Terminally Ill Cancer Patients." *European Journal of Cancer* 30A (1994): 764–66.

Mannheim, K. *Ideology and Utopia.* London: Routledge & Kegan Paul, 1936.

Martin, E. *Flexible Bodies: The Role of Immunity in American Culture from the Days of Polio to the Age of AIDS.* Boston: Beacon Press, 1994.

Mason, W. M., and S. E. Fienberg, eds. *Cohort Analysis in Social Research.* New York: Springer-Verlag, 1985.

Matthews, D. A., and C. Clark. *The Faith Factor: Proof of the Healing Power of Prayer.* New York: Viking, 1998.

Mauksch, H. O. "The Organizational Context of Dying." In *Death: The Final Stage of Growth,* edited by E. Kübler-Ross, 5–24. Englewood Cliffs, N.J.: Prentice-Hall, 1975.

Mauss, M. *A General Theory of Magic.* Translated by R. Brain. New York: Norton, 1972.

Maynard, D. W. "On 'Realization' in Everyday Life: The Forecasting of Bad News as a Social Relation." *American Sociological Review* 61 (1996): 109–31.

McClish, D., and S. H. Powell. "How Well Can Physicians Estimate Mortality in a Medical Intensive Care Unit?" *Medical Decision Making* 9 (1989): 125–32.

McHugh, P., S. Lewis, S. Ford, E. Newlands, G. Rustin, C. Coombes, D. Smith, S. O'Reilly, and L. Fallowfield. "The Efficacy of Audiotapes in Promoting Psychological Well-Being in Cancer Patients: A Randomised, Controlled Trial." *British Journal of Cancer* 71 (1995): 388–92.

McIntosh, J. "Patients' Awareness and Desire for Information about Diagnosed but Undisclosed Malignant Disease." *Lancet* 2 (1976): 300–303.

McKenney, M. G., and J. M. Civetta. "Iatrogenesis." In *Critical Care*, edited by J. M. Civetta, R. W. Taylor, and R. R. Kirby. 3d ed. Philadelphia: Lippencott-Raven, 1997.

McMillan, A., R. M. Mentnech, J. Lubitz, A. M. McBean, and D. Russell. "Trends and Patterns in Place of Death for Medicare Enrollees." *Health Care Financing Review* 12 (1990): 1–7.

Meissen, G. J., C. A. Mastromauro, D. K. Kiely, D. S. McNamara, and R. H. Myers. "Understanding the Decision to Take the Predictive Test for Huntington Disease." *American Journal of Medical Genetics* 39 (1991): 404–10.

Meissen, G. J., R. H. Myers, C. A. Mastromauro, W. J. Koroshetz, K. W. Klinger, L. A. Farrer, P. A. Watkins, J. F. Gusella, E. D. Bird, and J. B. Martin. "Predictive Testing for Huntington's Disease with Use of a Linked DNA Marker." *New England Journal of Medicine* 318 (1988): 535–42.

Merton, R. K. "The Ambivalence of Physicians." In *Sociological Ambivalence and Other Essays*, edited by R. K. Merton, 65–72. New York: Free Press, 1976.

————. "The Self-Fulfilling Prophecy." In *Social Theory and Social Structure*, 475–90. New York: Free Press, 1968.

————. "The Thomas Theorem and the Matthew Effect." *Social Forces* 74 (1995): 379–422.

————. "The Unanticipated Consequences of Purposive Social Action." *American Sociological Review* 1 (1936): 894–904.

Merton, R. K., and E. Barber. "Sociological Ambivalence." In *Sociological Ambivalence and Other Essays*, edited by R. K. Merton, 3–31. New York: Free Press, 1976.

Merton, R. K., G. G. Reader, and P. L. Kendall, eds. *The Student-Physician: Introductory Studies in the Sociology of Medical Education*. Cambridge: Harvard University Press, 1957.

Metcalf, P. *A Borneo Journey into Death: Berawan Eschatology from Its Rituals*. Philadelphia: University of Pennsylvania Press, 1982.

Meyer, A. A., J. Messick, P. Young, C. C. Baker, S. Fakhry, F. Muakkassa, E. J. Rutherford, L. M. Napolitano, and R. Rutledge. "Prospective Comparison of Clinical Judgment and APACHE II Score in Predicting the Outcome in Critically Ill Surgical Patients." *Journal of Trauma* 32 (1992): 747–54.

Miles, S. H., R. Koepp, and E. P. Weber. "Advance End-of-Life Treatment Planning: A Research Review." *Archives of Internal Medicine* 156 (1996): 1062–68.

Miller, R. J. "Predicting Survival in the Advanced Cancer Patient." *Henry Ford Hospital Medical Journal* 39 (1991): 81–84.

Mills, C. W. "Situated Actions and Vocabularies of Motive." *American Sociological Review* 5 (1944): 904–13.

Miyaji, N. T. "The Power of Compassion: Truth-Telling among American Doctors in the Care of Dying Patients." *Social Science and Medicine* 36 (1993): 249–64.

Mizrahi, T. *Getting Rid of Patients: Contradictions in the Socialization of Physicians*. New Brunswick, N.J.: Rutgers University Press, 1986.

Moinpour, C. M., and L. Polissar. "Factors Affecting Place of Death of Hospice and Non-Hospice Cancer Patients." *American Journal of Public Health* 79 (1989): 1549–51.

Mor, V., D. S. Greer, and R. Kastenbaum. *The Hospice Experiment.* Baltimore: Johns Hopkins University Press, 1988.

Mor, V., and J. Hiris. "Determinants of Site of Death among Hospice Cancer Patients." *Journal of Health and Social Behavior* 24 (1983): 375–85.

Mor, V., and D. Kidder. "Cost Savings in Hospice: Final Result of the National Hospice Study." *Health Services Research* 20 (1985): 407–21.

Morris, J. N., S. Suissa, S. Sherwood, S. M. Wright, and D. Greer. "Last Days: A Study of the Quality of Life of Terminally Ill Cancer Patients." *Journal of Chronic Disease* 39 (1986): 47–62.

Mosconi, P., B. E. Meyerowitz, M. C. Liberati, and A. Liberati. "Disclosure of Breast Cancer Diagnosis: Patient and Physician Reports." *Annals of Oncology* 2 (1991): 273–80.

Muers, M. F., P. Shevlin, and J. Brown. "Prognosis in Lung Cancer: Physicians' Opinions Compared with Outcome and a Predictive Model." *Thorax* 51 (1996): 894–902.

Mullins, R. J., N. C. Mann, J. R. Hedges, W. Worrall, M. Helfand, A. D. Zechnich, and G. J. Jurkovich. "Adequacy of Hospital Discharge Status as a Measure of Outcome among Injured Patients." *Journal of the American Medical Association* 279 (1998): 1727–31.

Murphy, D. J., D. Burrows, S. Santilli, A. W. Kemp, S. Tenner, B. Kreling, and J. Teno. "The Influence of the Probability of Survival on Patients' Preferences Regarding Cardiopulmonary Resuscitation." *New England Journal of Medicine* 330 (1994): 545–49.

Murray, L. S., G. M. Teasdale, G. D. Murray, B. Jennett, J. D. Miller, J. D. Pickard, M. D. M. Shaw, J. Achilles, S. Bailey, P. Jones, D. Kelly, and J. Lacey. "Does Prediction of Outcome Alter Patient Management?" *Lancet* 341 (1993): 1487–91.

Mushlin, A. I., C. Mooney, V. Grow, and C. E. Phelps. "The Value of Diagnostic Information to Patients with Suspected Multiple Sclerosis." *Archives of Neurology* 51 (1994): 67–72.

National Hospice Organization. "1992 Stats Show Continued Growth in Programs and Patients." *NHO Newsline* 3 (1993): 1–2.

Nelson, D. V., L. C. Friedman, P. E. Baer, M. Lane, and F. E. Smith. "Attitudes to Cancer: Psychometric Properties of Fighting Spirit and Denial." *Journal of Behavioral Medicine* 12 (1989): 341–55.

Nietzsche, F. *The Birth of Tragedy.* New York: Doubleday Anchor Books, 1956.

Nuland, S. B. *How We Die: Reflections on Life's Final Chapter.* New York: Alfred A. Knopf, 1994.

O'Connor, P., A. S. Detsky, C. Tansey, W. Kucharczyk, and the Rochester-Toronto MRI Study Group. "Effect of Diagnostic Testing for Multiple Sclerosis on Patient Health Perceptions." *Archives of Neurology* 51 (1994): 46–51.

O'Hara, J. J. *Death and the Optimistic Prophecy in Vergil's Aeneid.* Princeton, N.J.: Princeton University Press, 1990.

Olsson, B., B. Olsson, and G. Tibblin. "Effect of Patients' Expectations on Recovery from Acute Tonsillitis." *Family Practice* 6 (1989): 188–92.

Osler, W. *The Principles and Practice of Medicine.* 1st ed. New York: D. Appleton Company, 1892.

Osler, W., and T. McCrae, eds. *The Principles and Practice of Medicine*. 9th ed. New York: D. Appleton Company, 1924.

Oxenham, D., and M. A. Cornbleet. "Accuracy of Prediction of Survival by Different Professional Groups in a Hospice." *Palliative Medicine* 12 (1998): 117–18.

Paradis, N. "Making a Living off the Dying." *New York Times*, 25 April 1992, 23.

Parkes, C. M. "Accuracy of Predictions of Survival in Later Stages of Cancer." *British Medical Journal* 2 (1972): 29–31.

Parsons, T. *The Social System*. New York: Free Press, 1951.

Pearlman, R. A. "Inaccurate Predictions of Life Expectancy: Dilemmas and Opportunities." *Archives of Internal Medicine* 148 (1988): 2537–38.

———. "Variability in Physician Estimates of Survival for Acute Respiratory Failure in Chronic Obstructive Pulmonary Disease." *Chest* 91 (1987): 515–21.

Perkins, H. S., A. R. Jonsen, and W. V. Epstein. "Providers as Predictors: Using Outcome Predictions in Intensive Care." *Critical Care Medicine* 14 (1986): 105–10.

Petersen, A., and R. Bunton, eds. *Foucault: Health and Medicine*. London: Routledge, 1997.

Peterson, C., and M. E. P. Seligman. "Explanatory Style and Illness." *Journal of Personality* 55 (1987): 237–65.

Pfefferbaum, B., P. M. Levenson, and J. van Eys. "Comparison of Physician and Patient Perceptions of Communications Issues." *Southern Medical Journal* 75 (1982): 1080–83.

Phillips, D. P., and D. G. Smith. "Postponement of Death until Symbolically Meaningful Occasions." *Journal of the American Medical Association* 263 (1990): 1947–51.

Placek, J. T., and T. L. Eberhardt. "Breaking Bad News: A Review of the Literature." *Journal of the American Medical Association* 276 (1996): 496–502.

Plomin, R., and J. C. DeFries. "The Genetics of Cognitive Abilities and Disabilities." *Scientific American* 278, no. 5 (1998): 62–69.

Polak, F. *The Image of the Future*. New York: Oceana Publications, 1961.

Polzer, K. "The Role of Risk Adjustment in National Health Reform." *Academic Medicine* 69 (1994): 445–51.

Pompei, P., M. E. Charlson, and R. G. Douglas Jr. "Clinical Assessments as Predictors of One Year Survival after Hospitalization: Implications for Prognostic Stratification." *Journal of Clinical Epidemiology* 41 (1988): 275–84.

Popper, K. *The Open Universe: An Argument for Indeterminism*. London: Routledge, 1982.

Poses, R. M., C. Bekes, F. J. Copare, and W. E. Scott. "The Answer to 'What Are My Chances, Doctor?' Depends on Whom Is Asked: Prognostic Disagreement and Inaccuracy for Critically Ill Patients." *Critical Care Medicine* 17 (1989): 827–33.

———. "What Difference Do Two Days Make? The Inertia of Physicians' Sequential Prognostic Judgments for Critically Ill Patients." *Medical Decision Making* 10 (1990): 6–14.

Poses, R. M., C. Bekes, R. L. Winkler, W. E. Scott, and F. J. Copare. "Are Two

(Inexperienced) Heads Better than One (Experienced) Head?" *Archives of Internal Medicine* 150 (1990): 1874–78.

Poses, R. M., D. McClish, C. Bekes, W. E. Scott, and J. N. Morley. "Ego Bias, Reverse Ego Bias, and Physicians' Prognostic Judgments for Critically Ill Patients." *Critical Care Medicine* 19 (1991): 1533–39.

Potter, J. F. "A Challenge for the Hospice Movement." *New England Journal of Medicine* 302 (1980): 53–55.

Prigerson, H. G. "Socialization to Dying: Social Determinants of Death Acknowledgment and Treatment among Terminally Ill Geriatric Patients." *Journal of Health and Social Behavior* 33 (1992): 378–95.

"Prophets and Prophecy." In *Encyclopedia Judaica* (New York: Macmillan, 1971), 13:1150–81.

Quaid, K. A., H. Dinwiddie, P. M. Conneally, and J. I. Nurnberger Jr. "Issues in Genetic Testing for Susceptibility to Alcoholism: Lessons from Alzheimer's Disease and Huntington's Disease." *Alcoholism, Clinical & Experimental Research* 20 (1996): 1430–37.

Quirt, C. F., W. J. Mackillop, A. D. Ginsburg, L. Sheldon, M. Brundage, P. Dixon, and L. Ginsburg. "Do Doctors Know When Their Patients Don't? A Survey of Doctor-Patient Communication in Lung Cancer." *Lung Cancer* 18 (1997): 1–20.

Radecki, S. E., J. G. Nyquist, J. D. Gates, S. Ahamson, and D. E. Henson. "Educational Characteristics of Tumor Conferences in Teaching and Non-Teaching Hospitals." *Journal of Cancer Education* 9 (1994): 204–16.

Raines v. State Compensation Commissioner, 108 S.E.2d 519, 144 (W.Va. 430, 1959).

Ravdin, P. M., I. A. Siminoff, and J. A. Harvey. "Survey of Breast Cancer Patients Concerning Their Knowledge and Expectations of Adjuvant Therapy." *Journal of Clinical Oncology* 16 (1998): 515–21.

Reiser, S. J. *Medicine and the Reign of Technology.* Cambridge: Cambridge University Press, 1978.

———. "Words as Scalpels: Transmitting Evidence in the Clinical Dialogue." *Annals of Internal Medicine* 92 (1980): 837–42.

Rhoden, N. K. "Treating Baby Doe: The Ethics of Uncertainty." *Hastings Center Report* 16 (1986): 34–42.

Rich, B. A. "Prospective Autonomy and Critical Interests: A Narrative Defense of the Moral Authority of Advance Directives." *Cambridge Quarterly of Healthcare Ethics* 6 (1997): 138–47.

Robert, S. A. "Community-Level Socioeconomic Status Effects on Adult Health." *Journal of Health and Social Behavior* 39 (1998): 18–37.

Rosenberg, C. E. "The Therapeutic Revolution: Medicine, Meaning and Social Change in 19th-Century America." In *Sickness and Health in America,* edited by J. W. Leavitt and R. L. Numbers, 39–52. Madison: University of Wisconsin Press, 1985.

Rossi, P. H. "Vignette Analysis: Uncovering the Normative Structure of Complex Judgments." In *Qualitative and Quantitative Social Research: Papers in Honor of Paul F. Lazarsfeld,* edited by R. K. Merton, J. S. Coleman, and P. H. Rossi. New York: Free Press, 1979.

Rossi, P. H., and A. B. Anderson. "The Factorial Survey Approach: An Introduction." In *Measuring Social Judgments: The Factorial Survey Approach*, edited by P. H. Rossi and S. L. Nock. Beverly Hills, Calif.: Sage, 1982.

Roter, D. L., and J. A. Hall. *Doctors Talking with Patients/Patients Talking with Doctors: Improving Communication in Medical Visits*. Westport, Conn.: Auburn House, 1992.

Rothman, B. K. *The Tentative Pregnancy: Prenatal Diagnosis and the Future of Motherhood*. New York: Penguin, 1986.

Rothman, D. J. *Strangers at the Bedside: A History of How Law and Bioethics Transformed Medical Decision Making*. New York: Basic Books, 1991.

Russell, L. B. *Educated Guesses: Making Policy about Medical Screening Tests*. Berkeley: University of California Press, 1994.

Ryan, C. M., D. A. Schoenfeld, W. P. Thorpe, R. L. Sheridan, E. H. Cassem, and R. G. Tompkins. "Objective Estimates of the Probability of Death from Burn Injuries." *New England Journal of Medicine* 338 (1998): 362–66.

Saffle, J. R. "Predicting Outcomes of Burns." *New England Journal of Medicine* 338 (1998): 387–88.

Sankar, A. *Dying at Home: A Family Guide for Caregiving*. Baltimore: Johns Hopkins University Press, 1991.

Schachter, S., and J. E. Singer. "Cognitive, Social, and Physiological Determinants of Emotional State." *Psychological Review* 69 (1962): 379–99.

Scheff, T. J. "Decision Rules, Types of Error, and Their Consequences in Medical Diagnosis." *Behavioral Science* 8 (1963): 97–107.

Scheier, M. F., and C. S. Carver. "Dispositional Optimism and Physical Well-Being: The Influence of Generalized Outcome Expectancies on Health." *Journal of Personality* 55 (1987): 169–210.

Schneider, E. C., and A. M. Epstein. "Use of Public Performance Reports: A Survey of Patients Undergoing Cardiac Surgery." *Journal of the American Medical Association* 279 (1998): 1638–42.

Schneiderman, L. J., and N. S. Jecker. "Futility in Practice." *Archives of Internal Medicine* 153 (1993): 437–41.

———. *Wrong Medicine: Doctors, Patients, and Futile Treatment*. Baltimore: Johns Hopkins University Press, 1995.

Schneiderman, L. J., N. S. Jecker, and A. R. Jonsen. "Medical Futility: Its Meaning and Ethical Implications." *Annals of Internal Medicine* 112 (1990): 949–54.

Schneiderman, L. J., R. Kronick, R. M. Kaplan, J. P. Anderson, and R. D. Langer. "Effects of Offering Advance Directives on Medical Treatments and Costs." *Annals of Internal Medicine* 117 (1992): 599–606.

Schoenfeld v. Buker, 114 N.W.2d 560, 262 (Minn. 122, 1962).

Schonwetter, R. S., R. M. Walker, D. R. Kramer, and B. E. Robinson. "Resuscitation Decision Making in the Elderly: The Value of Outcome Data." *Journal of General Internal Medicine* 8 (1993): 295–300.

Schrag, D., K. M. Kuntz, J. E. Garber, and J. C. Weeks. "Decision Analysis—Effects of Prophylactic Mastectomy and Oophorectomy on Life Expectancy among Women with BRCA1 or BRCA2 Mutations." *New England Journal of Medicine* 336 (1997): 1465–71.

Schweiger, A., and A. Parducci. "Nocebo: The Psychologic Induction of Pain." *Pavlovian Journal of Biological Science* 16 (1981): 140–43.

Scott, M. B., and S. M. Lyman. "Accounts." *American Sociological Review* 33 (1968): 46–62.

Seale, C. "Communication and Awareness about Death: A Study of a Random Sample of Dying People." *Social Science and Medicine* 32 (1991): 943–52.

Seale, C., and A. Cartwright. *The Year before Death.* Brookfield, Vt.: Ashgate Publishing, 1994.

Seckler, A. B., D. E. Meier, M. Mulvihill, and B. E. Paris. "Substituted Judgement: How Accurate Are Proxy Predictions?" *Annals of Internal Medicine* 115 (1991): 92–98.

Seeman, I. *National Mortality Followback Survey: 1986 Summary, United States.* National Center for Health Statistics, Vital and Health Statistics, 1992.

Seligman, M. E. *Helplessness: On Development, Depression, and Death.* New York: W. H. Freeman, 1975.

Seneff, M., and W. A. Knaus. "Predicting Patient Outcome from Intensive Care: A Guide to APACHE, MPM, SAPS, PRISM, and Other Prognostic Scoring Systems." *Journal of Intensive Care Medicine* 5 (1990): 33–52.

Shapiro, A. K. "Iatroplacebogenics." *International Pharmacopsychiatry* 2 (1969): 215–48.

Sheikh, K., and S. Mattingly. "Investigating Non-Response Bias in Mail Surveys." *Journal of Epidemiology and Community Health* 35 (1981): 293–96.

Sherden, W. A. *The Fortune Sellers: The Big Business of Buying and Selling Predictions.* New York: John Wiley & Sons, 1998.

Shweder, R. A., N. C. Much, M. Mahapatra, and L. Park. "The 'Big Three' of Morality (Autonomy, Community, Divinity) and the 'Big Three' Explanations of Suffering." In *Morality and Health,* edited by A. M. Brandt and P. Rozin, 119–69. New York: Routledge, 1997.

Siegler, M. "Pascal's Wager and the Hanging of Crepe." *New England Journal of Medicine* 293 (1975): 853–57.

Siegler, M., S. Amiel, and J. Lantos. "Scientific and Ethical Consequences of Disease Prediction." *Diabetologia* 35 (1992): S60–S68.

Siminoff, L. A., J. H. Fetting, and M. D. Abeloff. "Doctor-Patient Communication about Breast Cancer Adjuvant Therapy." *Journal of Clinical Oncology* 7 (1989): 1192–1200.

Smedira, N. G., B. H. Evans, L. S. Grais, N. H. Cohen, B. Lo, M. Cooke, W. P. Schecter, C. Fink, E. Epstein-Jaffe, C. May, and J. M. Luce. "Withholding and Withdrawal of Life Support from the Critically Ill." *New England Journal of Medicine* 322 (1990): 309–15.

Social Security Act 1861(dd)(3)(A).

Sontag, S. *Illness as Metaphor.* New York: Vintage Books, 1977.

Sox, H. C., M. A. Blatt, M. C. Higgins, and K. I. Marton. *Medical Decision Making.* Boston: Butterworth Heineman, 1988.

Starr, P. *The Social Transformation of American Medicine.* New York: Basic Books, 1982.

Stefanek, M. E. "Bilateral Prophylactic Mastectomy: Issues and Concerns." *Journal of the National Cancer Institute* 17 (1995): 37–42.

Steiner, J. F. "Talking about Treatment: The Language of Populations and the Language of Individuals." *Annals of Internal Medicine* 130 (1999): 618–21.

Steinhauser, K. A., E. C. Clipp, M. McNeilly, N. A. Christakis, L. M. McIntyre, and J. A. Tulsky. "In Search of a Good Death: Observations of Patients, Families and Providers." Unpublished manuscript.

Stern, S. "Managed Care, Brief Therapy, and Therapeutic Integrity." *Psychotherapy* 30 (1993): 162–75.

Sternbach, R. A. "The Effects of Instructional Sets on Autonomic Responsivity." *Psychophysiology* 1 (1964): 67–72.

Stevens, R. *In Sickness and in Wealth: American Hospitals in the Twentieth Century.* New York: Basic Books, 1989.

Stokey, E., and R. Zeckhauser. *A Primer for Policy Analysis.* New York: W. W. Norton, 1978.

Strahan, G. W. "An Overview of Home Health and Hospice Care Patients: Preliminary Data from the 1993 National Home and Hospice Care Survey." *Advance Data* 256 (1994): 1–11.

Sudnow, D. *Passing On: The Social Organization of Dying.* Englewood Cliffs, N.J.: Prentice-Hall, 1967.

SUPPORT principal investigators. "A Controlled Trial to Improve Care for Seriously Ill Hospitalized Patients: The Study to Understand Prognoses and Preferences for Outcomes and Risks of Treatments (SUPPORT)." *Journal of the American Medical Association* 274 (1995): 1591–98.

Surbone, A., and M. Zwitter, eds. *Communication with the Cancer Patient: Information and Truth. Annals of the New York Academy of Sciences,* vol. 809. New York: New York Academy of Sciences, 1997.

Svarstad, B. L., and H. Lipton. "Informing Parents about Mental Retardation: A Study of Professional Communication and Parent Acceptance." *Social Science and Medicine* 11 (1977): 645–51.

Tambor, E. S., G. A. Chase, and R. R. Faden. "Improving Response Rates through Incentive and Follow-Up: The Effect on a Survey of Physicians' Knowledge of Genetics." *American Journal of Public Health* 83 (1993): 1599–1603.

Taylor, C. A., and R. H. Myers. "Long-Term Impact of Huntington Disease Linkage Testing." *American Journal of Medical Genetics* 70 (1997): 365–70.

Teno, J. M., J. Lynn, R. S. Phillips, D. Murphy, S. J. Younger, P. Bellamy, A. F. Connors Jr., N. A. Desbiens, W. Fulkerson, and W. A. Knaus. "Do Formal Advance Directives Affect Resuscitation Decisions and the Use of Resources for Seriously Ill Patients?" *Journal of Clinical Ethics* 5 (1994): 23–30.

Teno, J. M., D. Murphy, J. Lynn, A. Tosteson, N. Desbiens, A. F. Connors Jr., M. B. Hamel, A. W. Wu, R. Phillips, N. Wenger, F. Harrell Jr., and W. A. Knaus. "Prognosis-Based Futility Guidelines: Does Anyone Win?" *Journal of the American Geriatrics Society* 42 (1994): 1202–7.

Thomas, K. *Religion and the Decline of Magic.* New York: Scribner's, 1971.

Thomas, W. I., and D. Thomas. *The Child in America: Behavior Problems and Programs.* New York: Alfred A. Knopf, 1928.

Tulsky, J. A., G. S. Fischer, M. R. Rose, and R. M. Arnold. "Opening the Black Box: How Do Physicians Communicate about Advance Directives." *Annals of Internal Medicine* 129 (1998): 441–49.

Turner, V. W. *The Forest of Symbols: Aspects of Ndembu Ritual.* Ithaca, N.Y.: Cornell University Press, 1967.

Uhlmann, R. F., R. A. Pearlman, and K. C. Cain. "Understanding of Elderly Patients' Resuscitation Preferences by Physicians and Nurses." *Western Journal of Medicine* 150 (1989): 705–7.

United Nations. "World Population Prospects: Estimates and Projections as Assessed in 1982." In *Population Studies*. New York: Department of International Economic and Social Affairs, 1985.

U.S. Bureau of the Census. *Historical Statistics of the United States (1900–1970)*. Washington, D.C.: Government Printing Office, 1975.

———. *Statistical Abstract of the United States, 1976*. Washington, D.C.: Government Printing Office, 1976.

U.S. Fidelity & Guaranty Company v. Wilson, 120 S.E. 2d 198, 103 (Ga. App. 674, 1961).

Unschuld, P. *Medical Ethics in Imperial China*. Berkeley: University of California Press, 1979.

Wagg, A., M. Kinirons, and K. Stewart. "Cardiopulmonary Resuscitation: Doctors and Nurses Expect Too Much." *Journal of the Royal College of Physicians of London* 29 (1995): 20–24.

Waitzkin, H. *The Politics of Medical Encounters: How Patients and Doctors Deal with Social Problems*. New Haven: Yale University Press, 1991.

Walczak, T. S., D. T. Williams, and W. Berten. "Utility and Reliability of Placebo Infusion in the Evaluation of Patients with Seizures." *Neurology* 44 (1994): 394–99.

Wallston, K. A., C. Burger, R. A. Smith, and R. J. Baugher. "Comparing the Quality of Death for Hospice and Non-Hospice Cancer Patients." *Medical Care* 26 (1988): 177–82.

Walter, T. *The Revival of Death*. London: Routledge, 1994.

Walters, V., and N. Charles. " 'I Just Cope from Day to Day': Unpredictability and Anxiety in the Lives of Women." *Social Science and Medicine* 45 (1997): 1729–39.

Wasson, J. H., H. C. Sox, R. K. Neff, and L. Goldman. "Clinical Prediction Rules: Applications and Methodological Standards." *New England Journal of Medicine* 313 (1985): 793–99.

Watts, C. M., and W. A. Knaus. "The Case for Using Objective Scoring Systems to Predict Intensive Care Unit Outcome." *Critical Care Clinics* 10 (1994): 73–89.

Webb, M. *The Good Death: The New American Search to Reshape the End of Life*. New York: Bantam Books, 1997.

Weber, M. *The Protestant Ethic and the Spirit of Capitalism*. London: Unwin Hyman, 1930.

———. *The Sociology of Religion*. Boston: Beacon Press, 1993.

Weeks, J. C., E. F. Cook, S. J. O'Day, L. M. Peterson, N. Wenger, D. Reding, F. E. Harrell Jr., P. Kussin, N. V. Dawson, A. F. Connors Jr., J. Lynn, and R. S. Phillips. "Relationship between Cancer Patients' Predictions of Prognosis and Their Treatment Preferences." *Journal of the American Medical Association* 279 (1998): 1709–14.

Weinstein, N. D. "Optimistic Biases about Personal Risks." *Science* 246 (1989): 1232–33.

Weinstein, N. D., K. Kolb, and B. D. Goldstein. "Using Time Intervals between

Expected Events to Communicate Risk Magnitudes." *Risk Analysis* 16 (1996): 305–8.

Weisman, A. D., and T. P. Hackett. "Predilection to Death: Death and Dying as a Psychiatric Problem." *Psychosomatic Medicine* 23 (1961): 232–56.

Weisz, G., ed. *Social Science Perspectives on Medical Ethics*. Philadelphia: University of Pennsylvania Press, 1990.

Welch, H. G., and W. Burke. "Uncertainties in Genetic Testing for Chronic Disease." *Journal of the American Medical Association* 280 (1998): 1525–27.

Wertz, D. C., and J. C. Fletcher. "Fatal Knowledge? Prenatal Diagnosis and Sex Selection." *Hastings Center Report* 19 (1989): 21–27.

White, P. D. "Principles and Practice of Prognosis, with Particular Reference to Heart Disease." *Journal of the American Medical Association* 153 (1953): 75–79.

Wiggins, S., P. Whyte, M. Huggins, S. Adam, J. Theilmann, M. Bloch, S. B. Sheps, M. T. Schechter, and M. R. Hayden. "The Psychological Consequences of Predictive Testing for Huntington's Disease." *New England Journal of Medicine* 327 (1992): 1401–5.

Wilkins, W. E. "The Concept of a Self-Fulfilling Prophecy." *Sociology of Education* 49 (1976): 175–83.

Williams, R. B., J. C. Barefoot, R. M. Califf, T. L. Haney, W. B. Saunders, D. B. Pryor, M. A. Hlatky, I. C. Siegler, and D. B. Mark. "Prognostic Importance of Social and Economic Resources among Medically Treated Patients with Angiographically Documented Coronary Artery Disease." *Journal of the American Medical Association* 267 (1992): 520–24.

Wilson, J. D., E. Braunwald, K. J. Isselbacher, R. G. Petersdorf, J. B. Martin, A. S. Fauci, and R. K. Root, eds. *Harrison's Principles of Internal Medicine*. 12th ed. New York: McGraw-Hill, 1991.

Wilson, W. C., N. G. Smedira, J. A. McDowell, and J. M. Luce. "Ordering and Administration of Sedatives and Analgesics during the Withholding and Withdrawal of Life Support from Critically Ill Patients." *Journal of the American Medical Association* 267 (1992): 949–53.

Wineburg, S. S., and L. S. Shulman. "The Self-Fulfilling Prophecy: Its Genesis and Development in American Education." In *Robert K. Merton: Consensus and Controversy*, edited by J. Clark, C. Modgil, and S. Modgil, 261–81. Bristol, Pa.: Falmer Press, Taylor & Francis, 1990.

Wu, A. W. "The Measure and Mismeasure of Hospital Quality: Appropriate Risk-Adjustment Methods in Comparing Hospitals." *Annals of Internal Medicine* 122 (1995): 149–50.

Wu, A. W., A. M. Damiano, J. Lynn, C. Alzola, J. Teno, C. S. Landefeld, N. Desbiens, J. Tsevat, A. Mayer-Oakes, F. E. Harrell Jr., and W. A. Knaus. "Predicting Future Functional Status for Seriously Ill Hospitalized Adults: The SUPPORT Prognostic Model." *Annals of Internal Medicine* 122 (1995): 342–50.

Wulfsberg, E. A., D. E. Hoffman, and M. M. Cohen. "Alpha-1 Antitrypsin Deficiency: Impact of Genetic Discovery on Medicine and Society." *Journal of the American Medical Association* 271 (1994): 217–22.

Zawacki, B. E., S. P. Azen, S. H. Imbus, and Y. T. Chang. "Multifactorial Probit Analysis of Mortality in Burned Patients." *Annals of Surgery* 189 (1979): 1–5.

Zborowski, M. "Cultural Components in Responses to Pain." *Journal of Social Issues* 8 (1952): 16–30.

Zellner, A. "Bayesian Estimation and Prediction Using Asymmetric Loss Functions." *Journal of the American Statistical Association* 81 (1986): 446–51.

Zimmerman, J. E., D. P. Wagner, E. A. Draper, and W. A. Knaus. "Improving Intensive Care Unit Discharge Decisions: Supplementing Physician Judgement with Predictions of Next Day Risk for Life Support." *Critical Care Medicine* 22 (1994): 1373–84.

Zussman, R. *Intensive Care: Medical Ethics and the Medical Profession.* Chicago: University of Chicago Press, 1992.